D1327419

African Healing Strategies

African Healing Strategies

EDITED BY

Brian M. du Toit
&
Ismail H. Abdalla

TRADO-MEDIC BOOKS
A Division of Conch Magazine, Limited (Publishers)
Owerri   New York   London
1985

First published 1985

Printed in the United States of America

Library of Congress Cataloging-in-Publication Data
Main entry under title:

African healing strategies.

Based on a conference held Mar. 1984 under the
auspices of the Center for African Studies at the
University of Florida.
Includes bibliographies.
1. Medicine—Africa—Congresses. 2. Medicine,
Arabic—Africa—Congresses. 3. Folk medicine—Africa—
Congresses. I. Du Toit, Brian M., 1935- .
II. Abdalla, Ismail Hussein. III. University of
Florida. African Studies Center. [DNLM: 1. Health
Services—Africa—congresses. 2. Islam—congresses.
3. Medicine, Traditional—Africa—congresses.
4. Religion and Medicine—congresses. W 84 HA1 A2 1984]

R651.A35 1985   610'.96   85-20695
ISBN 0-932426-35-2
ISBN 0-932426-36-0 (pbk.)

TABLE OF CONTENTS

ILLUSTRATIONS

PREFACE

This volume stems from a conference on "African Healing Strategies" held under the auspices of the Center for African Studies at the University of Florida during March 1984. Most of the papers presented and discussed at the conference have been included here, while two papers by du Toit have been added because they related specifically to the topic. The first, dealing with isangoma, appeared originally in *Anthropological Quarterly* (44:2. 1971) and the second in *Urban Anthropology* (9:1.1980). We appreciate permission from the editors to reproduce these papers in this volume.

A conference and its proceedings are always the result of a great deal of hard work, sharing of burdens, and support personnel. This one was no exception. We would like to express our sincere thanks to the University of Florida departments and other administrative units and their heads which in addition to the Center for African Studies provided financial support for the conference: Public Foundations, Policy and Lectures Committee; College of Medicine; College of Liberal Arts and Sciences; Department of Pediatrics; Department of Anthropology; Department of Psychiatry; Department of Religion. In particular we need to thank R. Hunt Davis, Jr., Director, Center for African Studies personnel, especially Carol Lauriault, and various graduate students; Muriel Burks who typed much of the manuscript, and Richard L. Harris, who was responsible for final preparation of this manuscript for publication.

We also need to thank Sunday Anozie and Lynda Anozie at Trado-Medic Books for their guidance and their patience while the manuscript was being prepared for publication.

PART I
HEALING AND RELIGION

Researchers on African therapy agree that modern allopathic or cosmopolitan medicine which is described by some as "Western in orientation, naturalistic in approach, and positivistic in methodology" (Coe 1970: 125) reaches only a small portion of Afican population. It represents a rather small element in the available resources of health delivery in the Third World in general and in Africa in particular.

On the other hand, indigenous medical practice was and continues to be the only sources of therapy available to the majority of African peoples. This is because the indigenous system is logical and grounded deep in the vernacular culture and ecology. Indigenous medical practices, however, are not uniform because they are based on disease definition. Thus they are not only relative in their definition and classification of what a diseased state is but also aim at a return, through treatment, to what is seen as a non-diseased state. "Health" then may include malaria, cycle cell anemia and a variety of conditions defined as "disease" by other and especially allopathic medicine. Indigenous systems, also have different classifications of categories, various etiologies for illnesses and often asymetrical remedial procedures. These pluralistic medical systems range from the ancient Greco-Islamic medicine, a highly systemaized, codified and organized medical practice associate largely with literate societies, to medical systems which are greatly diversified, locally circumscribed and ethnically bounded, and which are prevelant among all preliterate African communities (Abdalla 1981:124).

That there is today in Africa a codified, systematized and, in the past, even an organized and centrally controlled medical system may be a surprise to those accustomed to the convenient though inaccurate classification of health care delivery systems into two only: the western and the traditional. This unfortunate methodological oversimplication has always blinded

1

researchers to the irreducible fact that Islamic medicine practiced in Africa is distinct from the local
healing art of the various African societies. It operates from different philosophical assumptions about the
universe and the place of man within it. While the
Greek humoral theory remains central to its approach to
disease and cure, Islamic medicine has incorporated
Indian and Iranian ideas as well as those of other
societies about health diet and human ecology that have
rendered it more responsive to the physical and psyhco-
logical needs of Muslims throughout the Islamic world.
It has thus a universal applicability which is absent
in other ethnic therapeutic practices in Africa.
Furthermore, Islamic medicine is mainly a written
science transmitted by the written word. Its custodians
are therefore those who can decipher the written word,
that is any one who reads and writes. On the other
hand, indigenous African therapy is committed to memory
and is orally transmitted customarily, by specialized
individuals (Abdalla 1981:120). Islamic medicine which
is based essentially on books often perceived to be
immutable and lasting, is therefore conservative in
nature. African indigenous practice, by the very
nature of its mode of transmission - orality - is flexible and receptive to change. This important difference prompted us to include one section in this volume
which deals exclusively with Islamic-Arabic influences
in African healing systems.
     One of the critical differences between allopathic
medicine and the indigenous therapeutic systems is
their view of the disease-person relationship. The
first is "oriented to combating pathologies one by one
in a relatively atomistic manner" (Janzen 1981:185)
while usually dealing only with the sickness in a
clinical sense. Indigenous therapeutics view the
individual who is not in a state of health as a total
person with a social-familial context who needs to be
restored to a healthy state. This includes a balance
in the cosmological sense. For this reason researchers, and especially anthropologists, have in the past
usually given indigenous medicine an ethonological set-
tiny as they described religion, magic, ethnobotany,
psychotherapy and related topics. Fabrega (1982:238)
clarifies the interest of the social scientist as
follows: "The medical domain tends to the one about
which people have a great deal of concern. Central
premises about social life are forged through individual and group adaptation, which partly involves coping
with illness and disease. In the medicine of a people,
then, social scientists have a very rich domain for the
discovery of basic aspects of social structure and process, and the study of them can contribute richly to
social theory."

To heal the whole person the therapist operates within the realm of the physical, and social, and the super-natural. For this reason we have separated the two major field of influence namely the religious and the scientific.

REFERENCES CITED

Abdalla, Ismail H. Islamic Medicine and its influence on traditionally Hausa Practitioners in Northern Nigeria. Ph.D. Dissertation. University of Wisconsin, Madison. 1981.
Coe, R.M. Sociology of Medicine, New York: McGraw Hill, 1970.
Fabrega, Horacido. Commentary on African Systems of Medicine. P. Stanley Yoder (ed.) African Health and Healing Systems. Los Angeles: University of California Press, 1982.
Janzen, John M., The Need for a Taxonomy of Health in the study of African Therapeutics. Social Science and Medicine, 15: 3. 1981.

A. ISLAMIC AND ARABIC INFLUENCE

Islamic medicine is not confined to those regions in North Africa which are culturally and historically identified with the Middle East and the Arab world. Indeed, in many Islamized societies in Africa south of the Sahara; from Senegal on the Atlantic coast to Somalia and Zanzibar on the Indian Ocean; Islamic medicine has been adopted and, in varying degrees, adapted to meet local needs, customs and conditions. There is today hardly a village containing a sizeable Muslim community without its own Muslim medical practitioner who consults as a matter of course some Arabic medical treatises in his daily practice, or who has read these tracts at one stage or anoter in his career.

The Isalamic medicine administered now in Africa south of the Sahara is representative of the medical practice once prevalent in Muslim countries further to the north during medieval times. After the twelfth century of the Christian era classical Islamic medicine, like many other aspects of Islamic culture and civilization, was in decline. (Ibn Khaldun 1958:125). It lost its impressive clinical approach to diagnosis and, more seriously, its scientific interpretation of disease causation and cure. Instead of mastering the renowned medical works of classical physicians like Al-Razi (d.925 A.D.) or Ibn Sina (d. 1039 A.D.) aspirant practitioners strove to become proficient in the quasi-scientific writings of the Algerian mystic, Al-Buni ((d. 1225 A.D.) or the Egyptian theologian, Al-Suyuti (d. 1505 A.D.). The emphasis had shifted from the didactic method in medicine in which cause and effect of disease, symptoms and cure are locked in a predictable calculable relationship to one that emphasize supernatural elements beyond human control.

Medical practitioners in Muslim societies had by and large limitied their profession to dealing with disease religiously interpreted and diagnosed and to cures spiritually perceived and administered.

4

It was this type of quasi-scientific medical thought and practice that crossed the desert and flourished eventually among Muslim communities in the Bilad al-Sudan. There are however additional factors that probably explain why clinical scientific Islamic medicine failed to take root here. The lack of developed urban centers (Tarikh AL-Fattash: 1964:146, 180, and Barth: 1857: Vol 1: 150) of the type common in North Africa and Egypt in the pre-colonial era is one. The absence of medical institutions--hospitals, infirmaries, sanatoriums, schools and the like as a result perhaps of the economic weakness of a mercantile class in the area that would endow them as it did elsewhere is another (Barth 1857: Vol 3: 367).

The problem is complicated further by the limited information we have regarding the introduction and the development of Islamic medicine in the Bilad al-Sudan. Little research on this important topic has been done. The three articles in this section concerning various aspects of Islamic medical practices among Islamized populations in the region are therefore a welcome contribution.

Brenner's article on the esoteric sciences in West African Islam gives the general cultural and intellectual framework in which the 'ulama or the religious clergy functioned in the past as healers and, more importantly, as intermediaries between the seen and the unseen worlds. It also highlights the rather subtle relationship between sufism and the esoteric sciences in West Africa and underscores the secrecy involved in transmitting them.

Perhaps the most important contribution the articles makes to the general historical studies of Islam in Africa is the call for a closer look at the sciences of numerology, geomancy and divination as a "manifestation of Islamic culture in the process of growth and development". The adaptive nature of these sciences to local needs and ideas, the limited requirement they have of a working knowledge of orthodox Islam, and, finally the comparative ease with which some of these sciences may be learned, account for their popularity and their wide-spread use in Africa. A close examination of the role of the 'ulama and the shaikhs of the turuq in the delivery of health services and the protection of peoples' well-being to which Brenner's article draws our attention will prove extremely valuable to the general understanding of Islam and Islamic culture in Africa.

In his article on the medical literature of the 1804 Fulani jihad in Northern Nigeria, Abdalla argues for a medically oriented investigation of the history of this crucial period in Hausaland. By examining the medical treatises compiled by leading Fulani scholars in nineteenth century Sokoto, Abdalla has shown that health and medical concerns were high in the agenda of the jihadists, who considered the religious reform incomplete without a concomitant reform of the existing health care system in Hausaland. In his view, there was a strong relationship between medical authority and political authority in nineteenth century Hausaland. This was why the jihadists set out diliberately to destroy the power of all pre-Islamic medical practioners, although they met with only partial success.

Abdalla has also stressed the significance of the introduction and adoption of the technology of writings to medical practice in Hausaland. He argues that once medical knowledge had been preserved on paper rather than being secured in the memory, major changes occurred. Hausa men came to dominate the healing profession to the exclusion of women who then became the main patronizers of the bori spirit possession cult.

Stock's article brings us to contemporary health problems in Northern Nigeria, and gives a rather unexpected twist to Abdalla's contention that Hausa malams are knowledgeable in Islamic medicine. Based on his recent field work among a sampling of practitioners in Hadejia Emirate Stock has shown that malams practicing Islamic medicine are less articulate about matters of health and disease than their counterparts who practice non-Islamic therapy. Nevertheless, he seems to reaffirm the point made by Abdalla on the centrality of the Prophetic medicine in the Hausa medical practice as opposed to indigenous or even Western medicine. Stock has found that for the Hadejia malams the medicine of the Prophet Muhammad remains their first choice for the treatment of common symptomatic illnesses, unknown illness or for problems stemming from social tension. Stock also makes the significant observation that more women than men depend on the Prophetic medicine for treatment. However, it is not clear from this whether women in Hadejia still patronize the bori cult as Abdalla would argue, or whether the utilization of this type of Islamic medicine precludes them from dependence on spirit-related treatment.

A fourth article, which focuses on the fate of Islamic medicine in North Africa and the Middle East in the face of an increasingly dominant western culture during the latter part of the nineteenth century, rounds off this section on Islamic and Arabic influences. In this articles, Gallagher suggests that Galenic-Islamic medicine had not declined to the extent that shcolars of this tradition generally concluded. Nor, was it simply a matter of Western medicine being more efficacious than the indigenous tradition and thus displacing it through winning acceptance by the people.

Rather, Gallagher argues, the emergence to dominance of
western medicine in North Africa and the middle East
rested with political factors that favored the Western
over the Galenic-Islamic medical tradition. In recent
times the two forms of revival of the Galenic-Islamic
tradition have emanated from Western-trained medical
personnel and not from the hakims who were the practitioners of the older tradition. Islamic medical
thought and practice in the Bilad al-Sudan drew heavily
on the Galenic-Islamic tradition of North Africa and
the Middle East and thus was affected directly by its
decline.

REFERENCES CITED

Barth, H. Travels and Discoveries in North and Central
    Africa. 5 vols 2nd ed. London. 1857-8.
Ibn Khaldun, Abdul Rahman. The Muqaddima (translated
    by Franz Rosenthal). London: Cambridge
    University Press. 1958.
Tarikh al-Fattash (translated into French by O. Houdas
    and M. Delafosse). Paris. 1913-14.

CHAPTER 1

THE ULAMA OF SOKOTO
IN THE NINETEENTH CENTURY: A MEDICAL VIEW
Ismàil H. Abdalla

The role of the Ulama or Muslim clerics in the preservation and the dissemination of Islamic sciences in tropical Africa hardly needs emphasis. This article explores the contribution some of the Ulama of Soko-to[1] made in the nineteenth century in the area of medicine and health care, and argues for more emphasis in the study of Islam in Africa on the function of Muslim clerics as medical practitioners in the expansion of Islam in the continent.

The importance of a medically oriented inquiry into the history of Islamized Africa has long been overlooked (Fisher 1973:2). Most of us are familiar with the frequent references to the role of the Muslim trader and the itinerate cleric in African conversion to Islam. Such generalizations as "black Islam is a trader's Islam" are not uncommon in the literature. Although the function of the trader in spreading the new faith has been more or less satisfactorily explain-ed (Bovil 1933:12-69, Adamu 1978:10-64, Newbury 1966: 233-246 and Hasan 1967:50), that of the cleric is only partially understood (Lewis 1966: 58-75, Trimingham 1968:148-59, Last and AL-Hajj 1965:232-43), even though it was he and not the trader who eventually brought about reforms and established caliphates. It has often been suggested that his function as a secretary to African kings, and his involvement as a go-between in times of tribal conflict account for his success as a proselytizer (Lewis 1966:62, Fisher 1971: 3913). This may well be true, but it only partially explains his importance. Insufficient attention in the studies of Islam in Africa has been given to the significance of of the itinerate cleric as a medical practitioner, as a dispenser of medicine in the broadest sense of the word, and as an intermediary not only among men, but more importantly, between them and their Creator; between the seen and the unseen; the known and the unknown. When the role of the Muslim cleric as a doctor in Islamized African societies is fully investi-

8

gated and understood, we will perhaps better comprehend
the process of conversion in Africa, and be able to
explain, more convincingly, the influence of Islam on
the life of the ordinary African. We shall also understand the reasons why the Muslim cleric occupied a
primary social and political position in the past, and
continues to do so at present. I hope to clarify the
strong association between clerics and medicine as
understood and practiced by one African group, the
Hausa of Northern Nigeria, in my discussion of the
medical writings of some of the leaders of the Sokoto
jihad.

From its start, the leaders of the Fulani reform
movement in Hausaland made serious efforts to model the
society on that of the pristine community of classical
Medina, and fashion their governing institutions after
those established by the Prophet Muhammad and his immediate successors. Accordingly, Shari'a became the
established law of the land, while the vizier, the qadi
(the magistrate), the qa'id al'jaysh (the Commander of
the Army), and the sahib al maal (the Secretary of the
Treasury) were entrusted with the difficult task of
carrying out the letter of that law.

Modeling Hausa society on that of Medina involved
more than mere adoption of Arabic names for state
offices, and Arabic titles for the people who held
them. In one area at least which concerns us here,
that of medicine, the jihadists faced a number of difficult problems. In the first place, Hausa society, like
many other African societies in the past, had not developed any centrally controlled administrative machinery
to organize and standardize medical care in the pre-
jihad period, be it at the regional or township level.
Medical care in those times was left to private medical
specialists - the boka (the medicine man), the yar bori
(the medium of the bori or spirit possession cult), the
mai magani (the herbalist), and the malam or the religious scholar among the Muslim Hausa. The lack of central
control in this important profession made the task of
the jihad leaders to reform the health care system
extremely difficult, if not impossible. Secondly, there
were two competing therapeutic systems in Hausaland; the
pre-Islamic Maguzawa or 'pagan' therapy, and a version
of Islamic medicine which was, from the reformers' point
of view, corrupt and misused. Corrupt, that is, because
of the tendency on the part of Muslim practitioners to
employ divination, astrology, and numerology for diagnosis and treatment, as well as for the foretelling of
the future (Bello c. 1832:folio 6). Thirdly, there was
the difficulty of acquiring original works on Islamic
medicine in Hausaland.

Several courses of action were open to the rulers
and the Ulama of Sokoto. One was to accept the medical

system that existed before the coming of Islam, with no
interference on their part in how the practitioners
conducted their business. Another was to make a compromise by adopting the Maguzawa medical system with
some modifications so as to comform to Islam. Lastly,
they could reject non-Islamic health care in toto, and
replace it with a medical system of their own creation,
or, one based on orthodox Islamic medicine (2).

For obvious reasons the leaders of the jihad could
not tolerate pre-Islamic medical practice which was
centered around spirits and spirit worship, for it
contradicted basic Islamic principles. Invoking supernatural beings to bring about cure or to remove hard-
ship contravenes a cardinal belief in Islam that
supplication and prayer can only be made to Allah and
to Him alone. Prayer to any other force is shirk or
unbelief. But the rejection by the jihadists of non-
Islamic Hausa therapy stemmed also from a genuine fear
of the conflict of interests on the political level
between themselves and the non-Muslim medical practitioners. The rulers of Sokoto were acutely aware of
the social and political importance of the boka and the
yar bori among the Maguzawa as well as among the newly
Islamized Hausa. It was incompatible, even politically
dangerous, to have a politico-religious system that
advocated that power lies with Allah, and Allah alone,
and a medical system like that of the Maguzawa in which
the boka and the yar bori invoked the help of iskoki or
"pagan" spirits. Allegiance needed to be undivided if
the Islamic ideal, and the jihadist control over the
destiny of the Hausa people, were to be realized. The
pre-Islamic medical system, like most other aspects of
Maguzawa culture, was therefore severely condemned and
its legitimacy undermined in the jihad literature.

The leaders of the jihad were quick to realize the
central place of the pre--Islamic practitioner in the
social and political fabric of his community, and the
incompatibility of his role with theirs. It was a
conflict not only between the elite of two religious
systems, but between two incongruous cosmologies; one
cyclical and particularistic--microcosmic, the other
linear and cosmopolitan--macrocosmic.

It is no surprise, therefore, that the Ulama of
Sokoto, and its leaders, were bitterly opposed to the
medical system represented by the boka and the yar
bori, and fought against it with the same determination
and courage as they did against the Habe kings. The
only difference was that their struggle to abolish the
Maguzawa medical system was intellectual and not physical. The jihadists used the written word and not the
sword against non-Islamic medical practice. They wrote
many treatises condemning pre-jihad Hausa customs and
traditions before and, for a long time, after the

establishment of the Caliphate. Uthman ibn Fudi, his brother Abdullahi, and his son Muhammad Bello, but especially the latter, attacked in their writings non-Islamic therapeutic practice associated with Hausa spirits and labelled it sihr or magic, hence haram or unlawful and therefore reprehensible in Islam (Bello 1957:57).

One of the options open to the reformers, as we have seen, was to make a compromise: to adapt Maguzawa practice to Islam. But this is exactly what they had, all along, been accusing the Habe kings and their Ulama of, namely the mixing of Islamic and non-Islamic practice. The jihadists could not accept the Maguzawa medical system as a whole, nor even in a modified form as long as the efficacy of herbs and plants was believed to have been derived from the spirits.

Equally, they could not tolerate marginal or unorthodox Islamic medicine for the same reason. It gives too much power to the jinn and Satan, while its preoccupation with the unveiling of the hidden and the foretelling of the future, known only to Allah, contradicts basic Islamic beliefs. Such unorthodox Islamic medicine seems to have been extensively used by the less educated malams or religious leaders, as the poem Shurb al-Zulal clearly shows (Hiskett 1962:120). As we shall see, the reformers were not successful in eliminating non-Islamic practices from Islamic medicine, and failed to eradicate the profession of the boka and the yar bori.

As a replacement for both Maguzawa therapy and marginal Islamic medicine, the leaders of the jihad offered the medicine of the Prophet Muhammad (3). This final choice was dictated to them by a number of important considerations. In the first place, the Fulani reformers, because of the very nature of their reform movement, could not develop an entirely new medical system for Hausa society. Such an endeavor on their part would perhaps lead, in the end, to the very rejection of Islamic medicine, an eventuality which would be counter-productive to their efforts at reform, and would compromise the spirit of the jihad itself. Again, developing a new medical system would involve innovation and change, which were anathematized by the conservative Malikite school of law to which the reformers belonged. Innovation and independent judgement in legal matters, and by extension, in all matters dealing with daily life in Muslim societies, was suspended early in medieval times when the 'door of ijtihad' or the re-interpretation of religious dogma had been closed (Ibn Khaldum 1900:284). It must be observed that the Fulani movement was a revivalist movement, and its leaders were muqallids in Islamic legal terms, or imitators, and not mujtahids or inde-

pendent thinkers. They were faithful to the Islamic
heritage, and strongly felt that it was incumbent upon
them as Muslims to revive orthodox Islam in its pure
and unadulterated form. This is why the Sokoto leaders
shunned innovation and strongly condemned nonconformity
(Bello 1957:146).

Compilers of medical works in the Caliphate exploited to the full the technology of writing which
came with Islam in order to disseminate orthodox
Islamic medicine among fellow Muslims in Hausaland and
beyond, and to attack and undermine the non-Muslim
Hausa medical system. Let me digress here, therefore,
to explain the importance of the technology of writing
in the history of Islam and Islamic medicine in this
region.

The ability to read and write in nineteenth century Hausa society not only predetermined the type of
medical knowledge which was derived from traditional
Islamic sources, but also the audience for whom this
knowledge was to be reproduced. It was for the literate among the Hausa people that such medical compilations were made. The literate had therefore a special
role to play in the process of the dissemination of
medical knowledge in Hausaland. They read medical
compilations, interpreted them, and applied appropriate
sections to the various situations of combatting
disease or alleviating suffering. This elite group
consisted of the malams and their students who would
eventually take their masters' place.

The malam was an important figure in society. In
his capacity as educator, political advisor, secretary,
a leader of social and religious functions and ceremonies, and above all, as a judge and interpretor of
the Shari'a or the Divine Law, the malam wielded considerable power among the Hausa. When a child was
born, it was the malam who formally accepted it into
the membership of the group by giving it a name and a
blessing. He also guaranteed its protection and that
of its mother during and after birth by charms, medicine, or by recitation from the Quran. From the time
he was born to the hour of his death, the individual
was in constant need of the malam's protection, advice,
instruction, and guidance. The individual's health,
security, and spiritual and material well-being, as
well as all the critical stages of life; birth, circumcision, marriage, and death, were sanctified, guaranteed and rendered free of danger through the intervention of the malam. He was also the diviner without
whose prediction and blessing no business, trade,
journey or marriage was considered safe or desirable.
This considerable power which the malam was able to
weild in the past, and in many instances does so still
today, was made possible because of his ability, real

or assumed, to control space-time events by manipulating the Word. This control, I suggest, could only be achieved through literacy in Arabic which was an important instrument of social mobility in Hausa society.

As far as the history of medicine in Hausaland was concerned, the introduction of the technology of writing was a water-shed. In non-Muslim Hausa society, medical knowledge passed down from one generation to the other orally. In the case of Muslim Hausa society, on the other hand, such knowledge was transmitted mainly through writing. Even when oral communication was used to convey medical advice or a prescription, it is likely that that advice and prescription were originally taken from a medical book or a treatise. As we have noticed before, the role of the malam-practitioner in this respect was crucial. He effectively bridged the gap between the oral and the written medicine, and in doing so helped diffuse Islamic medicine among the illiterate masses. This in turn, re-inforced his own position of leadership in the community.

Literacy in Arabic made medicine more accessible, more unified, rich, and practical. In the form of a book, a treatise, or even a simple letter, medical knowledge could easily be transmitted from place to place, and from one community to the other in Hausaland or beyond. After the introduction of writing in Hausaland, it became no longer necessary for an aspiring medical practitioner to undergo a psychological trauma or actual physical illness as was the case with Maguzawa therapy connected with the _bori_ spirit cult (Greenburg 1941;57). Medicine was no longer the exclusive domain of specialists who knew the secret of communicating with the supernatural, but also of those who could decipher letters; not only of those mediums who could interpret the language of the _iskoki_ or spirits, but of malams who could read and write Arabic.

Medicine became also less awesome and frightening compared to the practice of _bori_ adepts. To be able to minister to for the sick, the Hausa malam-practitioner needed only a medical book which he could store in his house and could consult when necessary: not _bori_ spirit that would come uninvited to live with him or in him, and to whose whims, likes and dislikes he would often have to sacrifice some of his own freedom of action, or compromise his faith.

Unlike the _bori_ spirit which can only exist _in_ a specialist, the medical book has a physical existence of its own outside the body of the practitioner. In terms of geographical locality, seasonal changes, and ethnic diversity, the medical book or treatise is much more flexible than the traditional spirit which is often associated with a certain clan or a particular locale. The medical book could and did cross political

and ethnic boundaries, while its efficacy applied
equally in the different seasons of the year. On the
other hand, spirits with strong ethnic or cultural
traits tend largely to retain these distinctive characteristics wherever they are transplanted, precluding,
thereby, non-members of the group from joining in the
cult. This is perhaps why the Hausa bori cult and
spirits failed to attract Nupe worshippers (Nadel
1954:160). In North Africa, the adherents of the bori
were descendents of Hausa emigrants only (Tremearne
1914:120).
     Literacy profoundly affected medical practice in
Hausaland in another way. It brought about a sharper
division in the medical profession according to sex.
In non-Muslim Huusa society, women play an important
role in the management of illness (Ibid:150, Last
1976:40-41). With Islam and its concomitant technology
of writing, which became men's specialty, men not only
dominated the profession of medicine of the written
word to the total exclusion of women, but used their
own special position to exploit the craft to their own
advantage, so to speak. No one who reads the many
medical treatises extant in Nigeria will fail to
observe the strong emphasis the authors have placed for
example on matters such as male sexual virility, or
devices to restrict womens' extra-marital activities
(Tuker c. 1826: folios 3-4). On the other hand,
womens' complaints connected usually with pregnancy,
nursing or menstruation have attracted but the slightest attention on the part of the Hausa compilers of
medical works. This explains, perhaps, why Hausa women
took to bori, probably as a compensatory measure for
the neglect, often deliberate, they suffered under the
male dominated, male oriented Hausa Muslim therapy.
     The preceeding paragraphs give us some idea of the
cultural and political environment in which the leaders
of the jihad, more especially Muhammad Bello, compiled
their medical works, and the audience for which these
compilations were intended. The relationship between
literacy, Islam and jihad, on the one hand, and between
these and Islamic medicine, on the other, conditioned
Bello's writings and pre-determined what he wrote, and
why he wrote on the subject of medicine.
     Sultan Muhammad Bello, who died in 1837, was
probably the most important writer on medicine in the
Sudan. Certainly he was in Hausaland. In addition to
his sixty-five or so works on Islamic sciences in
general, Bello could boast ten additional treatises on
the different aspects of medicine, hygiene, and related
topics (Bello c. 1827:folio 6). Beside these, several
extant treaties written by others that deal with medicine are attributed to him, a fact that shows that
Bello was a recognized authority in this field.

Like the rest of the leaders of the jihad Muhammed Bello was educated in the traditional Islamic educational system, with a strong bias toward Quaranic and hadith sciences. Like them, too, he was a muqallid, a traditionalist. As far as medicine is concerned, Bello was self-educated, and was well-read in Islamic sciences, including medicine. He once counted all the major works that he had read and found them to be in excess of two thousand books and articles (Bello c. 1827:folio 2).

Bello believed that good health care was essential for political stability. During the upheaval of the jihad and the inevitable shortages of food supplies, there were wide-spread famines and epidemics in the Sokoto area, and perhaps elsewhere (Bello 1957:8, 113). These catastrophies seemed to have made a strong and lasting impression on Bello, and in many ways influenced his policies later on. The threat of famine could only be avoided by greater agricultural productivity, and the danger of disease and the devastation of epidemics could only be stopped by an efficient medical system. Bello's interest in the development of a sound medical and agricultural system in Hausaland can not be separated from his overall commitment to the establishment of the ideal Muslim society in the land, which was the main aim of the jihad. The Islamic society which the leaders of this reform movement envisaged was a self-sufficient, self-sustaining politico-religious system whose sole purpose on earth was to carry out the Divine Will of Allah in preparation for the coming life. But the reformers knew better than anybody else that the intellectual ideals could easily be frustrated by sheer physical obstacles or human incapacity, and that the actual ability of any society to follow the word of Allah and implement His divine law, depended, to a large measure, on the society's capacity to overcome the problems of deprivation, hunger, and disease. For this reason, Bello paid special attention, from the beginning, to the development of a substantial infrastructure in the Caliphate. He saw to it that bridges were constructed, and roads were opened between major urban centers, and remained open even during times of unrest and revolt, so as to encourage trade. His record of establishing new towns and garrisons, to which the present city of Sokoto bears witness, is even more impressive. In these new centers, nomads as well as people displaced during the wars of the jihad were settled, and serious efforts were made to introduce them to agriculture, which had been greatly encouraged and improved.

In the field of medical care, Muhammad Bello was a pioneer in Hausaland. He realized the importance of improving the standard of hygiene in urban communities,

16

AFRICAN HEALING STRATEGIES

and accordingly planned and built the new towns and
garrisons with wide streets and in open airy surroundings. He even provided these and other settlements
with veterinary service, a fact that indicates Bello's
understanding of the importance of animals, especially
the horse, in the economy and the defense of the
Caliphate (Dan Lardi 1979: personal communication).
    Bello also appointed qadis or magistrates for the
proper execution of the Shari^ca law. It is important
to remember that the qadi in Hausaland, as elsewhere in
Dar al-Islam, acted as a muhtasib or overseer of the
market and public conduct, (Abdullahi Dan Fodio
1956:30) in addition to his normal duties as a judge.
In his capacity as a muhtasib, and in the spirit of the
all-embracing Islamic principle of upholding goodness
and condemning wrong-doing (al-'amr bil-ma'-rufi wal
nahyu 'an al-munkari), the qadi enforced measures he
deemed necessary to improve and guarantee the wellbeing
of the community, including those having to do with
health care.
    To be sure, there were no hospitals or other medi-
cal institutions in nineteenth century Hausaland. But
there were doctors who administered medicine to the
sick, and specialists who sold plants, herbs, and other
medical ingredients to the public. The qadi, under
whose jurisdiction these practitioners were, must have
exercised some kind of control over the medical profession, if only to insure that their practice conformed
to the letter of the Shari^ca law.
    That conformity to Shari^ca in medical practice
was an overriding concern to the leaders of the jihad
is evident in many of their writings. Muhammad Bello
in his Talkhis tibb al-Nabi, and again in 'Ujalat al-
Rakib emphasized this point. His uncle Abdullahi ibn
Fudi (d. 1829) reiterated the same concern when he
warned both practitioners and patients against using
haram or prohibited things for medication (Adullahi Dan
Fodio c. 1820: folio 36).
    The most significant contribution of Sultan Muham-
mad Bello in the area of medical care was, however, his
endeavor to improve the standard of public health
through education.
    Bello believed that the goal of reincarnating the
Medinese society in Hausaland could be achieved by
educating the masses in Islamic sciences, including
medicine, more particularly, the medicine of the Prophet Muhammad. For him, medicine was only a vehicle
for the realization of a much higher and nobler goal
than the temporary relief from pain or misery in man or
beast. Bello's immense political and religious authority gave Islamic medicine in Hausaland an enhanced
credibility. Islamic medicine, especially the medicine
of the Prophet Muhammad, became particularly important

in the poeple's life because it was the medicine of the
founder of Islam, but equally, because it was strongly
advocated by no less a personage than Amir-al-Mu'minin
or the Commander of the Faithful, Muhammad Bello himself.

     As we have seen above, a strong case can be made
for the relationship, even the interdependence of scho-
lastic authority and medicine in the Sokoto Caliphate.
It was a positive relationship in which political and
religious authority was used to establish a viable
orthodox Islamic medical system. Conversely, medicine
re-inforced the power of the political elite, since it
was they who advocated it, and remained its main custodians and interpreters.

     Loyalty was now to a universal ideology, and not
to a local diety, and allegiance was to the Caliph and
not to the ethnic group. The medicine of the deity of
the compound, the farmstead, or the ethnic group was
replaced at least on the official level, by Islamic
medicine which had as its central focus the Quran and
the hadith and not the iskoki or the ancestral figure.

     Did the leaders of the jihad succeed in their
struggle to abolish Maguzawa therapy and eradicate non-
orthodox Islamic medicine in Hausaland? The answer to
this question is no. Among the Hausa of Northern Nigeria today, the boka, the yar bori and the non-orthodox
Muslim practitioner still dominate the profession of
traditional health care. There are several reasons for
this. First, these medical specialists performed, and
continue to perform a useful role in traditional
therapy which could not be discontinued easily, more
especially since the Fulani reformers did not come up
with a ready medical system of their own. Secondly,
the nonorthodox malam-practitioner rightly thought that
he had as much claim to the medicine of the Prophet as
the orthodox Fulani reformers. He was often unaware or
unwilling to admit any contradiction between his type
of medicine and that advocated by the jihadists.
Thirdly and more importantly, was the fact that after
the establishment of the Caliphate on firm ground, the
reformers themselves became more tolerant and were more
willing to accept certain Hausa customs and traditions
that they once condemned and out-lawed (Abdalla
1979:89).

     The jihad leaders did not totally fail either. In
one area at least, their success was complete. For all
practical purposes, they eliminated the boka and the
yar bori from whatever political authority these
practitioners had enjoyed in the past.

NOTES

[1] Sokoto is a metropolis in the northwestern part of Nigeria and the capital of a state by the same name. It was founded in 1812 by Amir Al-muminin Muhammad Bello, the second caliph of the Fulani Empire that lasted from 1804 till the British occupation of Northern Nigeria in 1903.
[2] I am using the term "orthodox" here to distinguish the type of medicine advocated by the jihadists - the medicine of the Prophet Muhammed - from the then widespread medical practice of divination, astrology and numerology which the reformers strongly condemned, at least in the beginning of the jihad.
[3] The medicine of the Prophet Muhammad is essentially the therapy of pre-Islamic Arabia coupled with a few notions on drugs and herbs borrowed from the Indian or Iranian materia medica while the Koran provides the broad base of hygiene and nutrition.

REFERENCES CITED

Abdalla, Ismail H.   Medicine in Nineteenth Century Arabic Literature in Notheren Nigeria. Kano Studies, n.s. 4:91-99. 1979
Adamu, Mahi.   The Hausa Factor in West African History. Zaria, Nigeria: Ahmadu Bello University Press. 1978.
Al-Tunisi, Muhammad ibn Omer.   Tashhidul Adhhan bi Siati Bilad Al-Urb wal Sudan. H.S. Umar ed. and transl. Kano: Bayero University. 1975
Bello, Muhammad Shifa' Al Ghalil. MS in Bayero University Archives, unnumbered. c. 1827.
Talkhis, Tib Al-Nabi. MS in Bayero University Archives, unnumbered. c. 1832.
Bello, Muhhammad. Infaq al-Mysuri. C.E.J. Whiting, ed. London: Luzzac and Company. 1957.
Bovill, E.W. Caravan of the Old Sahara: An Introduction to the History of the Western Sudan. London. International Institute of African Languages and Culture. 1933
Dan Fodio, Abdullahi. Masalih AL Insan Aluta-Muta'alliqa bil Adyan wal Abdan. MS in _____. Bayero University Archives, unnumbered. c. 1820.
Diya'u AL-Hukkam. Zaria, Nigeria: Government Press. 1956.
Fisher, Humphrey. Hassebu: Islamic Healing in Black Africa. In M. Brett ed. Northern Africa: Islam and Modernization. London: Frank Cass. 1973.
Greenberg, J. Some Aspects of Negro-Mohammadan Culture Contact among the Hausa. American Anthropologist, n.s. 41:51-61. 1941.

Hasan, Y. Fadl. The Arabs and the Sudan. Edinburgh:
    Edinburgh University Press. 1967.
Hiskett, M., and Bivar, A. Arabic Literature in Nigeria
    to 1804: A Provisional Account. Bulletin of the
    School of Oriental and African Studies,
    24:1:104-148. 1962.
Ibn Batuta, Muhammad. Tuhfat al-Nuzzar fi Ghara'ib
    Al-Amsar wa Aga'ib al-Asfar. Cairo: Bulaq.
    1870.
Ibn Khaldun, Abdul Rahman. Al-Muquddima: Beirut,
    AL-Matb'a AL-Adabiyya. 1900.
Junaydu, Wazir. Nail Al-Muram. Manuscript in author's
    possession. 1960.
Last, Murray. The Sokoto Caliphate. London:
    Longmans. 1967.
_____. A Note on Attitudes Toward the Supernatural
in the Sokoto Jihad. Journal of the Historical Society
of Nigeria. 4, 1:3..
Last Murray and M.A. AL-Hajj. An Attempt to Define a
    Muslim in Nineteenth Century Hausaland and Bornu.
    Journal of the Historical Society of Nigeria. 3,
    2:231-243. 1965.
Lewis, I.M. (ed.) Islam in Tropical Africa. London:
    Oxford University Press. 1966.
Nadel. S.F. Nupe Religion. London: Routledge and Kegan
    Paul. 1954.
Newbury, D.W. North African and the Western Sudan
    Trade in the Nineteenth Century. Journal of
    African History. 7:233-256. 1966
Tremearne, A. J. M. The Ban of the Bori: Demons and
    Demon Dancing in West and North Africa. London:
    Cranton and Ousley Ltd. 1914.
Trimingham, H.S. The Influence of Islam Upon Africa.
    London: Longmans. 1968.
Tukur, Muhammad. Mu'unatal Ikwan fi Mu'asharatal Nis-
    wan. Manuscripts in author's possession. c. 1882

CHAPTER 2

THE "ESOTERIC SCIENCES" IN WEST AFRICAN ISLAM

Louis Brenner

Ibn Khaldun devotes a sizeable section of his
Muqaddimah to a discussion of man's capacity for what
he calls "supernatural perception" (Ibn Khaldun 1958:
184 ff). That human beings can perceive the supernatural is not a question for Ibn Khaldun; the existence of prophetic revelations are proof enough for him.
His concern is more with how such perception is achieved and who can in fact achieve it. In examining these
questions, he investigates numerous sorts of practices
and practitioners ranging from Sufis to diviners and
soothsayers in order to test the validity of their
claims. In his view, the possibility for supernatural
perception resides in the subtle nature of the "soul",
which can perceive not only the visible world through
the organic senses, but also, potentially, the hidden
spiritual world directly without the aid of the senses.
This latter capacity requires that somehow the soul
becomes liberated from the limitations of the organic
body. In very general terms, the distinction being
drawn by Ibn Khaldun is between perception of the
visible, manifest world (al-zahir) and the hidden,
esoteric world (al-batin). His discussion of these
phenomena is a subtle combination of doctrinal, sociological and psychological observations and insights.
        For the purposes of the present article, I wish to
enlarge Ibn Khaldun's concept of supernatural perception to embrace what might be called the "esoteric
sciences." We are here concerned not only with man's
supposed ability to perceive the hidden world of
al-batin, but also with his capacity to contact and to
manipulate its esoteric, spiritual powers. This shift
in emphasis is significant because it removes certain
doctrinal limitations from the discussion. Indeed, one
of our major interests is to examine the complex relationships in West Africa between doctrine, as it is
narrowly defined in Qur'an, hadith, and shari'a, and
belief, which is a much more broadly based cultural and
sociological phenomenon. For example, the strict doc-

20

trinal view of holy men in Africa was as passive agents
of spiritual power, as perceivers or transmitters of it
(of baraka, for example). Amongst the people at large,
however, holy men were seen as active agents and manip-
ulators of spiritual power. What is significant is
that, regardless of the varieties of interpretation,
all Muslims, and many non-Muslims as well, seem to have
believed that certain individuals could acquire the
capacity to transmit or control supernatural powers for
the benefit of others. So widely accepted was this
belief that it does not seem unwarranted to suggest
that historically Islam in West Africa has been perceived by Africans themselves more in terms of these
cultural attributes than in terms of specific doctrine.
But even if one does not wish to accept such an extreme
point of view, it is clear that a study of the manifestations of such beliefs reveals aspects of the development of Islam in West Africa in a very different light
to studies which are more doctrinally oriented.
     We can take the writings of the Sokoto jihadists
as an example. Shaikh Uthman in particular expended'
considerable effort to condemn the practitioners of
certain esoteric sciences not only because of their
"venality," but also because preoccupation with them
was diverting students from the study of the basic
texts of the religious sciences (Last: 1967: 3-13, and
Last and Al-Hajj: 1965: 231-9). But if we look at
these same practices from the perspective of the practitioners themselves, we can see that these clerics
were also enhancing the reputation of Islam as an
effective and practical religion which was responsive
to everyday human needs, such as healing, avoidance of
illness or disaster: aid in acquiring children, and so
forth. In the process, they were "Islamizing" numerous
non-Islamic practices, if not in a doctrinal, at least
in a cultural sense. Similarly, Shaikh Uthman attacked
the narrow and sectarian interpretations of the
mutakallimun; but their dogmatic teachings seem to have
been originally designed, and were widely spread in
Africa, as a means to instruct non-literate Muslims in
the tenets of their religion (Brenner: 1984b:79 ff).
These more popular practices, often pursued by less
learned clerics, must be studied in their own right in
order to understand their role in the diffusion of
Islam in Africa. But it should not be thought that
such practices were limited only to the less learned;
we now have ample evidence to suggest that this was not
so. Certain esoteric sciences, known collectively as
tasrif, were an important element in the Jakhanke
religious studies curriculum (Sanneh: 1979:158-9); the
same seems to have been true among the seventeenth-and
eighteenth-century scholars of Borno and Baghirmi
(Brenner: 1984a).

What were the esoteric sciences?

The following attempt at definition or description
makes no claim to being definitive; indeed, the very
attempt raises numerous questions. So far as I know,
no Arabic term exists in the literature which would
denote the esoteric sciences as such; nor do I think
that West African Muslim scholars would have grouped
all the practices which are listed here under one head-
ing. But as explained above, we are examining a
cultural pheomenon based on Ibn Khaldun's concept of
supernatural perception, broadened to include the various forms of man's attempts to treat with supernatural
power. I would suggest that these beliefs and practices fall into three broad categories in West Africa.

(1) Those thought to be related to prophecy and
to prophetic revelation. These include visions and
dreams, as well as the concept of wilaya (sainthood)
and Karamat (the wonders or miracles which give evidence to the sainthood of an individual). All of these
manifestations of supernatural perception and power
have played a central role in West African Islam for
centuries. Even sainthhood and miracles, rather
closely associated with Sufism and the turuq (Sufi
brotherhoods), preceded the widespread diffusion of the
brotherhoods in West Africa.

(2) Those based on the esoteric significance and
power of words, letters and numbers. These include the
repetition of the beautiful names of God (al-asma'
al-husna); and especially knowledge of the great or
secret name of God (al-ism al-akbar); the esoteric
interpretation of the verses of the Qur'an ('ilm
al-ta'wil); the science of letters ('ilm al-huruf) and
its related numerological practices, the science of
magic squares ('ilm al-awfaq) and the use of phrases,
letters and numbers in the manufacture of amulets and
talismans. All of these sciences seem to be included
in what the Jakhanke call tasrif.

(3) The predictive sciences such as astrology and
geomancy ('ilm al-raml or Khatt al-raml, or sandwrit-
ing) and other forms of divination and soothsaying.

Several comments must be appended to this cursory
list. First, this division into categories, even if
justified from an analytical perspective, is somewhat
arbitrary and tends to gloss over the fact that the
esoteric sciences were an integral part of the larger
fabric of Islamic belief and practice. An emphasis on
words and letters is related to beliefs about the
Qur'an as a revealed text and also about the efficacy
of prayer or the repetition of certain words and
phrases; such beliefs were endorsed by the most orthodox of scholars. On the other hand, when the same
beliefs were extended to the writings of talismans,

some scholars questioned their legitimacy. For example, al-Maghili was opposed to the manufacture of
talismans, whereas al-Suyuti, with certain reserva-
tions, was not (Hunwick:1970:29). In spite of the
complexity of such questions, I would suggest that the
order of the above listing reflects in very general
terms a nineteenth-century orthodox view of the legitimacy of the esoteric sciences: visions, miracles and
sainthood reflect the most respectable face of these
sciences, whilst the predictive sciences reflect the
least respectable. Having said that, the point should
be re-emphasized that evidence exists that all of these
sciences, including Khatt al-raml, are known to have
been studied by at least some learned scholars of high
reputation. We do not yet know the extent to which
this kind of study took place, but at one time it may
have been far more extensive and more respectable than
today appears to have been the case.
     To a certain extent we are forced to argue this
position by analogy. During the eighteenth-and
nineteenth-centuries, Sufi forms of Islam, as mediated
through the Qadiriyya and Tijaniyya brotherhoods,
became widespread and highly respected in West Africa.
The hierarchies of the brotherhoods, with their saints,
shaikhs, and muqaddamun dominated much of Islamic
belief and practice. Today in various parts of Africa,
the Sufi interpretation of Islam is under attack by
fundamentalist Muslims who condemn Sufism on doctrinal
grounds. What was considered in the nineteenth-century
a most hightly respectable and orthodox form of Islam
is today being condemned by other Muslims who conform
to different interpretations. This development clearly
shows how the interpretation of Islamic doctrine is
affected by changing social factors. Given such evidence, there is no reason to doubt that other forms of
esoteric Islam might also have achieved great respec-
tability among some Muslims. Such acceptance had in
part to do with proving that these sciences were
possessed of proper religious legitimacy. Examples of
literature which sought to establish such legitimacy
are not abundant, but they do exist. For Tijani Sufism
we have al-Hajj Umar al-Futi's Rimah, a polemical
defense of the Tijaniyya Sufi order, the precepts and
practices of which were said to have been transmitted
from the Prophet to Ahmad al-Tijani in a series of
visions (Beirut: c.1960). For 'ilm al-huruf we have
Muhammad al-Katsinawi's Bahjat al-afaq, (Bibliothèque
national, Paris: Arabe 2635) in which he traced the
transmission of the "secrets" of the science of letters
from the prophet Adam through Muhammad, Ali, and the
saints of Islam to his own teachers. For Khatt al-raml
no comparable West African treatise has come to my
attention, but certain North African authors ascribed

the origins of this science to a revelation from the
Angel Jibril to the prophet Idris, whose practices were
subsequently endorsed by Muhammad himself (Bibliothèque national: Arabe 2699). In all these cases, ultimate legitimacy of the practices in question rests upon
information or techniques which were first made available to human beings in the form of visions or revelations, and which were subsequently transmitted via a
reputable chain of scholar-saints and practitioners.
The analogy with the revelation of the Qur'an and the
transmission of the <u>hadith</u> is evident.

<u>What are the characteristics of the esoteric sciences?</u>
In principle the esoteric sciences are secret and
initiatic. Despite their analogy in origin and transmission to the Qur'an and <u>hadith</u>, they propose no alternative to orthodox doctrine; rather their role is
explained as supplementary to, or supportive of, this
doctrine. The Sufis claim that they seek to move beyond
the letter to the spirit of Islam, thereby implying that
they play a special role in sustaining Islamic doctrine.
The more learned practitioners of other esoteric sciences sought to conceptualize their practices as much as
possible in accordance with generally acepted doctrinal
tenets, as suggested by the literary examples cited
above. These sciences were transmitted in secret
through varying forms of initiation (<u>talqin</u>, implying transmission of secret knowledge); and the organizational structure of their transmission was separate
from, if similar in structure to, that of the exoteric
religious sciences. This separate structure is most
visible in the Sufi brotherhoods where the <u>muqaddam</u> who
authorizes recitation of the <u>wird</u> or of other prayers of
the order was very often not one's teacher of religious
sciences. Of course, the exoteric and esoteric systems
could merge with powerful effect; many of the leading
Muslim figures of the last two centuries in West Africa
were learned scholars as well as Sufi shaikhs (Stewart:
1973).
But if the structure of Sufi orders in West Africa
became visible in the nineteenth-century, one should
not lose sight of their essentially secret nature.
Initiation into a <u>tariqa</u>, the authorization to recite
certain specified prayers, was a private affair between
individuals (the <u>muqaddam</u> and the acolyte). Beyond
that, Sufis seem to have been in the habit of exchanging
secrets among themselves, the precise nature of which
are not very clear. But what of Sufism in West Africa
before it went public in the eighteenth-and nineteenth-
centuries? Was a Sufi influence present, transmitted
individually and in secret, with little public recognition of the fact? Such a practice would have been in
conformity with the concept of <u>tariqa</u> as a "religious

rule" comprised of special prayers and spiritual exercises rather than as a corporate organization. It is
difficult to imagine that such a Sufi influence could
not have been present, given its significance in North
Africa. Certainly many associated aspects of Sufism
were present, including belief in wilaya and Karamat.
Perhaps we should be looking for Sufism in earlier
centuries not so much in the form of turuq as in certain religious practices and beliefs, particularly
those of a private devotional nature.
     There is no suggestion here that all private,
devotional exercises were necessarily esoteric in
nature, but many of them certainly were. It also seems
clear that even if the esoteric sciences were thought
of as separate from the exoteric sciences, the two were
often closely linked. One example, already mentioned,
is to be found among the Dyula/Jakhanke scholars who
boast a centuries-old tradition of leadership in
studies of fiqh and other religious sciences, but who
were also important practitioners of the esoteric
sciences known collectively as tasrif. Some studies
have implied that this prominence of tasrif is the
result of a latter-day decline of scholarship among the
Dyula; but there is no reason to believe that such
esoteric practices were not always a part of standard
studies among these groups. The discovery of Maliki
asanid for the study of fiqh which reveal considerable
historical depth, and their absence for the esoteric
sciences, is not adequate proof of any such decline,
because the esoteric asanid were generally not recorded.
     An interesting exception to this rule is to be
found in the Bahjat al-afaq of Muhammad al-Katsinawi,
referred to above, who recorded his own isnad for 'ilm
al-huruf. It would seem that al-Katsinawi wrote all of
his works on the esoteric sciences after he had left
West Africa. It has been suggested that he might have
done so under the encouragement of students and scholars in the east who were interested in these subjects;
but does his failure to write these treatises in West
Africa also suggest any local constraint against such
writings there? Muhammad al-Katsinawi's career also
sheds light on other aspects of the esoteric sciences.
One of his close colleagues in West Africa was Muhammad
al-Wali b. Sulaiman al-Fullani, whose father was a
noted seventeenth-century scholar of 'ilm al-huruf.
Muhammad al-Wali himself wrote numerous works which
were widely distributed in West Africa, none of which
was directly concerned with the esoteric sciences,
although many of them presented what might be called an
acceptable public face of these sciences, for example,
works on the names and attributes of God and various
aspects of tawhid and Kalam.

The study of tawhid, prticularly in the form of
commentaries on Muḥammad b. Yusuf al-Sanusi's al-Aqid
al-Sughra, became closely associated with the transmission of certain esoteric sciences. The reasons for
this are not entirely clear, but may be related to the
idea that the al-Sughra claimed to explain the esoteric
meaning of the shahada, primarily in the form of the
attributes of God and the prophets. Al-Sanusi also
asserted that those who recite properly the shahada
might perceive "boundless secrets and wonders." Cerno
Bokar of Bandiagara taught a version of this commentary
on tawhid, and initiated a number of persons into an
associated form of 'ilm al-huruf. These initiations
were completely separate from those of the Tijaniyya
Sufi order, in which Cerno Bokar was also a muqaddam
(Brenner: 1984).

One final, isolated example of the secret nature
of the esoteric sciences should be mentioned here.
Early this century, a Muslim scholar in Porto Novo told
a European researcher that while pursuing Qur'anic
studies with his own father, he had also been "under
the order" of an Alfa, a Tukolor from Futa Toro, who
had taught him geomancy (katt al-raml). According to
this informant, one was not allowed to reveal the name
of ones's Alfa, (Maupoil: 1943) thus implying that this
aspect of his religious training was not public knowledge.

The changing status of the esoteric sciences among the
'ulama.
The significance of the esoteric sciences in West
Africa can be fully understood only in the social and
political context in which they were practiced.
Practitioners may have sought their legitimacy with
reference to accepted Islamic doctrine, but they also
functioned in response to the needs of ordinary people
as well as to the demands of political authorities, all
of whom sought the aid of persons who were seen to
exercise "supernatural" power. These sciences were
practiced by all manner of clerics, from the highly
educated to the barely literate. Nor do we need to
reject as completely invalid the charges levelled
against certain pactitioners (their exploitation of
popular credulity, or their venality) in order to suggest that there was also a positive side to their
efforts as a sincere response to human needs of all
sorts. The esoteric sciences were a particular manifestation of Islamic culture in the process of growth
and development; they played a vital role in extending
that culture over vast areas. One of the best examples
of this process is to be found in Islamic divination,
which seems to have spread throughout the African continent wherever Muslims had travelled, and which also

enjoyed considerable influence on the European coasts
of the Mediterranean (Tannery: 1921). The origins of
this form of divination are almost certainly non-Islamic, and all the efforts to "Islamize" it never managed
to convince any but a few 'ulama of its validity as a
technique; Ibn Khaldum concluded that geomancy was
"based on arbitrary notions and wishful thinking." (Ibn
Khaldun: 1958: 1:226). But if researchers accept
this doctrinal rejection of divination, which is in
effect the present situation, and refuse to consider it
a part of Islam in Africa, then we cut ourselves off
from the study of one of the most dynamic elements in
the diffusion of Islamic culture on the continent.

In the past, many West Africans perceived the
value of Islam in the ability of its clerics to manipulate supernatural power. It might be said that many
practitioners of the esoteric sciences were "innova-
tors," with all the ambivalence that this term implies.
Non-Islamic practices were adopted which could be condemned as bid'a; but much of the process of borrowing
and experimentation can also be understood as a search
for those techniques which might prove effective in
responding to practical, everyday human needs. Studies
of doctrinal confrontations over these issues contribute to our understanding of Islamic history in West
Africa. But we must also attempt to study the esoteric
sciences on their own terms in order fully to appreciate their role in the diffusion of Islam in Africa.

REFERENCES CITED

Brenner, Louis. Three Fulbe Scholars in Borno. The
    Maghreb Review, XI, no. 3-4. 1984a.
    _____. West African Sufi. The Religious
    Heritage and Spritiual Search of Cerno Bokar
    Saalif Taal. London: C. Hurst & Co., 1984b.
Hunwick, John. Notes on a Late Fifteenth Century
    Document concerning 'al-Takrur'. In C.H. Allen
    and R.W. Johnson, eds. African Perspectives.
    Oxford: Oxford University Press. 1970.
Ibn Khaldun. The Muqaddimah. Tr. from the Arabic by
    Franz Rosenthal. London, 1958.
Ibrahim ibn Sha'ban ibn Nafi' al-Salihi, Kitab Tamtam
    al-Hindi. Bibliothèque Nationale, Paris. MS
    Arabe 2699.
Last, Murray. A Note on Attitudes to the Supernatural
    in the Sokoto Jihad. Journal of the Historical
    Society of Nigeria, IV, 2: 3-13. 1967.
Murray Last and Al-Hajj, M.A. Attempts at Defining a
    Muslim in Nineteenth Century Hausaland and Bornu.
    Journal of the Historical Society of Nigeria 3.
    2:231-39. ;1965.

Maupoil, B. Contribution à l'étude de l'origine
    musulmane de la géomancie dans les bas Dahomey
    Journal de la Société des Africanistes, XIII:
    3-4. 1943.
Muhammad ibn Muhammad al-Fullani al Katsinawi
    al-Barnawi: Bahjat al-afaq wa-idah al-labs wa
    'l-ighlaq fil'ilm al-huruf wal'awfaq.
    Bibliothèque Nationale. Paris: Arabe 5635,
    folio 3b-112b.
Sanneh, Lamin. The Jakhanke. London: International
    African Institute. 1979.
Stewart, C.C. Islam and the Social Order in
    Mauritania. Oxford: The Clarendon Press. 1973.
Tannery, P. Le Rabolion. In Memoiresd Scientifiques.
    Paris and Toulouse, IV: 297-411. 1921.
Umar ibn Sa'id al-Futi. Ramah hizb al-rahim 'ala nuhur
    hizb al-rajim. Printed in the margins of 'Ali
    Harazim, Jawahir al-Ma'ani. Beirut: Dar al-Fikr,
    No date.

This paper was first presented at the conference: Islam in Africa: The Changing Role of
the 'Ulama', held at Northwestern University, March 28-31, 1984.

CHAPTER 3

ISLAMIC MEDICINE IN RURAL HAUSALAND
Robert Stock

ABSTRACT

This study examines the healing activities of
ordinary rural Hausa malamai, or Koranic scholars.
They are important providers of protective and curative
medicines for individuals and overseers of community
health. Malamai use both prophetic and herbal medicines, often in combination. The therapies used by
malamai to treat various health-threatening problems
are described, and the utilization of prophetic cures
is assessed. The results are preliminary and show the
need for additional research on contemporary Islamic
medical systems in Africa.

Hausaland is blessed with a great diversity of
skilled medical practitioners. Hausa healers, particularly herbalists, barber-surgeons and Islamic scholars, practice medicine far beyond Hausaland and are
widely respected for their therapeutic skills. Hausa
medical traditions may be subdivided into those which
are essentially secular and those which involve spiritual models of healing. The former include various
kinds of herbalists, as well as others with special
skills in bonesetting, midwifery and bloodletting.
Their skills are based on personal and family secrets
and craftsmanship, transmitted from one generation to
the next. Spiritual healers, or intercessionists
(Abdalla 1981: 111), ultimately attribute their healing prowess to their privileged access to some supernatural power. This permits them to learn about potent
medicines unknown to others and to act as intermediaries on behalf of patients, approaching the supernatural
sources of affliction and of potential relief. The
bori spirit possession cult is the primary example of a
therapy based on intercession with spirits (Nicolas
1967; Besmer 1983). The bokaye are herbalists who
likewise depend upon the guidance of spirits in their
medical practice.

The malam, or Islamic scholar also practices a
type of intercessionist medicine, only one which is
based on the healing power of Allah. Malamai adopt a
highly antagonistic stance toward the traditional
spiritualists, the masu bori and bokaye, whose medical
practice they claim to be unIslamic. In contrast,
there is generally supportive relationship between
malamai and the various secular healers such as masu
ganye (herbalists), wanzamai (barber-surgeons), mad'ora
(bonesetters), and ungozomai (midwives). These practitioners are generally considered to be Muslims in good
standing.   In fact, there is considerable overlap
amongst the various types of medicine.   Thus, the
mad'ora and wanzamai incorporate selected Islamic elements in their therapies, while many malamai dispense
herbal as well as Islamic medicines.
     This paper focuses on malamai, practitioners
specifically following the Islamic model of prophetic
medicine, and excludes other types of Muslim Hausa
healers who have in certain ways been influenced by the
Islamic heritage. Despite the many resources available
for the study of Islamic medicine in Hausaland-- practitioners who are to be found in every Hausa city, town
and village, historical and contemporary medical texts
and comparative studies from other parts of the Islamic
world-- very little has been done to study Islamic
medicine in Hausaland. The only significant exceptions
are works by Murry Last on attitudes are towards the
supernatural inthe Sokoto jihad (Last 1967) and by
Ismail Abdalla (1979; 1981), on the impact of Islam on
Hausa medicine, based on the study of historical and
contemporary manuscripts on Islamic medicine, and on
discussions with several prominent Hausa healers and
scholars.
     The present study provides a preliminary sketch of
the medical acitvities of "ordinary" practitioners of
Islamic medicine in rural Hausaland.   It presents a
contrast to the studies of Abdalla which focused on the
elite, learned tradition in Hausa Islamic medicine.
The data in this study mostly relate to curative medicine provided by malamai. Nevertheless, it is recognized that their provision of preventative and protective medicines and their role as primary guardians of
community health are at least as important as their
curative activities.
     Data for the study are from two surveys conducted
in Hadejia Emirate in the North-eastern part of Kano
State, Nigeria. Interviews were conducted in Bulangu
District with 29 healers who identified themselves as
malamai, as well as with 51 other traditional practitioners. They were questioned about their training,
their conceptualization of matters related to illness
and its treatment, their areas of specialization, and

their preferred treatments for selected health problems. Secondly, data on the prior utilization of
Islamic medicine were extracted from interviews with
some 5,000 patients attending a health center or dispensary. The sample is not a random one excluding,
for example, those who were unable or unwilling to seek
Western-type therapy at a health facility. Nevertheless, these responses provide preliminary information
on the utilization of Islamic prophetic medicine for
curative purposes.

Malamai in Hausa Society

Islamic influence in Hausaland dates back to the 14th
century when the religion of Islam was first introduced
(Hiskett 1984:73). Islam became much more influential
and widespread following the reformist jihad of Uthman
dan Fodio early in the 19th century. It became the
religion, at least in a formal sense, of a steadily
increasing proportion of the talakawa (the masses),
rather than merely of masu sarauta (the ruling classes). Uthman dan Fodio's successor as Sultan of Sokoto,
Mohammed Bello, studied and actively promoted Islamic
medicine as a means of spreading Islam and establishing
the hegemony of the Sokoto Caliphate (Abdalla 1981:23).
As a result, the traditional spiritual healers such as
the bokaye and masu bori lost much of their influence
while the malamai rose to prominence as the dominant
healers.

A malam is a literate person and a teacher (Abraham 1946:650). Yet, malamai vary considerably in terms
of education and influence. Some are very learned and
possess extensive libraries on a variety of subjects,
while others have limited education. Some are considered to be influential and powerful--"big" in Hausa
terminology--while others are "small" and unimportant.
Malamai are present in all Hausa communities.
Some villages are essentially composed of malamai,
their families and their students (almajirai). The
conduct of Islamic education is a primary duty of
malamai, and is central to their role as guardians of
Islamic principles and overseers of community morality.
From an early age, Hausa children are entrusted to a
malam for education. For serious students of Islam,
studies last a lifetime; advanced students may specialize in a variety of fields ranging from law to
medicine.

The apprenticeship of almajirai often takes them
to several destinations, often far from home. Most of
the malamai interviewed in Hadejia Emirate had pursued
their education away from their place of birth. Over
half of them mentioned destinations to the east of
home, reflecting both the attraction of the highly-
regarded Islamic education of eastern Kano State and

Borno (Hassan 1980:165), and the lure of traveling in
the direction of Mecca.
   A second specialization of malamai, integrally
related to the first, is the maintenance of community
and personal health. Malamai provide individuals with
a variety of medicines designed to restore health, to
prevent illness and to bring good fortune. Malamai act
as guardians of community morality, speaking out
against tendencies which they see as unIslamic, and
leading the community in prayer in times of crisis.
The educational activities of malamai underpin their
health-related functions, since education provides
individuals with guidelines for healthy living within a
society of fellow believers.
   The powers which malamai utilize in order to safeguard health may potentially be turned toward evil
ends. Unscrupulous practitioners may sell medicines
designed to bring harm to one's rival. One example is
jifa in which a curse is literally hurled at the con-
jured image of the victim, often using a needle as the
symbolic medium of delivery. Rumours abound about such
unscrupulous "black" malamai; they remain a shadowy
minority whose activities do not meaningfully tarnish
the image of the scholarly profession as a whole.

Medical Practice
Malamai employ, either separately or in combination,
two major types of medicines, namely Koranic or prophetic medicines and herbal medicines. A few practitioners may also use certain non-Islamic practices and
medicines.
   The herbal remedies used are essentially the traditional Hausa pharmacopea, which malamai administer in
the same way as other healers. Thus, herbal remedies
may be given as an infusion to be drunk and/or rubbed
over the body, or fermented for several days prior to
use (tsimi), or put into a fire so the vapors (turare)
may be inhaled, or rubbed onto the body in its raw
state. In addition, malamai commonly combine the se of
herbal remedies with some aspect of prophetic medicine.
For example, rubutu (Koranic ink medicine) may be mixed
with plant materials, or prayers may be said in connection with the dispensing of medicine.
   The Islamic medicine which reached Hausaland was
not the scientific medicine which had flourished during
the first centuries of Islamic civilization (Abdalla
1981:58). The original Islamic medicine, based ultimately on the medical legacy of ancient Greece, was
highly developed and scientific in its approach. The
vigor of Islamic medical science gradually waned, and
prophetic medicine came to the fore. Instead of promoting scientific investigation, prophetic medicine
emphasized absolute conformity to the fundamental

tenets of Islamic law. The instructions and sayings of the Prophet Mohammed assumed a new role of absolute dominance in this new conformist medical tradition. Also important was the status of the healer, since it was believed that some were blessed with greater baraka (mystical powers derived from Allah or the Prophet Mohammed) than others (Darrah 1980:16).

In present-day Hausaland, Islamic prophetic medicines are administered in a variety of ways:
(a) Rubutu (literally writing), the most common Islamic remedy, is prepared by writing appropriate verses from the Holy Koran on a writing board and then drinking the ink washed from the board. Rubutu may be used as a curative medicine, but is more often employed as a tonic to preserve health and bring good fortune (Last n.d.).
(b) Laya are amulets worn on the body or placed in an appropriate place in the house. They contain pieces of paper with Koranic verses believed to confer protection. These are normally preventative medicines, and are particularly employed to protect children from the many diseases threatening them. Headaches are often treated by tieing laya to the forehead.
(c) Tofi (spitting) involves transfering the power of the therapeutic spoken word by rubbing the malam's saliva on the center of pain. Tofi is used for headaches and scorpion stings, among other problems.
(d) Kamun Kai is used to treat headaches; the patient's held is grasped by the malam while the therapeutic passages are recited.
(e) Addu'a refers to the invocations which follow the five-times daily laudatory prayers (Abraham 1946:7), or specifically to medical invocations in these prayers.
(f) Rokon Allah (supplication, "begging" Allah) is commonly employed when the malam does not know the actual treatment for some condition.

Table 1 summarizes the ways in which the interviewed malamai use prophetic, herbal and "other" techniques in their medical work. Approximately two-thirds of them prescribe herbal remedies for certain illnesses. A significant number combine two or three distinct types of medicine in a simple therapeutic procedure. While this may be represented as a clear case of cultural convergence along the interface between indigenous and prophetic medicine, it can also be interpreted as evidence that Islamicization remains incomplete, despite the fact that the study population has been Muslim for several generations at least.

Each practitioner was asked to list the illnesses he specialized in healing, and to describe the usual treatment employed. The mean number of specialties identified was three. Approximately half cited stomach problems, headache and iskoki (spirits) as areas of

specialization. Table 2 lists the major areas of
specialization. These fall into three main categories,
namely common symptomatic illness, more serious conditions associated with spirit attack, and social
problems. This last category included the one example
encountered of "black" medicine; a malam claimed that
he could provide medicine to forcefully seize a rival's
property.
        Among healers who are amenable to giving either
prophetic or herbal medicines (Categories 3 and 4 in
Table 1), the therapeutic strategy employed varies
significantly according to the problem being treated.
This is the most fundamental message of Table 3, which
shows the treatments used by the interviewed malamai
for nine selected problems. The examples chosen include three common symptomatic illnesses, three spirit-
related conditions, two social problems and "unknown
illness". These examples have been ranked to show the
importance of prophetic medicines relative to other
therapies, particularly those using herbal medicines.
        It is apparent that prophetic medicine is very
dominant in the treatment of common symptomatic illnesses, unknown illness and non-biomedical (i.e.,
social) problems. In fact, there was not a single
example of a malam using a herbal remedy alone to treat
any of the six conditions of the above types. There
were rare cases in which prophetic and herbal medicines
were combined or used interchangeably for the treatment
of these generally minor problems. The infrequent
prescription of herbal remedies ls surprising since the
Hausa have several commonly-known remedies ior measles
(the thistle dayi in particular) and stomach upsets
(notably jar kanwa (red potash), sabara (Guiera
senegalensis), ganyen carbi (leaves of Azodirachta
indica) and toka (ash). However, herbal remedies
assume the dominant role in the treatment of spirit-
related illness. Herbal remedies were used exclusively
or jointly with prophetic medicines by half of the
malamai treating spirit attack, by two-thirds of those
treating jaundice, and by three-quarters of those giving snakebite medicines. Snakebite falls within the
spirit category since the Hausa regard many types of
wildlife, including snakes, as probably being physical
manifestations of spirits.

Common symptomatic illness
        Prophetic medicines are heavily dominant in the
treatment of these conditions by malamai (see Table 3).
Virtually all treat headaches and stomach disorders,
although actual therapeutic strategies vary. For headaches, laya tied to the forehead with thread and kamun
kai are most important. Rubutu, sometimes used in combination with non-prophetic medicines, is most often

used for stomach problems. An interesting example of
the sometimes subtle merging of prophetic and herbal
traditions concerns the preference for toka (ash) taken
from the hearths of Koranic schools to "ordinary" ash,
for treating stomach complaints. A third example of
common symptomatic illness is measles, surprisingly
treated by only 42% of those questioned. Prophetic
medicines were indicated by all of these healers; none
mentioned the various herbal remedies commonly utilized
by the Hausa to treat measles. The focus on curative
medicines in Table 3 obscures the fact that two-thirds
of those questioned said that they make laya (protective amulets) for children who are susceptible to
measles. Conjunctivitis is another common illness
which malamai often treat. Rubutu is prepared and used
to wash out the patient's eyes. However, many of the
other common illnesses of Hausaland seem to be treated
infrequently by malamai. Curative medicines for
fevers, diarrhea, schistosomiasis and skin rashes, for
example, do not seem to be areas of expertise for
malamai. Nevertheless, many provide protective laya
for these conditions.

In summary, some common symptomatic illnesses are
the specialties of malamai while others are treated by
them only sporadically. Prophetic medicines may be
administered in a number of ways for curative purposes.
However, the preparation of protective amulets (laya)
for children and others at risk no doubt constitutes
the most important function of malamai with respect to
these illnesses.

Social problems

Malamai administer medicines for a variety of
general social problems, not directly related to biomedical disease. This reflects the very broad, holis-
tic Hausa conceptualization of health (lafiya) and
likewise of medicine (magani). Lafiya encompasses a
full range of relationships with family, with community, and with Allah. Thus, the absence of the
symptoms of disease constitutes only one component of
lafiya. Magani is anything which brings about a
desired effect, generally by counteracting some undesirable state or affliction with its opposite (Ryan
1974:vii). All magani, whether taken primarily for
curative, health-maintaining or protective purposes,
has as its objective the promotion of individual and
communal health. Thus, "social" problems are treatable
essentially as "medical" problems, with the malamai,
guardians of community health, taking the leading role.

Two examples of social problems have been included
in Table 3, namely fighting involving co-wives and
finding lost property. The most common approach in
treating such problems was rokon Allah (supplication),

apparently indicating that these malamai didn't know
specific suras for the preparation of rubutu or performance of addu'a. The malamai questioned were able to
be specific more often about their medicines for fighting wives than for the recovery of property. Some
prepare rubutu which is then surreptitiously added to
the food or water of the combatants. Others prepare
laya for burial at strategic locations within the
compound.

Married women are important consumers of protective social medicines. They feel themselves to be very
vulnerable since divorce, which causes mothers to be
separated from their much-loved and desired children,
is very common (Fleischer 1974:155). Thus, women in
purdah obtain laya and rubutu in order to retain the
love of their husbands and to protect themselves from
the machinations of jealous co-wives and meddlesome
in-laws.

As the recognized guardians of community health,
malamai are looked to for leadership with respect to
diverse social issues affecting the community. For
example, malamai led the grassroots opposition to
Nigeria's Universal Primary Education scheme (Clarke
1978:135). Despite apparent setbacks in the early days
when U.P.E. seemed successful, the malamai have pre-
vailed and U.P.E. is now essentially dead in most of
rural Kano State. Malamai also take the lead in
responding collectively to environmental crises such as
drought. Communal prayers are held and prostitutes are
frequently driven from town. In pre-colonial times,
the annual Islamic grain tithe provided food reserves
to insure that the impact of drought was minimized
(Watts 1983:138).

Spirit-related illness

Iskoki (spirits) and aljannu (djinns) are invisible
creatures which share the world with human beings --
there are urban and forest spirits, good(="white") and
bad (="black") spirits, each with its own distinctive
personality traits. The Hausa conceptualization of the
spirit world has resulted from the merging of the
pantheon of iskoki, which were central to pre-Islamic
Hausa religious beliefs, with aljannu, the spirits or
djinns which are mentioned in the Holy Koran. While
there are many variations in individual's conceptualization of the spirit world, iskoki are generally
considered to reside primarily in rural areas and to be
potentially dangerous if not malicious, while aljannu
are usually believed to inhabit towns and to bring good
fortune.

Spirit-related diseases may be treated by several
different healers. In addition to malamai, the bokaye,
and masu bori provide medicines to ward off spirits.

But whereas the cures of the malamai invoke the power of
Allah to protect those at risk or to drive off the
offending spirit, bokaye, and masu bori rely on their
privileged contacts with the spirit world to learn the
secret remedies needed, or to intervene with the
health-threatening spirit on behalf of the patient.
    Table 3 lists three conditions normally attributed
to spirits. The first category is a general one for
healers claiming to have maganin iska (medicine for
spirits). Whereas most of the non-Islamic spirit healers spoke of their speciaiizations in terms of remedies
for counteracting specific spirits and for the particular diseases they cause, most malamai spoke only of
spirit attack in general. Whole the majority used
prophetic medicines exclusively, 48% of those claiming
to have medicines for spirit attack, prescribed herbal
remedies, used either exclusively or jointly with
prophetic cures. In addition to the provision of curative medicines for spirit attack, malamai often prepare
laya for the protection of those at risk. These laya
may be worn, or may be strategically placed within the
house to keep iskoki at bay.
    Shawara and bayamma are terms for jaundice which
most people use interchangeably. Not only is it a very
common illness but one about which the Hausa are always
aware. People are constantly on the lookout for
shawara medicines for themselves and family members.
Traditional herbal remedies for shawara usually make
the patient vomit; yellowish vomit is taken as a sign
that the disease has been expelled from the body and
that recovery is imminent. Two-thirds of malamai
treating shawara utilize herbal remedies, usually without prophetic additions.
    The persistence of indigenous, pre-Islamic beliefs
concerning shawara was evident. Some malamai recommended gwazarma (crushed white grubs from a dung heap)
as a treatment for shawara. This practice relates to
an indigenous Hausa belief that the ingestion of filth
can be therapeutic. "Desperate diseases require
desperate remedies" (Darrah 1980:108).
    An even more striking example of a pre-Islamic
treatment for shawara came from one malam, the chief
imam in a large community. He identified three types
of cures, namely addu'a (invocation), itace (wood) and
a ceremony involving the ritual slaughter of a chicken.
This ceremony begins with the selection and slaughter
of a young, pure white chicken. All feathers, bones,
intestines and blood from the chicken are put into a
hole which has been dug in the ground. The patient
washes thoroughly so that all blood is removed from
his body and goes into the hole. The contents of the
hole are then thoroughly burnt. The chicken meat is
cooked and eaten, but without any spices being used.

This ritual slaughter includes several symbols of
purification - the choice of a white chicken, the
thorough washing after slaughtering the chicken, the
burning of blood, bones, feathers, etc., and finally
consumption of the pure, "uncontaminated" meat.

A third example of a spirit-related condition is
snakebite. Snakebite medicines are more likely to come
from bokaye or maharba (hunters) than from malamai.
Vomiting is usually induced using the bulbous plant
gadali (crinum giganteum). Most of the malamai treating snakebite mentioned gadali, while a small minority
recommended prophetic medicine.

In summary, the treatment of spirit-related diseases is quite different from common symptomatic illness or social problems. It is evident that indigenous
herbal remedies remain the dominant medicines, even
among malamai. Moreover, certain indigenous, non-
Islamic concepts such as ritual slaughter and the
therapeutic value of filth, are still held by some
rural malamai. Nevertheless, many malamai utilize
prophetic medicines in treating spiritual illness. A
significant number were found to prescribe both herbal
and prophetic remedies, thus essentially combining the
two medical traditions.

Unknown Illness

Malamai were asked how they would treat an illness if
its cause was not clearly apparent. Only one mentioned
a herbal remedy; the others said they used prophetic
strategies, particularly rokon Allah and rubutu. The
popularity of rokon Allah (supplication) and experimentation with different medicines, shows that the treatment of an unknown illness is highly uncertain and
empirical.

Fractures and burns

The healing power of Allah is commonly invoked by the
Hausa in the treatment of injuries such as fractures
and burns. Prayers (addu'a) are always said after the
setting of a fracture by the bonesetter. Should the
fracture be slow to heal, additional prayers are offered. Addu'a may be performed by the bonesetter himself,
or a malam may be summoned to perform the task.
Prayers of this sort appear to be obligatory for the
treatment of fractures, but optional for other injuries
such as burns.

The discussion so far has focused on the medicines
provided by malamai, comparing in particular the use of
herbal and prophetic remedies. The focus will now
shift to the general population and evidence concerning
the relative importance of Islamic therapies.

Utilization of Islamic Prophetic Medicines

Hausa people have a clear range of therapeutic options at their disposal. Not only are there various types of medical practitioners, but there is an extremely widely known body of knowledge on maganin gida, namely home remedies comprised of common herbal medicines and other cures. These medicines are often used in the initial treatment of comparatively minor illnesses. Western scientific medicines may be obtained from various sources, including hospitals and dispensaries, the patent medicine stores found in larger towns and itinerant medicine hawkers. Thus, it is important to go beyond an investigation of medicines offered for sale by malamai in order to see how their medicines, and alternate therapies, are actually used by consumers.

The utilization data discussed in this section are derived from a survey of patients at hospitals and dispensaries which include questions about previously-obtained treatment for each patient's present illness. These data include counts of the reported frequency of prior use of prophetic medicines and so provide some indication of the influence of malamai as healers, with particular respect to curative medicine. In order to provide some comparative context for assessing the use of prophetic medicines, data on the prior utilization of herbal medicines and patent remedies have been included.

These data have some obvious deficiencies which necessitate a cautious interpretation of results. Firstly, this research was not undertaken with the specific intent of studying Islamic medicine. Since the data were collected at Western-type health facilities, healthy people and those unwilling or unable to utilize such health services were automatically excluded from the sample. Secondly, the probability of using some treatment prior to visiting a health facility increases with distance from the facility, reflecting the increasing temporal and monetary costs in respect to distance. Thus, the incentive to utilize Koranic remedies or another form of treatment as first-resort therapy increases in relation to distance. In order to reduce distance-related biases, the data have been disaggregated into 0-2 km, 2-10 km and over 10 km (from the health facility) distance categories. Thirdly, the data do not permit an assessment of the relative importance of malamai as providers of herbal medicines. Fourthly, the primary emphasis on curative medicine means that other important functions of malamai, especially the preparation of protective amulets, are excluded from these data. Finally, there is inevitably some under-reporting of traditional medicine use by respondents.

Table 4 shows the expected increase with distance
from a health facility in the proportion of patients
previously using Islamic medicine.   It appears that
female adults are the most likely to have utilized
Koranic remedies. While this may merely reflect male-
female differences in disease profiles, it may instead
result from women being confined to purdah and therefore having to overcome more obstacles in order to
reach a hospital (Stock 1983:566).   The apparently
greater frequency of use of Islamic medicine by women
is somewhat surprising since women are usually portray-
ed as less involved in and committed to Islam than men.
On the other hand, many of the interviewed malamai
reported that women used their medicines more often
than men.
Table 5 compares the reported prior utilization of
prophetic, herbal and patent medicines for selected
illnesses.   What is particularly striking is the extremely infrequent mention of prophetic medicines.
Utilization levels were generally below 10%, even at a
distance greater than 10 km from a health facility.
Complaints such as headache, stomach ache and conjunctivitis, which are considered by a large proportion of
malamai as among their areas of specialization, and
which consumers habitually cite as diseases for prophetic treatment in hypothetical-situation interviews, had
very surprisingly low utilization rates.   The highest
levels of reported utilization of prophetic medicines,
amongst the Table 5 examples, were for spirit attack
and kumburi (swelling, edema), which is also considered
to have a spiritual etiology.   Spirit-related diseases
are brought for hospital treatment only infrequently.
This accounts for the greater probability of initially
using non-Western medicine, but it also highlights the
danger of concluding too much from hospitalbased data.
After all, virtually all spirit-related conditions will
have been treated using non-Western medicine.   Only a
minority consisting of people whose symptoms persist in
spite of non-Western health care, or whose illness
seems life-threatening, actually seek help at a
Western-type health facility.
The findings point to a much greater utilization
of herbal and patent medicines than prophetic cures.
With the single exception of spirit attack, either herbal remedies or patent medicine or both are apparently
utilized several times as frequently as Islamic cures.
For common symptomatic illnesses like headache, malaria
and conjunctivitis, patent medicines (e.g., Aspirin
tablets and penicillin ointment) appear to have effectively supplanted rubutu, addu'a and kamun kai.   For
other illnesses, herbal remedies are apparently dominant.   A large proportion of measles patients had
previously used herbal remedies (60% of the 10-plus km

cohort); these would mostly be home remedies such as d-
ayi. For more serious, chronic complaints such as
gonorrhea, tropical ulcer and edema, the medicines of a
professional herbalist are likely to be sought at an
early stage. However, the use of prophetic cures
appears to remain quite peripheral, irrespective of tne
illness.

Discussion
The relatively low levels of utilization of prophetic medicines reported in the present study clearly
suggest that malamai play a comparatively minor role in
curative health care in Hausaland. The prior utilization of both herbal and patent remedies was reported as
being several times as great as prophetic cures. Yet,
malamai are commonly identified as being the most
important category of healers in Hausaland. While the
nature of the sample data, collected with a different
research question in mind, means that conclusions can
only be tentative, the magnitude of the disparities
suggests that malamai indeed occupy a peripheral position in Hausa curative medicine.
The focus on curative medicine is problematical
since malamai also dispense protective medicines and
assume a leading role in safeguarding community health.
Malamai prepare amulets (laya) which are used to confer
protection against specific health risks. Virtually
all children wear laya, some as many as ten of them.
Adults also obtain these amulets in order to achieve a
desired result. The consumption of rubutu as a general
tonic and potion for good luck is very common among
those able to afford it, and represents a significant
aspect of the broadly medical practice of many malamai.
If malamai are indeed the most important healers, it
must relate mainly to these preventative and prescriptive medicines rather than to curative health care.
There certainly are many individuals who rely very
heavily on prophetic medicine, resolutely believing
that "Alkur' ani kantia magani" - the Holy Koran is a
medicine shop. However, it seems that these people are
a relatively small minority, and that herbal medicines,
for the most part prepared at home, form the corner-
stone of rural people's therapeutic mindset. Patent
medicines are also becoming more important, to the
extent that the aspirin tablet has effectively supplanted prophetic and herbal cures for headaches and
fevers.
If the status of the malamai as healers has indeed
been over-emphasized, there are some possible explanations. Firstly, malamai are found in every village.
Not only are they very numerous but many are relatively
visible as community leaders. Secondly, their protective laya are always highly visible when worn by small

children; other healers' medicines are seldom readily
visible in the same way. Thirdly, strict religious
orthodoxy is expected in the close-knit Islamic society
of rural Hausaland. Few Hausa men will acknowledge,
for example, that contemporary bori (spirit possession)
is anything but play-acting. The opposite side of this
coin, namely the tendency to deny the persistence of
unIslamic practices, may be a tendency to exaggerate
for the importance of Islamic medicine. This is especially possible in conversations about behavior in
hypothetical situations.

The medicine discussed by the malamai interviewed
in this study is a rather different Islamic medicine
from that reported in Abdalla's studies. Abdalla refers to a very significant learned tradition in Islamic
medicine which dates back to the very founding of the
religion, and which incorporates not only manuscripts
produced in major centers of Islamic learning like
Cairo and Mecca, but also historical and contemporary
manuscripts on medicine by Hausa authors. Bulangu
District malamai were asked about books in their
possession which related to their healing activities.
Half reported that they only had a copy of the Holy
Koran. Ten of the 29 said that they also possessed
kundi, which are loose notes with indeterminate content. Only 5 were able to name specific works on
medicine in their possession. Without more information
on these books and kundi and in the absence of comparable data in other studies, little can be said except
to note the surprising scarcity of book ownership among
this group of Islamic scholars.

This conclusion should really be a beginning.
Very little is known about malamai and their healing
activities; the same can be said for other Hausa healers as well. We need to know about the differing roles
of "big" and "small" malamai, and of differences between urban and rural Islamic medicines. We need to
know how ordinary malamai combine prophetic and herbal
medicines, whether they have an explicit conceptual
basis for this, and whether trends may be discerned in
their preparation of medicines. We need to know about
who uses prophetic medicines and alternatives to them,
and the circumstances in which they are used. We need
to know whether malamai are generally becoming less
important as healers, or less important with respect to
selected conditions such as headache and conjunctivitis. There are plenty of other worthwhile questions
which likewise can only be answered after further
research, oriented specifically toward the study of
Islamic medicine in Hausaland.

ACKNOWLEDGEMENTS
The financial support of Social Sciences and
Humanities Research Council of Canada is gratefully
acknowledged. Research was made possible by the grant-
ing of Research Associateships by Bayero University and
by Ahmadu Bello University. The assistance of
Babangida Ahmed, Adamu Saleh and Alhaji Muhammadu,
Wamban Hadejia is gratefully acknowledged.

REFERENCES CITED
Abdalla, Ismail H. "Medicine in Nineteenth Century
  Arabic Literature in Northern Nigeria: a Report."
  Kano Studies n.s 4:55-67. 1979.
Abraham R.C. Dictionary of the Hausa Language. London:
  University of London Press. 1946.
Besmer, Fremont. Horses, Musicians and Gods: The Hausa
  Cult of Spirit-Possession. South Hadley, Mass.:
  Bergin and Garvey. 1983.
Clarke, Peter B. "Islam, Education and the Develop-
  mental Process in Nigeria." Comparative Education
  14: 133-141. 1978.
Darrah, Alan C. A Hermeneutic Approach to Hausa Thera-
  peutics: the Allegory of the Living Fire. Ph.D.
  dissertation, Northwestern University. 1980.
Fleischer, Luitgard M. Crises of Life and How They are
  Handled: a Case Study of Hausa Women in Jos. M.
  Phil. thesis, Edinburgh University. 1974.
Hassan, Usman. "The Provision and Content of Islamic
  Education in Kano." Kano Studies n.s.2:162-173.
  1980.
Hiskett, Mervyn. The Development of Islam in West
  Africa. London: Longman. 1984.
Last, D. Murray. "A Note on the Attitudes to the
  Supernatural in the Sokoto Jihad. Journal of the
  Historical Society of Nigeria IV: 3-13. 1967.
  _____. "Some Hausa Ideas Concerning Sickness.
  Unpublished paper, Ahmadu Bello University. No
  date.
Nicolas, Jacqueline. 'Les Juments des Dieux': Rites
  de Possession et Condition Feminine en Pays Huasa.
  Paris-Niamey: Etudes Nigeriennes. 1967.
Ryan, Pauline M. Aspects of Hausa Symbolism, with
  Special Reference to the Literature. D. Phil.
  dissertation, Oxford University. 1974.
Stock, Robert. Distance and the Utilization of Health
  Care Facilities in Rural Nigeria. Social Science
  and Medicine 17:568-573. 1983.

Watts, Michael. Silent Violence: Food, Famine and
    Peasantry in Northern Nigeria. Berkeley:
    University of California Press. 1983.

Table 1

Therapeutic Approaches Used by Malamai in
   Bulangu District, Kano State[a]

1. Prophetic medicines only		
(rubutu, addu'a, etc.)	9	(31%)
2. Herbal remedies only	1	(03%)
3. Prophetic and herbal Combined[b]	7	(24%)
4. Prophetic or herbal[c]	6	(21%)
5. "Other" and/or herbal and/or prophetic	6	(21%)

Source:
[a] Sample survey.
[b] In at least one of the cures described by each
    healer.
[c] Used some prophetic and some herbal remedies, but
    apparently does not use them in combination.

Table 2

Medical Specializations
Identifiend by Malamai

Usually common symptomatics illness		Usually relatively serious and spirit-related		Social Problems	
Stomach problems	16 (55%)	Spirit attack	13 (45%)	Domestic	
Headache	15 (52%)	Jaundice	6 (21%)	strife	1 (3%)
Fever	6 (21%)	Sorcery	4 (14%)		
Conjunctiv- itis	4 (14%)	Impotence	2 (0)	Seizing	
Measles	2 (07%)	Chest pain	2 (07%)	property	
Other	4 (14%)	Difficult birth	2 (07%)	by force	1 (3%)
		Others	12 (35%)		

Source: Interviews with 29 malamai, Bulangu District.

Table 4

Utilization of Prophetic Medicines as
Prior Therapy by Patients
at Hadejia-Area Health Facilities

		Distance (km)		
	N	0-2	2-10	10 Plus
Male child (0-14)	1310	1.5%	4.7%	6.8%
Male adult	1114	1.9%	8.5%	6.4%
Female child	957	2.1%	4.4%	14.6%
Female adult	854	3.7%	7.5%	13.2%

Source: Sample survey

CHAPTER 4

WHAT HAPPENED TO ISLAMIC MEDICINE?

Nancy Elizabeth Gallagher

When the first autopsy began in the new British medical school in Calcutta in 1835, Lord Macaulay ordered fifty cannon rounds fired off. He hoped to celebrate the end of indigenous, or Ayurvedic medicine which did not pemit dissection or surgery. Soon Indian medical students were anxiously seeking admission to the Western medical schools in India where they received scholarships, classroom supplies, and finally a prestigious and well-paid job (Gupta 1976:369-371). In 1841, a British surgeon in Bengal Medical Service found only four or five Ayurvedic practitioners who were able to read the Sanskrit medical texts (Leslie 1976:358). Yet by the end of the nineteenth century Indian medical practitioners were actively reviving and restructuring their medical traditions. Ayurvedic (Brahman) and Yunani (Muslim) doctors founded medical schools, associations, journals, and pharmaceutical companies that manufactured powders and pills and exported to European pharmacists (Gupta 1976:372-375). Soon the number of indigenous doctors had substantially increased and the professional organizations were working for governmental and popular recognition. In India this professionalization of indigenous medicine was an integral part of the cultural, religious, and nationalist revival of the late nineteenth- and early twentieth centuries that attempted to resist the challenge of British imperial and cultural domination. The Ayurvedic and Yunani organizations function until the present.

Why was there no similar indigenous medical professionalization accompanying the cultural, religious and nationalist revival in North Africa and the Middle East? Certainly much of the indigenous intellectual heritage was actively revived and restudied with new interest, new questions, and new purposes. Scholars of Shar'ia law, for example, often opposed the introduction of Western legal systems and sometimes organized themselves into very effective groups. Such

47

groups borrowed organizational forms from the Western
legal professions to better oppose them. One might expect <u>hakims</u> (physicians) or practitioners of Galenic-
Islamic medicine to have done likewise to resist losing
their position and influence in society. Yet indigenous medical practitioners in the Middle East and North
Africa did not organize themselves into professional
organizations unlike their medical counterparts in
India, Pakistan, or Bangladesh, or jurisprudents in the
Middle East and North Africa.

In this paper we will ask not how Galenic-Islamic
medical beliefs and practices came to accommodate, to
parallel, or to give way to Western medical beliefs and
practices but rather ask what happened to the hakims
outside the Indian sub-continent. Why were they unable
to revive their vocation by forming professional
associations to help resist their increasingly marginalized status and the increasingly dominant European
medical culture? The term revival is of course something of a misnomer because the formation of Ayurvedic
and Yunani professional associations, journals, medical
schools, and pharmaceutical manufacturing companies has
been something new. Indigenous medical practitioners
in reviving their medical traditions have borrowed
organizational forms from Western medical practitioners. The question is important because understanding
the role of the practitioners themselves can provide an
historical dimension lacking in the more customary
philological examination of medical texts. Political,
social, and economic forces that shape medical developments can be more easily traced through the practitioners' lives than through medical texts because they are
the actors who respond to these forces.

Scholars of Galenic-Islamic medicine seldom give
more than a word or two to developments in the tradition after the classical age, usually dated from the
ninth to the twelfth centuries.[1] Most dismiss the
later years with an observation that the great tradition had declined and fossilized and was finally
replaced with a more viable medical tradition. More
recently, scholars have at least begun to consider
continuities in the Galenic-Islamic heritage. After
summarizing the introduction of Western medical institutions into Egypt and Iran in the nineteenth century,
Manfred Ullmann for example suggests the "...coexist-
ence of traditional Arabic (i.e. Galenic-Islamic)
medicine and modern European medicine. When cholera
raged in Egypt in the summer of 1883, and the French
and German missions under Louis Pasteur and Robert Koch
came to Egypt to study the epidemic, the leading
doctors in Cairo and Alexandria were almost entirely
European. At the same time, however, Arabic medicine
was fully asserting its validity. The Bulaq editions

of the great works of Ibn-al-Baytar (1874), Avicenna and al-Mausi (both 1877) were not occcasioned by an interest in the history of medicine, but by the fact that they contained a living, practical medicine" (Ullmann 198:51-52). Many Galenic-Islamic medical texts have indeed been printed for popular use. In Tunis, for example, al-Suyuti's al-Rahma fi al-tibb wa al-hikma was printed and sold widely. The publication of these texts did not however signal a revival, re-organization, or professionalization of the Galenic-Islamic medical practitioners themselves. While this seems to have been the case throughout the Middle East and North Africa, we will take nineteenth- and twent-ieth-century Tunisia as one example of a Muslim state undergoing intense colonization and ask first if there was an indigenous medical system and second if so why it did not professionalize like its counterpart in India.

Through records in the Archives Générales du Gouvernement Tunisien, we can establish the existence of a rudimentary medical association in the early nineteenth century (Gallagher 1975:145-149). Generally the ruler appointed a bash hakim or head doctor who practiced at court and who issued certificates of competence to other medical practitioners. The bash hakim was also apparently chief doctor in the maristan or hospital of Tunis (Gallagher 1983:21). From at least the eighteenth century European doctors also served at court. The rulers apparently found them useful informants of European realities and felt they possessed more medical expertise than their local counterparts. This feeling was based on the recognition of the growing superiority of European military science, political strength, and commercial expansion. Western medicine at the beginning of the nineteenth century was as yet no more efficacious than GalenicIslamic medicine (the two systems shared common roots and were in fact quite similar). What mattered was the assumption of superiority which of course was colored by new political relationships.

The certificates of competence (ijazas) issued by the bash hakim contained in the government archives reveal a process of change. In the early part of the century the bash hakim himself wrote out the ijazas (Gallagher 1983:1617). His successors continued to do so until 1861 when new laws regarding public notariza-tion changed the procedure. The medical applicant followed a standard procedure of calling together local notables who then signed a document testifying to his competence. The document (fig. 1) was then notarized by a government 'adl or notary public (AGGT 713/1). In this document, Muhammad bin Nasr al-Farashishi al-'Alawi is certified a competent doctor on the testimony of the signatories who were men of reputation familiar with the applicant's work. The document could then be used as an ijaza or submitted to the government's head doctor, now usually of Italian or French origin. The head doctor would then issue a new ijaza allowing the applicant to practice medicine in his region. Figs. 2 and 3 show the Italian and Arabic versions of such an ijaza issued to Si Muhammad bin al-Hajj al-Harfawi of the Drid tribe in 1861 (AGGT 794/2 and 794/6). Alternatively the ruler himself could issue such a certificate. Fig. 4 shows an ijaza issued in 1861 by the ruler, Sadiq Bey, to Faraj bin Yaqub Shatbun who was by his name from the indigenous Jewish community (AGGT 793/8). In 1873, Hamda Tabal al-Masakini, the last officially appointed indigenous Muslim doctor, was replaced by an Algerian, Ahmad bin Qadur who had trained in a French medical school in Algiers.

In 1881 the French occupied Tunis and organized a colonial government which retained many procedures of the old bureaucracy. The certification system was continued by the new French government. In 1877 for example Vittorio Namia of Livornese Jewish origin received his ijaza from Dr. F. Gandolphe (Fig. 5, AGGT 794/18). In 1888 however the colonial government limited the practice of medicine by indigenous practitioners. At first hakims could acquire the status of médecin toléré, a secondary status that allowed practice in regions with no licensed doctor. Eventually the practice of indigenous medicine became nearly illegal (Gallagher 1983: 93-96). Indigenous practitioners of course continued to practice but unlike in India, they did not organize to resist the new policies. Sons of the head doctors worked as orderlies in new Western-style hospitals. One or two indigenous herb sellers sought training in Italian or French pharmaceutical schools and returned to open licensed pharmacies stocking Western medicines.

In the twentieth century, the indigenous medical system has not revived but many Galenic-Islamic medical concepts and practices continue to exist. A visitor to Tunis can easily walk to medicinal herb shops which enjoy a brisk business. Fig. 6 shows an herb seller located about a half kilometer from the Porte de France entrance to the madina (ancienne ville). Use of herbal remedies has increased in recent years. Outside the madina in a popular quarter barbers still cup or bleed patients, a practice advocated by the Galenic humoral system (Fig. 7).

Tunisian reformers have been enthusiastic advocates of Western science and medicine. The current Ministry of Health is entirely staffed by Western educated medical administrators. Virtually all Tunisian physicians regard indigenous practitioners with

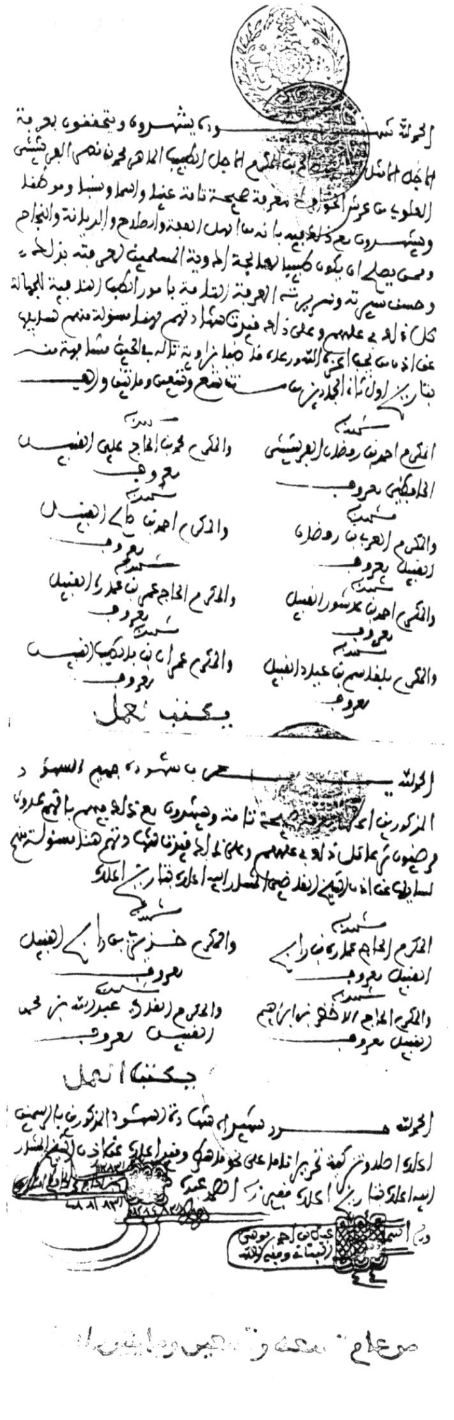

Figure 1: Document signed by local notables testifying to local medical practioner's competence.

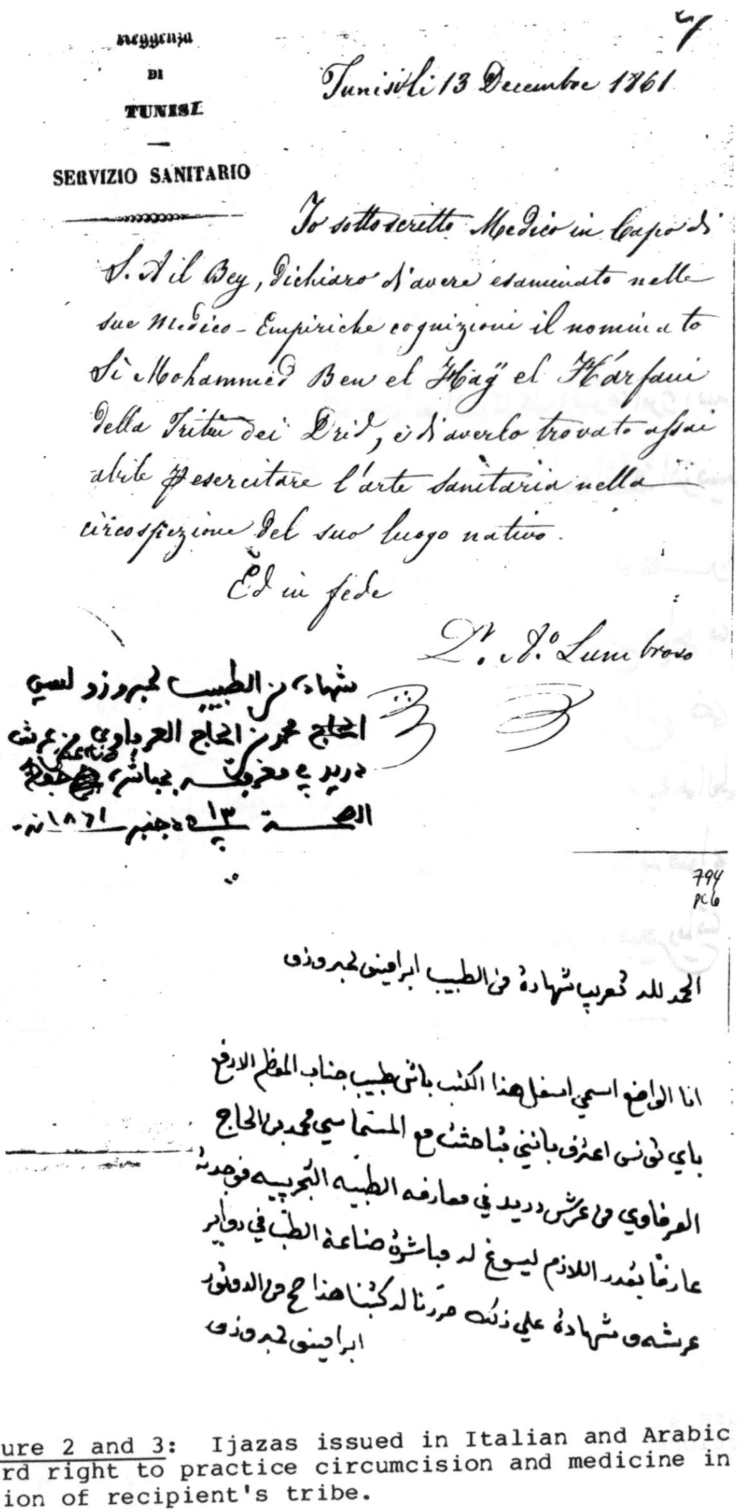

REGGENZA
DI
TUNISI

SERVIZIO SANITARIO

Tunisi li 13 Decembre 1861

Io sottoscritto Medico in Capo di
S. A. il Bey, Dichiaro d'avere esaminato nelle
sue Medico-Empiriche cognizioni il nominato
Si Mohammed Ben el Hağ el Kárfaui
Della Tribu dei Drid, e d'averlo trovato assai
abile ji esercitare l'arte sanitaria nella
circospezione Del suo luogo nativo.

Ed in fede

D. S. Lumbroso

شهادة من الطبيب لمبروزو لسي
الحاج محمد الحاج العرداوي ... عرش
درير ... محرك ... مباشر ...
الصـــــــــة ١٣ ديسمبر ١٨٦١ نه

794
pc66

الحمد لله تعريب شهادة من الطبيب ابراهيم لمبروزو

انا الواضع اسمي اسفل هذا الكتب باشي طبيب جناب المعظم الارفع
باي تونس اعترف باننى بحثت مع المسما سي محمد بن الحاج
العرداوي من عرش دريد في معارفه الطبيه التجربيه فوجدته
عارفا بقدر اللازم ليسوغ له مباشرة صناعة الطب في دواير
عرشه وشهادة على ذلك حررنا له كتابنا هذا حرر الدفنو
ابراهيم لمبروزو

Figure 2 and 3: Ijazas issued in Italian and Arabic
award right to practice circumcision and medicine in
region of recipient's tribe.

من عج ـــ ـــ لله سبحانه التوكل عليه الجبرص امرد ا به

الش ـــ ـــ م اداده باشا باي طحب الملكة التونسه

سرج الله اعماله وبلغه ته اعز از هزا انذهم . الماله اتى ته يقب كا هـــ زا
التشورت اخناصة راجمهورا اما بعد باندا اوليلا الكرم اتقكم بماجـ بن
يعفرح شتقيون طبا ما نيل بانطابيهه بحاض تذ الحميد ياتم احوال الم ضى
بلهها متقضى ما قهرنانه انفرانير وما عسا ه ان يحر ر راجم ياه . بخذا الم
جمى الطبل . اتاله واوصلام عبه واحتها ام وان اتفنا ت با بذا ت به صوا ه
الهام كلد الله ركتب جى رجب الصب من ـــــــــ نم تبع دبسرريا تنا
راهـ ـــــ ـــ

Figure 4: Ijaza issued by Ruler of Tunis to medical practioner.

50c

Figure 5: Ijaza issued by European chief doctor to European practioner in Tunis.

50d

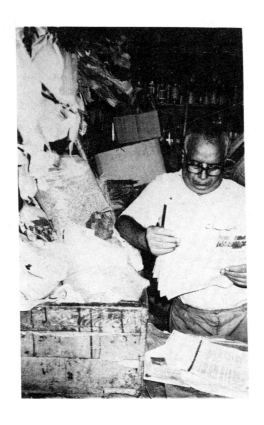

Figure 6: Medicinal herb seller in Tunis.

photographs taken
by Nancy E. Gallagher

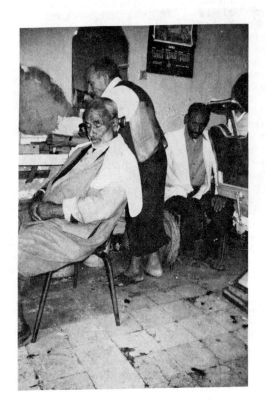

Figure 7: Barber bleeding patient in Tunis (hajjam practicing art of hija ma) in 1982.

photographs taken
by Nancy E. Gallagher

suspicion and contempt. Indigenous practioners are
carefully controlled. In her dissertation entitled
"Changing Health Beliefs and Practices in an Urban Setting: A Tunisian Example", Christina Hermanson Klein
notes that the government has taken great care to limit
popular indigenous healers (many of whom are women):
"The traditional beliefs and practices associated with
dwa 'arbi clearly have no place in the elite's vision
of a modern Tunisia. Indeed, dwa 'arbi is to be
replaced by the superior dwa suri (French or Western
medicine) which according to the national elite, is
based not on superstition and ignorance but on the
principles of modern science. (However)...unwilling to
isolate those segments of the population who continue
to place a great deal of faith in the practices associated with dwa 'arbi by taking extreme measures, the
government prefers generally to take a modified stance
with respect to traditional health care alternatives,
particularly so since the emergence in 1969 of a movement for the revival of Arab-Islamic culture." (Hermanson 1976:145-148). This movement however has not, at
least as of 1984 given rise to an active effort to
revive or reorganize the Galenic-Islamic medical
system.

We turn now to discuss possible explanations of
the lack of professionalization of indigenous practitioners in Tunisia and elsewhere in North Africa and
the Middle East in relation to the cultural revival
that accompanied the nationalist movements. Ralph
Croizier has suggested a tentative answer to this
question: "...only Arabic (Galenic-Islamic) medicine
could approach the Chinese or Indian tradition in richness and sophistication. The fact that it has not
assumed any vital role in modern Arab nationalism might
be related to the different character of Islamic culture, or more obviously, to the single truth that
Arabic medicine is closely related to pre-Renaissance
European medicine, making it much more difficult to
assert a unique value to it unknown in the West"
(Croizier 1968:7). Croizier is comparing the Islamic
with the Chinese medical tradition which also experienced a revival in the twentieth century. The Chinese
medical revival has been associated with the cultural
nationalist movement of the early twentieth century and
with the post-1949 revolutionary and anti-elitist movements. It may be that Chinese medicine did offer knowledge and experience unique to that known in the West.
Certainly Galenic-Islamic and Western medicine shared
common roots in Hellenic medical tradition though the
older theories had been overturned in Europe since the
nineteenth century. Ayurvedic physicians, like their
Chinese counterparts but unlike their Muslim Indian
counterparts, could feel that their medical system was

unique and offered knowledge over and above that possessed by Western trained physicians. In any case,
practitioners of all three medical systems became
professionalized in China and India.

Yunani medicine was of course Galenic-Islamic
medicine. Yunani in Arabic means Ionian or more generally Greek. The medical system may have been introduced into India beginning with the Turco-Afghan conquests
of the thirteenth century and intensifying wlth the
expansion of Persian culture in the fifteenth century.
Lahore, Agra, Delhi, and Lucknow became centers of
Islamic learning from which Yunani medicine spread.
Yunani or Galenic-Islamic medical texts were generally
written in Arabic and contained frequent citations to
Hippocrates, Aristotle, or Galen. Some of the texts
combined Galenic with Prophetic medicine, based on the
sayings and doings of the Prophet Muhammad and his
companions. Despite the origins of Yunani medicine,
its practitioners in India clearly throught it had
something unique to offer even when compared to Western
medicine with its similar roots.

Could it have been a religious association that
led Indian practitioners to organize? Ayurvedic medical texts form part of Hindu holy scripture. To many
Hindus, seeking the attention of a Western=trained
doctor violated religious principles (Gupta 1976: 368).
This may have encouraged Ayurvedic doctors to resist
Western medicine. Yunani medicine was also associated
with Islam and one might suppose that this may have
made Muslims unwilling to seek Western medical advice.
But this was not necessarily the case. Medical texts
such as Ibn Sina's Qanun or Ibn al-Nafis's or Jagh-
mimi's commentaries were not part of the holy scriptures as were the Ayurvedic texts part of Hindu
scripture.

Barbara Metcalf has observed that in Muslim India
on the one hand, "medicine was widely understood to be
not an obective science but an ancillary dimension of
religion." (The patient) was to turn, rather to the
shaikhs who were "healers of the body" as they were
"healer of the soul." Indeed, the two were interrelat-
ed....the value of practicing tibb was....great. It
was held to be a way of serving one's fellow creatures,
for the prime prerequisite for its practitoners was
compassion for the unfortunate, the quality above all
of God himself." On the other hand, Metcalf is careful
to note that medicine did not have the status of the
Islamic sciences. Medicine "in no sense enshrined the
truths of the religion, as did the fundamental studies
of Qur'an and hadis (hadiths).... There was an ambivalence about the place of medicine, not only as exemplified by those who favored simple trust in God in times
of illness, but also by those who felt it legitimate to

frequent practitioners of various systems, specifically Ayurvedic and allopathic, "as the Prophet used both the medicines of 'arab and 'ajam" (Metcalf 1982: 191-193). Could the non-Islamic character of Galenic-Islamic medicine be a possible explanation for the willingness to give way to the Western medical associations established by the colonial government in Tunisia? This is not likely because the Yunani practitioners were like their counterparts in North Africa well aware of the largely non-Islamic origins of their system. It may be that they organized following the example of the Ayurvedic physicians whose medical tradition did have a religious character (Bürgel 1976:44). Certainly Yunani practitioners may have wished to organize in order to rival Ayurvedic practitioners much as Islam rivals Hinduism. But similar motives might have caused practitioners of Galenic-Islamic medicine in North Africa to organize.

Historically the pattern of exposure of the West was quite different in India and North Africa. In India, intense exposure to Western medicine began in the early nineteenth century. In North Africa, it began considerably later, in the latter half of the nineteenth century. In India, the British first tried to combine the indigenous and European systems teaching both at schools they established in Sanskrit and in English. In North Africa the French also established schools but courses were taught entirely in French. There was no question of teaching Galenic-Islamic medicine in Arabic in French schools. So the British educational policy may have at least for a while legitimized the indigenous system while the French policy never acknowledged it.

North Africa was much closer to the metropole than was India and the intensity of cultural exposure may have been greater. Furthermore, the transfer of medical knowledge was sequentially different. By the time Tunisia for example was exposed to French medicine through colonial governmental policies, science had advanced considerably. Discovery of anesthesia, asepsis, and antisepsis for example made surgery far safer and more efficacious by the end of the nineteenth century than it had been at the beginning.

Finally, in North Africa the nominally Ottoman beylical government was accustomed to appointing the head of the medical order. There was no basis for organizing outside of state sponsorship. When the beys (Muslim rulers of Tunis) officially opted for Western medicine even before the establishment of the French Protectorate in 1881, indigenous practitioners lost their status with no means of protest outside of open resistance. This might have been possible had there been more hakims. But they were few in number, pro-

AFRICAN HEALING STRATEGIES

bably no more than 20 or 30 in Tunis and a few more in the provinces. Their numbers were probably not much greater than the number of European doctors at least in the capital city of Tunis. Most Tunisians probably sought home remedies or sought care from a saint or religious authority before seeking help from either a hakim who specialized in Galenic-Islamic medicine or a European doctor. Of course the medical tradition could have revived itself as in India where there were also very few trained practitioners in the mid-nineteenth century (see Mujeeb 1967:533-544 for a description of the founding of a Yunani medical school in India in the late nineteeneth century).

For any medical system to be accepted people must believe in its efficacity. Political, cultural, and religious beliefs of course influence the perception of efficacity. In North Africa, the Middle East, and India, Western medicine became the preferred system for most ailments if it was accessible. Even where indigenous medical personnel have professionalized they have remained in a secondary status. A Moroccan historian, Abdallah Laroui has noted the difference in patterns of cultural response to the Western cultural impact in his book Crisis of the Arab Intellectual and tends to dismiss the whole process with a sniff: "In passing, let it also be said that the Indians, whose intellectuals have gone even further in their nationalism and cultural pride than their Arab emulators, have failed to lend plausibility to a single one of their pretensions, whereas the Chinese, who seem to have more titles to glory and until recently were also given to displaying them, are exhibiting an unlooked-for humility in the very hour of their success" (Laroui 1976:8).

Laroui is correct in observing that the process of revival of indigenous science and culture has not got very far. After experience with indigenous and Western medicine, most people seem to prefer Western medicine for major diseases and injuries if it is affordable, accessible, high quality, and well-administered. These of course are important qualifications for peoples of nonindustrialized nations. The great sympathy for indigenous medicine shown by many nationalists often stops when the nationalists themselves need serious medical attention. Of course Western medicine cannot treat all diseases and many people feel better served by medicine they can understand. Many diseases have a cultural component which a local healer familiar with the problems and beliefs of the patient might understand better than a Western trained physician. Diseases partly caused by psychological states, such as eczema or lower back pain, can be effectively treated by indigenous medicine. This might have led hakims to form professional organizations with limited rights

such as homeopaths or chiropractors have done in the
West, perhaps on condition that serious cases be referred to Western-trained physicians. But to date this
has not happened.2

    There have been two forms of revival of Galenic-
Islamic medicine in the Arab world in recent years.
The first form of revival can be traced to a decision
taken by the World Health Organization. At the WHO
Conference at Alma Ata in 1978 it was decided to recognize the role played by indigenous healers for the 70
to 80 percent of the Third World population without
access to Western medicine. The WHO decided to work
for the establishment of traditional medical institutes
to study remedies in common use and to better train
local healers such as birth attendants. One such
institute has been established in Khartoum, Sudan,
under the direction of Dr. Ahmad al-Safi. The other
form of the revival of Islamic medicine is exemplified
by the government=funded Institute of Islamic Medicine
in Kuwait. It sponsors conferences on medical history
and supports scholarship in Galenic-Islamic medical
sciences. Both the WHO and Kuwaiti institutes are
established by experts educated in the West or in
Western-style schools. The local hakims did not organize the institutes as professional societies on their
own initiative, for their own professional recognition,
or for the revival of their medical tradition.

    Finally, we might consider the Islamic political
movements that have been increasingly influential in
North Africa and the Middle East. Many medical students and doctors trained in Western medical schools
support the movements. There is however no thought to
reviving Islamic medicine at the expense of Western
medical knowledge. Many point out that science has no
nationality but that the administration of medicine
should follow Shari'a (Islamic) law. This means in
practice that free clinics are attached to mosques or
provided by local Muslim societies where anyone can
receive free (Western) medical care (Sardar 1977:
21-36).

    To understand the reasons for the nonprofessional-
ization of indigenous medical practitioners in North
Africa and the Middle East, we must consider not the
foreign (Hellenic) component of Galenic-Islamic medicine, nor its association with religion but the role of
the Muslim state in sponsoring professional organizations, the time sequence and process of the introduction of Western medicine by Muslim reformers and by the
colonials government, and finally the social status of
the hakims in relation to the power of the Westernizing
elites. In conclusion, this paper is only an introduction, not a solution to the question. Virtually all of
the questions of current interest in the social history

of medicine have yet to be answered for the field of
Galenic-Islamic medicine in medieval, early modern, and
modern times.

REFERENCES

Gupta, Brahmananda. "Indigenous Medicine in
    Nineteenth- and Twentieth-Century Bengal. In
    Charles Leslie, ed., Asian Medical Systems.
    Berkeley: University of California Press. 368-38.
    1976.
Hermanson Klein, Christina. "Changing Health Beliefs
    and Practices in an Urban Setting: A Tunisian
    Example. Ph.D. thesis, New York: New York
    University. 1976.
Laroui, Abdallah. The Crisis of the Arab Intellectual.
    Berkeley: University of California Press. 1976.
Leslie, Charles. "The Ambiguities of Medical
    Revivalism in Modern India." In Charles Leslie,
    ed., Asian Medical Systems, 356-368. 1976.
Metcalf, Barbara Daly. Islamic Revival in British
    India: Deoband, 1860-1900. Princeton: Princeton
    University Press. 1932.
Mujeeb, M. The Indian Muslims. Montreal: McGill
    University Press. 1967.
Sardar, Ziauddin. Science, Technology, and Development
    in the Muslim World. London: Humanities Press:
1977.
Thomson, Robert. Natural Medicine. New York:
    McGraw-Hill Book Company. 1978.
Ullmann, Manfred . Islamic Medicine. Edinburgh:
    Edinburgh University Press. 1978.

FOOTNOTES

I would like to thank my colleague, Stephen Hay,
for help with paper.

1. For further this information on Galenic-Islamic
medicine see the comprehensive bibliographical review
by Emilie Savage-Smith in Pietro Corsi and Paul
Weindling, eds., Information Sources in the History of
Science and Medicine (London, 1983): 436-455. This
sourcebook also contains very useful bibliographical
reviews of studies on Indian and Chinese science and
medicine.
2. There is an Islamic Medical Association in Pitts-
burg, which publishes the Journal of the Islamic
Medical Association. Robert Thomson, a descendent of
Samuel Thomson who founded Naturopathy, is a member of
the association. He thinks Persian (i.e. Galenic-
Islamic) medicine can provide new and valuable medical
insights to Westerners (Thomson 1978:1-19).

LITERATURE CITED

AGGT. Archives Générales du Governement Tunisien

Bürgel, J. Christoph "Secular and Religious Features of Medieval Arabic Medicine," in Charles Leslie, ed., Asian Medical Systems. Berkeley: University of California Press, 44-62. 1976.

Croizier, Ralph. Traditional Medicine in Modern China. Cambridge; Harvard University Press. 1968

Gallagher, Nancy Elizabeth "The Arab Medical Organization in Nineteenth-Century Tunisia," in Revue d'histoire maghrebine, 4:145-149. 1975

_____. Medicine and Power in Tunisia. Cambridge: Cambridge University Press. 1983

B. CHRISTIAN AND WESTERN INFLUENCE

Indigenous African societies have been influenced, incidentally or administratively, by Europeans for many centuries. As colonies of Western nations, their traditional beliefs were questioned, their native practices criticized, and their indigenous systems replaced by alien ones. This applies both to systems of religions and belief, and to related systems such as healing which were very closely related. In spite of these attempts to recast Africans into the image of European administrators traditions persisted and today a new appreciation is experience for indigenous knowledge and practices. While centuries of culture contact have left their mark, the continuity of these traditions permit us to study and record them within a wider context that is uniquely African.

Health, or a local cultural definition of it, is a universal value. All persons wish to live in as healthy a condition as possible and utilize practices and behavior available to them to achieve this goal. These healing strategies will include avoidances, communication with supernaturals, rituals, and the use of various materia medica. They may be based on individual action and private performance or the use of specialists. The latter includes the ngoma therapy discussed by Janzen and illustrated by du Toit with a study of urban Zulu.

One of the most important features which mark African healing is the role of the patient's family. In his study of therapy among the Kongo, Janzen (1978) speaks of the "therapy managing group", usually close kin, who assist a patient in decisions concerning choices of healers to consult and therapies to follow. We find this theme again in contributions to this volume. Sargent, while mentioning that pregnancy is not considered abnormal or a disease, nevertheless describes the role of female members of the household who act as an advice and support group.

58

The role of religion in healing can be found in almost every contribution. While some societies rely more heavily on a religious causation explanation, supernatural forces are invariably partially responsible for a lack of health. "Illness" says Comaroff, "was perceived as an expression of social conflict or cosmic disorder, revealed in disruptions in the normal relation of men, spirit and nature" (1981:371). If negative relations resulted in ill-health then health could be restored by normalizing these relations. The diagnostician, frequently the ngoma or ngaka in this part of Africa established which norms had been breached, and which of three therapeutic systems should be utilized. "They use allopathic medicine for relief of disabling physical symptoms, indigenous healing for signs of interpersonal conflict, and Zionist healing for what appears to be spiritiual intrusion" (Comaroff 1981:375).

The importance of formal religious institutions, and especially Zionist and other independent churches, has been remarked on by various researchers. Frequently healing is at the core of the independent church. Sanneh emphasizes this in his discussion of conversion where ecological harmony in the traditional and the modern is the aim. This aspect of religion is also treated by du Toit in his discussion of urban Black South Africans.

Closely related to this aspect of new religions is the role of women. They often play a critical role in both healing and new religious organizations, as they do in healing and traditional ngoma rituals. Spring deals with this in her discussion.

Most of the contributions in this section deal in one regard or another with, what Kroeger call, "pathway models" (1983). They describe different steps in the decision making process and in the continuum of illness behavior. This may involve the support of the "group"; it may result from consulting a diagnotician; it may find expression in a religious organization; and it may serve as avenue for role expression by women. The latter will depend on social structural and related factors, e.g. Islam. We should always keep in mind that illness concepts as much as illness behavior form part of an everchanging process. As concepts of illness causation change so will behavior aimed at treating it. As health services are introduced, a further analysis and redefinition of type, cause and cure will be made. Sickness, after all, despite its varied cultural definitions, is a departure from health and the latter is the aim.

AFRICAN HEALING STRATEGIES

REFERENCES CITED

Comaroff, John L. Healing and Cultural Transformation:
     The Tswana of Southern Africa. Social Science and
     Medicine (B). 15(3B)367-78. 1981.
Jansen, John M. The Quest for Therapy in Lower Zaire.
     Berkeley: University of California Press, 1978.
Kroeger, Axel. Anthropological and Socio-Medical
     Health Care Research in Developing Countries.
     Social Science and Medicine. 17:3. 1983.

CHAPTER 5

CHANGING CONCEPTS OF AFRICAN THERAPEUTICS: AN HISTORICAL PERSPECTIVE

John M. Janzen

I. Introduction

The historical perspective on African therapeutics is long overdue; writing on the subject has only recently begun (Janzen & Feierman 1979; Janzen & Prins 1981). In the present context, two aspects of the subject will be stressed: the changing concepts of scholars who have considered African therapeutics, and the changing concepts and realities "in the field" on the part of practitioners, the populace, and policy-makers.

In launching a discussion on these issues of African therapeutic strategies, we do well to make explicit our purpose for this project. As far as I am concerned, it is first and foremost to enhance the health of the broadest spectrum of people. As an officer in the Swaziland Ministry of Health queried in discussing the government's criteria for being interested in, and supportive of, particular therapeutic practices: "Do they improve the survival rate of children?" We dare not be content merely to chase the colorful butterflies of African healing customs.

Our theoretical approach to African therapeutics will therefore emphasize health concepts or ideals toward which various healing strategies aim or aspire. These concepts, ideals, and strategies may co-exist and change over time; yet they provide the bases for the evaluation of a therapeutic strategy's efficacy.

The present paper will first consider several characteristic health profiles in historic and contemporary African society; then it will present a spectrum of health concepts, both ethnograpic or historic, and analytical; these are held up to concrete therapeutic realities: first, the "marketplace" of contemporary health care uses and decision-making in many African settings; then, in examining one widespread therapeutic tradition of Central and Southern Africa, the supportive network-forming, song-dance ritual institution

which I shall call ngoma therapy, after the central
term or concept that accompanies it from Western Zaire
to the coast of Tanzania, and from the Equatorial for-
ests to the Cape. In this wise theoretical, methodological, and substantive issues will be covered in the
hope of advancing our understanding of health issues in
Africa, and in making the most effective use of available therapeutic alternatives.

II. The Socioeconomic Context of Health and Medicine
     The approach I advocate emphasizes the historical
background of contemporary analysis of health and
medical systems; both are situated in the social and
economic order which offers distinct demographic and
disease profiles varying over time and regionally.
Distinctive socioeconomic orders shape health status
and therefore determine the character of therapeutic
interventions, although these latter are always conditioned by cultural traditions, scientific modes and
religious assumptions. Four major socioeconomic settings, with numerous variants, have been identified in
recent literature, each with a distinct health profile
(Polgar 1975:1-14).
     Africa's hunting and gathering societies, in both
forest and desert settings, portray relatively "level"
population rates, based on moderate death rates and
fertility rates, with a great deal of emphasis on
childbirth spacing. The disease and health profile of
these societies before they are engulfed by other
socioeconomic modes reveals relatively few, and only
episodic, epidemic diseases because of the small population sizes. In the desert settings, there are very
low microbial rates. These factors are tied to a keen
knowledge and awareness of food and related health
resources, yielding a rather distinctive, although
vulnerable, health profile in the hunting and gathering
society.
     The transition to agriculture, where we have
access to population and epidemiological trends, demonstrates rapid increases in mortality, then fertility
rates, with the introduction of endemic contagious
diseases whose hosts are often animals living in, or in
symbiotic relationship with, the human community (Faris
1975). Therapeutic practices emerge having to do with
the maintenance of fertility, the assurance of crops
and food, and the protection of sedentary populations
and their social structures. In Africa, such societies
are know to us largely through archeological and infer-
ential evidence.
     These autonomous horticultural societies become
peasant societies when they come in contact with larger
societal systems such as empires, trade routes, cities
and, in Africa, colonialism. As this occurs, there is

an increase of epidemic levels in contagious diseases, resulting in cycles, or continuous high levels, of death and devastation, with the attendant increase in fertility. Therapeutic systems become more elaborate, often requiring semi-specialized practitioner roles, in an attempt to deal with both physiological disorders and societal stresses. In Africa, divination and possession therapies, midwifery, bone-setting, herbalism on a larger scale than before, evidence of innoculation against some of the contagious diseases such as smallpox, and a variety of specialized sacred medicines focusing on pandemic stress points, emerge.

The African scene is rendered to some extent unique by the history of the slave trade and its impact on health. Heightened chronic levels of contagious disease, and depopulation, are the most recognizable results of the Atlantic trade (and probably of the Indian ocean trade). One careful examination of Congo coast societies has stated that population levels declined by half from the sixteenth to the early twentieth century (Sautter 1966). This finding can be extended to other West African regions, although sometimes higher fertility appears to have offset the forced migration of slaves and the ravages of diseases and social dislocation. Coupled with the forced migrations and labor conditons of early colonialism, the late nineteenth and early twentieth century has been described as the unhealthiest moment in all of African history (Hartwig & Patterson 1978). In one West African city where demographic data are available for part of this period, mortality outstripped fertility to such an extent that constant in migration from the countryside was necessary to maintain a steady population level (Patterson 1979). Early industrial capitalism, and its political-economic setting, colonialism, provided little basis for "health". Early colonial medicine began to strike effectively however at certain contagious diseases such yaws, smallpox, and sleeping sickness.

It was not, however, until better housing, restored adequate diet, and public health measures were begun, that mortality rates in the colonial industrial setting began to decline. In the West African city mentioned above, Accra, Ghana, installation of a pure water system raised health levels significantly by eliminating water-borne diseases(Patterson 1979). In Africa generally, mortality rates have declined in this century from about 50/1000 to below 20/1000, indicating the real health progress that has been made (WHO Annuals). Infant mortality rates remain the highest for any continent, at 142/1000 live births, but significantly down from about 350/1000.

This trend replicates the first part of the well-
known "demographic transition" to lower mortality and
fertility rates begun in the last century in Western
Europe, and in Asia in this century, giving rise to
unprecedented population increases. In Africa, the
continent with the world's highest population growth
rates (around 3%), this phenomenon has roused considerable debate amongst medical planners and development
experts. Some believe it is an impediment to development and should be halted or lowered by birth control
measures, whatever its cause, whom these advocates
often attribute to "tradition", or irrational beliefs.
Others see it as a logical consequence of development
which will in due course bring about a decline in
growth rates, as has occurred in Europe, Asia and the
Americas, as the perceived need for large families
recedes through better social security measures, and
through genuine economic development. Yet others
(Gregory & Piche 1982) argue that the seeming failed
decline of fertility, i.e., the continued general
desire for large families, is a measure of the economic
peripheralization of Africa in the world capitalist
economy. The only rational reaction of parents is to
increase offspring to maximize their opportunities in
what remains of a peasant or horticultural economy,
while at the same time hedging their bets for a stake
in the very precarious, and exploitative labor market
where they are increasingly driven by land loss, disad-
vantageous market conditions, and inflation.
    It is clear, then, that the socioeconomic setting,
and the forces shaping it, play a greater role in
health status than therapeutics or medical care. Measures to affect health levels must be seen in this
light.

III. The Varied Meanings of Health
    Therapeutic systems, of whatever type, are orient-
ed by cocepts and values also present in the socioeconomic and cultural systems which harbor them. This
is true of the varied African therapies no less than
those imported from the Islamic East and the Euro-
Christian West. These therapeutic systems may be
identified initially by implicit and explicit criteria
of health to which they aspire, and which they aim to
instill in individuals and communities. Evaluative
criteria of health are useful for the same reason in
development and health policy planning. Therefore it
is useful here to identify several common sets of
health concepts as a basis for the study of therapeutics. This approach to the analysis and evaluation of
therapeutics has been recently popularized by the Well-
ness Movement; however it has a history of scholarship
in the philosophy of medicine and science (Boorse

1977), as well as history of medicine (Temkin 1973;
Kohler 1978), and to some extent in medical anthropology (Janzen 1981).

"Health is what physicians do." This notion
underlies a certain stereotypic North American view of
the basis of health, as well as--perhaps for related
reasons--a common perspective on the study of African
health. Just as in North America some people leave
their health up to the physician, who is expected to
patch up their body machines when they are ill, so
commonly in the past many Western scholarly studies of
African therapeutics concentrated on the customs of
healers. This assumption as to the origin of health
also has pervaded ministries of health in their common
tendency to grant a major share of their budgets to
centralized hospitals and the training of physicians,
in lieu of preventive, public health, and broadly based
nutritional assessment, or standard-of-living surveys,
or such important measures as Well Baby Clinics, or
primary health care, including the recognition of
African therapy's part in a community.

"Health as the absence of disease" is a view that
can be traced to classical antiquity in Western medicine, although it came into primacy in the nineteenth
century with the discovery of the bacterial causes of
the major contagious diseases, and related techniques
for their elimination. This view of health served
agencies well in Africa in the twentieth century, during the heroic pursuit of cures for, or the total
elimination of, scourges such as malaria, smallpox,
cholera, typhus, measles, and sleeping sickness. The
focus on pathology that this view entails, and which
has governed biomedicine in Africa during much of the
twentieth century, may however obscure some of the
social and economic sources of poor health that actually precipitate or exacerbate these contagious diseases.
It may lend support to the erroneous policy that there
are "magic bullets" or quick fix medical technological
solutions to diseases that respond also to improved
work and living conditions. The epidemiology of tuberculosis in Southern Africa, related to mining and
deplorable living conditions in reserves and slums, is
a case in point.

"Health as functional normality" is a theoretical
concept that has been proposed by philosophers of medical science to overcome some of the disadvantages of
the above negative definition of health. "Normality"
however proves difficult to define in a way that is
both measurable and managable. Also, what is "normal"
is not always healthful. Taken in a strictly statistical sense, the norm may include high levels of malaria
infection, or intestinal parasites, of TB positives.
This may also be seen by members of the community as

"normal", even if not acceptable, but it should not be a justification for inaction on the part of authorities or scholars. The health norm, according to some writers, must be seen in terms of cohort groups defined by gender, age, and possibly occupational roles. Thus, functional normality of the elderly would include some disability; that of chilren, some childhood diseases; or of work-related roles, certain unique physiological hazards or phychological stresses. Philosophers also raise the issue of teleology in connection with functional normality, that is the function of an organism as being defined by its goal, its typical developmental course. A teleological, or circular definition of goals and functions, of ends and means, characterizes many social states, especially in health. The notion of "risk" in a given social or biological role has grown out of the implicit "end state"; further, goal-oriented health programs seek to achieve an end product. Without a degree of teleology, health policies and programs would not be possible.

"Health as adaptation" is another orientation, based on the ecological perspective, that has seen currency in studies of African health and health care. Certainly much research has benefited from this perspective; for example, the understanding of defenses against malaria in West Africa. However, the same problem arises here as in the foregoing definition of health. Not all that is adaptive, is healthful.

"Positive health" and "health utopias" are proposed by some scholars to openly recognize the role of value-charged goals in health programs and interventions. Certainly the World Health Organizations's call of "Health for all by the year 2000" is such a goal; the WHO's definition of health as the "well-being of body, mind and society", in a related way, invokes a utopian image of perfection. These approaches to health are recognized to be value-related, goal-oriented, and often particularistic; they correspond to advocacy stances. Many of the indigenous African health definitions would seem to fit here, with such over-riding notions as "balance", "purity", "harmony", or "coolness", propagated by therapeutic acts and attitudes that address the quality of life in the community.

"Social reproduction as health" is a final concept to be considered here; it refers to the perpetuation of a particular social order or social formation in terms of the quantity and quality of health indicators. The notion of social reproduction is used by some Marxist scholars to refer exclusively to the reproduction of labor in the interest of those who control the means of production. These writers see the continuing high rate of fertility, and the attendant rise in population in

Africa, in such a light, attributing it to the dilemma
of increasingly marginalized African laborers who
strive to cover both their peasant productive base,
usually family-oriented, as well as that of the capitalist wage giver, to make ends meet. From that
vantage point, numbers of offspring are important.
However, it seems necessary to go beyond mere biological reproduction in defining "health", and to include
measures of the quality of related social and economic
settings, the ability of social institutions and cultural patterns to perpetuate themselves. This wider
definition of social reproduction as health will be
used below to examine the ngoma therapeutic practices
in Central and Southern Africa.

   In evaluating particular therapies, one or a
combination of the foregoing health criteria may be
used. Although there may be no single "correct" set of
criteria for a given therapy, all types of therapeutic
interventions reflect a range of intended aims. Innoculation campaigns aim to reduce particular diseases,
to achieve health as the absence of disease. Possession therapies probably strive to reproduce segments of
the society, to channel legitimate sanctions and
resources toward a particular constellation of values.
Therapeutic systems need to be examined, then, against
the most appropriate set of health concepts and goals.

IV.   **Medical Pluralism, or the Marketplace of African
         Therapeutic Systems and Settings**
   Going beyond the health paradigms examined above,
therapeutic practices may also be characterized as
behavioral traditions, used selectively and in combination, in relationships that vary over time. African
therapeutic strategies, in the past and today, seen in
the context of communities, regions, and social strata,
present a stunning variety of such traditions, a willingness to try almost anything available. An important
perspective in the study of African therapeutics
includes attention to the total combination of therapeutics alternatively utilized in an on-going context
(Janzen 1978a, 1978b); that is, it must be a historical
perspective, and therefore one which focuses on individual and group practices. Several illustrations from
the contemporary African scene suggest what a
researcher or practitioner might encounter.
   There is simultaneous support for multiple therapeutic traditons, by trained practitioners and lay
clients alike. In Dar es Salaam, a survey conducted by
a Tanzanian medical doctor revealed that the majority
of trained biomedical health workers in the city's
clinics "believe in witchcraft", that is, they find it
a plausible and recurring problem for their clientele,
in need of attention.

Accordingly, there is very widespread crossing-over, or parallel utilization, of two or more therapeutic traditions. This has been identified in field studies within single African communities (Janzen 1978). But it also characterizes the broadest social spectrum that includes highly differing ethnic identities. A well-known Swazi diviner (sangoma) related to this author in 1982 that a significant number of her clients are whites, particularly Afrikaners from the Republic of South Africa.

Similarly, there is extensive technological borrowing in African therapeutics. Many herbalists and doctors of African medicine utilize stethoscopes, microscopes to examine blood, stool, and urine, and injection needles; diviner-psychotherapists increasingly read texts in psychology and psychotherapy. One pharmacy in Swaziland, to illustrate this trend, sells local herbs and plant preparations, dried and packaged, alongside imported German homeopathic medicines. A Zairian pharmacologist is running a series of tests on anti-diarrhoeal medications prepared from herbalists' prescriptions in collaboration with several clinics and hospitals.

The integration, or at least juxtaposition, of multiple therapeutic and medicinal traditions in individual cases, in consultation patterns, and in practitioners' repertoires, is unexceptional because the philosophical basis of African, like most medical, thought, is universalistic. Medicine has usually been eclectic; healers and physicians borrow what works, or what their clients request. In this sense African medicine is typical. African medical thinking is unique in the exceptional degree of its openness. Throughout much of Central and Southern Africa, at least, diagnosis, divination, and therapeutic practice allows for both naturalistic afflictions and cures, as well as for human-caused, and spirit-related, afflictions and cures. In the few settings where we have historical documentation regarding this diagnostic perspective, such as the Congo coast, every indication is that it is a very old perspective (Janzen 1979). This means that not only the present, but the past as well of African therapeutics must be described in terms of innovation, borrowing, parallel consultation, and continual change.

Not suprisingly, African governments are striving to define what licensing, legitimation, and quality control may mean in the face of such medical pluralism. Few countries have as yet really resolved the issues at stake; there continues to be keen interest in the questions, and a desire for research of the "secrets" of African medicine. As research continues, more and more segments of African medicine will be brought under the banner of scientific legitimation, and will be accepted as an official part of the national trust. The implications of these observations for scholarship and practice are several. First, it is not useful, nor theoretically accurate, to distinguish between "traditional" and "non-traditional" African medicine. The dichotomy, derived from Modernization theory, and used in much North American social science during the fifties and sixties, and in a few areas to the present, ignores the evolving nature of all therapeutic traditions, not just "Western", or Islamic", but that originating within African civilization as well. The perspective must be historical; attention must be paid to the relationship between traditions—in clients' use patterns, in practitioners' borrowings, in legitmation policies.

A second implication, related to this, is that therapeutics in Africa—perhaps everywhere—cannot be entrapped in "tribal" categories. There are as great internal variations in medical custom among speakers of Zulu, Kongo, or Yoruba as between these language communities. Many distinctive patterns in African therapeutics are regional, or they relate to historic economic, social structural and environmental characteristics, rather than to language groupings. This is not to say that local, community and area studies are inappropriate. Rather, that the conceptual isolation of "tribal" therapeutic and health variables is usually irrelevant, and misleanding.

Thirdly, it is highly unlikely that an outside, detached, and fully objective perspective exists from which the diversity of health concepts and therapeutic practices may be studied. The ethnoscience dichotomy "emic" and "etic", referring respectively to the "native" understanding, and to the "analyst's" objective account, so commonly used in a generation of Western social science study of African culture, is misleading and often inaccurate. We have seen above how the perspective that health is what the doctor does, common in earlier decades in the United States, pervaded much so-called "etic" social science in Africa. So-called observer neutrality and objectivity are notoriously prone to slippage over time. The study of health and therapeutics in Africa is best served by admission that health traditions have their own expert, or inside theoretical modes which must be grasped in order to interpret or explain them. It is of course possible and appropriate to test therapeutic paradigms and related practices from other health orientations. Certainly, one would wish to examine the incidence of hepatitis in the use of herbal injections; also, one should examine the efficacy of innoculation campaigns in terms of decreases in new cases of the disease in

question; or well-baby clinics in terms of declines of
infant mortality. These are straight forward interventions readily measured by epidemiological and demographic variables. Many therapies are not as strictly
tied to specific health concepts or criteria of testing. For these a combination of criteria must be
selected.

In the case of ngoma possession therapies, to
which I turn next, a variety of criteria may appropriately be applied, including demographic, positive
health, and social production factors.

V. The Historical and Comparative Study of
    Therapeutic Traditions: The Case of Ngoma
        Therapy in Central and Southern Africa
    To illustrate some of the foregoing theoretical
and methodological approaches, and to test them on my
own research, I shall briefly introduce one particular
therapeutic tradition widespread in Central and Southern Africa: ngoma therapy, named after the term
usually used to identify the drum type, rhythm, song,
dance, or a combination of all these, in a therapeutic
setting. This therapy was introduced to scholarship
most forcefully by Victor Turner's work The Drums of
Affliction (1968), an indepth study of several therapies of the ngoma type among the Ndembu of Zambia. The
therapy's existence over a much wider region has been
substantiated by this writer's review of the literature, and by a field survey in Western Zaire, coastal
Tanzania, Swaziland, and the Western Cape in 1982-3. I
am using the term "ngoma" to identify this therapy type
because it seems to be the most widely-used indigenous
term, although there are many variations in this connection. Across the mid-continent the term refers to
"drum" generically, as well as a specific type of drum,
an elongated wooden cylinder with a single leather
membrane at one end, affixed with pegs; this instrument
type is the most frequently used drum in the therapeutic rituals, and is accompanied by shakers, other
drums, and song. From the Swahili East African area
down to Southern Africa, the term also refers to
musical groups, often in a secularized, entertainment
derivation from the therapeutic idiom. Among Southern
African Nguni speaking groups, the cylindrical drum
type with pegged membrane is absent, the cowhide-over-
metal-barrel now being used. Here ngoma refers to the
therapeutic song; the practitioners isa-ngoma, "those
who do ngoma" (except for the Xhosa, who call them
amagqira).
    This introductory sketch suffices to make the
point that all therapeutic traditions have in common a
number of characteristics. (1) Therapy is always
embedded in a wider cultural tradition--whether religi-

ous, scientific, or intellectual--with values and
perspectives that carry over from the society to the
therapeutic function. (2) Therapeutic traditions have
a focus of affliction types regarded as appropriate to
them, a classification of the "epidemiology" of disease
treated. (3) They have a set of therapeutic specifics,
a kit of techniques considered necessary for this
focus. (4) They legitimate these features in terms of
an ideology or worldview. (5) Finally, they are
socially organized either as loosely affiliated individuals, or into a more tightly incorporated association
or group with a social status. Because of the wide
variability from one therapeutic tradition to another,
and in all traditions over time, it is advisable not to
use the concept of "system" too hastily in a comparative study. "Tradition" implies an on-going cluster of
values, classifications, behaviors, and organizational
attributes with ever-changing relationships between
them. I shall further characterize ngoma therapy in
these terms, with especial attention to some of the
areas of continuity, and change or variation.
     Ngoma therapy is an important part of the health
and healing perspective of Central African classic culture, perhaps even several millenia old. Linguistic
similarity throughout the region where the term ngoma
exists, suggests that it is consonant with much of the
Bantu language speaking region. The space of this
paper permits only a restricted presentation of the
ideas and values that accompany the Bantu-speaking
cultural region. Central ideas are suggested by common
cognate terms for "illness", "wound", "health" (coolness), the verbal, or thought-directed, sources of
sickness and misfortune (witchcraft, sorcery), the role
of ancestors in sickness and healing, numerous therapeutic ingredients and techniques, and terms for the
roles of healers, as well as for concepts that reflect
a systematic understanding of diagnosis (Janzen 1983).
Each of these notions, and the applications made of
them, reflect extensive, and continuing, adaptation and
evolution, in the light of ecomonic, political and
social changes over the centuries. Some societies have
become pastoral nomads, others sedentary cultivators;
in recent decades, urbanization has introduced major
changes. Nevertheless, a common cultural core, reflected in the terminology of health and healing, is
clearly in evidence.
     Ngoma, as other therapeutic traditions, addresses
a focused taxonomy of afflictions in the total spectrum
of afflictions of Central and Southern African people.
Generally, it is considered more appropriate for chronic, spirit-or human-originated affliction than for
episodic, natural affliction. It is thus often considered a "final-recourse" therapy that assists the

sufferer or the society at large in adjusting to a
life-long relationship to the condition. Within this
broad rubric, a wide range of particular conditions may
be noted. In societies such as the Lunda-Ndembu, where
during Turner's study in the fifties, hunting was still
an important economic activity, chronic hunting failure
was regarded as an ngoma-appropriate problem. In more
industrialized settings, chronic inability to retain a
job may become a "syndrome" appropriate for ngoma
therapy. In many societies, impotence in men and
infertility in women is directed toward ngoma therapy,
as is the parenting of twins or triplets. Epilepsy and
other chronic or debilitating handicaps may, similarly,
be included. An important dimension of ngoma appropriate affliction concerns not just the individual, but
also the collective social institution. In Western
Kongo society, the segmentary lineage, at the time of
segmentation, is seen to be the appropriate object of
the Nkita therapeutic rite, individual members of the
lineage, particularly sick children, being the symptoms
of an Nkita disorder. Children's sickness, of whatever
type, seen in clusters during or after segmentation, is
considered caused by the lineage's disorganization and
lack of authority of its heads. One part of Nkita
therefore entails the reconsecration of lineage authority emblems, or the re-connection of new segments to
lineal ancestral shrines. Another historic Kongo therapeutic rite named Lemba emerged in the mid-seventeenth
century along coastal and inland trade routes, with
special concern addressed to the role of merchants
involved in the great trade, and the impact of the
trade, through them, upon their domestic communities.
Lemba, structurally, assumed many of the functions of a
regional governing order (Janzen 1982). Somewhat
later, an East African rite, the Beni-Ngoma, emerged
along trade and migration routes with a somewhat
similar role (Ranger) 1975).
     Across the region, there is a wide variation in
the scope of afflictions addressed. Some are extremely
specific, such as hunting disorders, or, in Tanzania,
snake bite remedies, or smake handling; in other
instances the focus of affliction includes all chronic,
unresolved, human or spirit originating difficulties.
This latter is especially true in South Africa, where
any and every symptom may potentially qualify for an
undifferentiated mode of therapy. The underlying
reasons for this classificatory variability from
specific to generalized are too involved to analyze in
this paper; I have discussed them elsewhere (Janzen
1982; 1983).
     The therapeutic techniques in ngoma bear a number
of common features throughout the region. Although
specific therapeutic measures for a particular

syndrome--epilepsy, segmentation of a lineage,
twinning--may be unique, everywhere the therapy is
associated with an initiation process whereby the subject or subjects are, at least prospectively, recruited
to the role of healer. As the therapeutic course continues, counselling gradually gives way to training of
the novice. If the therapy is successful, the subject
graduates as a full-fledged healer of the affliction
originally suffered. This therapeutic-initiatory
course may vary in duration from a few days to many
years, depending on the nature of the affliction.
    Another important feature of the therapeutic rites
is the refashioning of the sufferer's identity through
the testing of dreams or visions, as expressed in
songs. The use of music in the therapeutic rites
heightens affect and provides a performance structure
through which inchoate feelings and contradictory
emotions may be sorted out, given negative or positive
valence, and "moved" from a less, to a more desired,
state. All ngoma therapy is thus psychotherapeutic;
however, labelling is not singled out as specifically
psychic or physical. Frequently the subject literally
composes a new song-identity which is picked up by the
ritual partners; one's new identity is thus mirrored
back and tested by one's therapist-teachers and fellow
patient- students. The strong rhythm of drumming and
dancing which always accompanies the singing undoubtedly affects brain patterns, facilitating dissociation
and psychic and cognitive rearranging. A rich cluster
of therapeutic techniques is brought together in ngoma
to achieve a forceful approach to healing.
    The therapeutic techniques and approaches taken to
illness identification in a therapeutic tradition are
usually "anchored" ideologically in a wider system of
beliefs, values, and cognitive realities. This may be
spoken of as legitimation. The theory of legitimation
with regard to medical practices is often traced to Max
Weber in sociology, Temkin in medical history, and
other writers in medical ethics (Janzen 1978b; Schipperges 1978; McCormack 1981). In the African setting,
ngoma is legitimated by the religious, ideological, and
scientific underpinnings that the practitioners and
their public use to validate their work. In this
sense, ancestors provide the single, most widespread,
but by no means exclusive, ideological grounding for
the therapy. Victor Turner's presentation of ngoma
among the Ndembu portrays them as exclusively ancestor-
related; specific ancestors are said to possess specific members of the living community, recruiting them
into particular cults, thus drawing them back into a
normative lifestyle. Elsewhere many other types of
spirit personages appear in connection with ngoma, so
that it is not accurate to limit this dimension to

ancestors alone. Very widely, nature spirits are associated with ngoma, as are a variety of alien spirits.
This may be a recent development reflecting the breakdown of lineage and kin-based communities, and to the
opening up of cultural categories to include the wider,
plural society in the cognitive worldview of people
(Werbner 1977). Other writers see the relationship
between norm-reinforcing ancestors and nature and alien
spirits as evidence that ngoma spirit logic differenti-
ates the quasi-sickness of recruitment to healing from
that due to psychopathology, the former being in the
orbit of ancestors, the latter other spirits (Sibisi
1975).
    The picture of spirits as legitimation symbols in
African therapeutics is rendered more complicated by
the fact that the spirits present themselves in terms
of named communities or fields, not necessarily by
these labels as "ancestor", "nature", or "alien".
Often an entire constellation of spirits will be held
to be derived from an ancient kingdom. Thus the Buc-
wezi complex of the lake region of Uganda, Burundi,
Rwanda, and Tanzania is a well-known ngoma spirit
group, with its own character differentiations, derived
from the legendary Cwezi kingdom (Berger 1973). Spirit
movement in relation to therapeutic communities is
exceedingly dynamic, with much borrowing across political, language, and ethnic lines. The Swahili-speaking
coast of East Africa has taken over the Arabic term for
spirit (Sheitani) to describe the African-derived
spirits in ngoma groups; Islamic-specific spirits, the
majini, are organized into ancestral, water and land
groupings, these again specialized according to named
ngoma groups. The same spirits, controlled or approached by orthodox Muslims, relate not to ngoma
communities, but to Sufi brotherhoods. As complicated
are the lines of articulation between ngoma and
Christianity. There are reports of Christian ngomas
(Ranger 1979) which are inspired by the Holy Spirit;
many lines of continuity may be found in Central and
Southern African independent Churches from the ngoma
tratition.
    Legitimation theory establishes the type of inspi-
ration which justifies therapeutic practitioner roles.
Following Weber's several types of legitimation, it is
readily apparent how "charismatic" authority along with
"traditional" authority would be the main types of
legitimation of the ngoma system. "Rational-legal"
authority, Weber's third type of legitimation, is
emerging in some ngoma settings. This type of authority applies mainly to scientific theory inspiring
therapy or research; legal legitimation applies to a
scientific or therapeutic tradition's support by the

state. As suggested in an earlier section, therapeutic
traditons need to be explained, and understood, in
terms of their own theories. Ngoma is no exception.
Some of the ngoma orders have developed highly intri-
cate divination and diagnostic routines; others have
developed medicinal knowledge for specialized diseases
whose "legitimacy" rests on popular and expert understanding of its efficacy. Most striking in this regard
is the lore, techniques, and pharmacopoeia of Tanzanian
snake-handling and snake poison antidotes in the Mun-
gano ngoma. Pharmaceutical research is providing these
old techniques and recipes a rational scientific legitimacy. State support through research and training
programs extends legal legitimacy to ngoma in a number
of African countries. Thus, a technique which in its
popular and widespread form was legitimated by spirit
possession, may come to be legitimated by entirely
other sets of symbols. The comparative case of
acupuncture is instructive. Originally explained by
demon theory, it then came to be explained by bodily
meridians which expresses Ying-Yang and the five
forces. Today neurological theory is replacing these,
although the technique remains very similar (Unschuld
1980).

     All therapeutic systems are organized socially.
Such organization may be one in which the therapeutic
function is embedded in other institutions or is
separately incorporated. Ngoma therapeutics is no
exception; across the Central and Southern African
region its organizational modes vary widely from being
a loose network of independently operating individuals,
to being tighter cell communities, to being a hierar-
chical professional corporate group recognized by the
state. The variation from the one extreme of loose
networks to centralized hierarchy is so pronounced that
many observers have not put the two extremes into the
same rubric at all. Yet utilizing the criterion
announced earlier of the use of the term "ngoma" to
describe therapeutic song, dance, counselling, and
professional initiation in the same context, activities
as widely diverging as divination on the one hand, and
cults of twinship and hunting on the other must be
included. A helpful analytical notion to evaluate
diverse ritual modes within the same rubric is Mary
Douglas's concept of "gird" and "group" (Douglas 1970).
Across the region, "gird" would be represented in an
emphasis on cognitive ordering, "group" in an emphasis
on interpersonal relations. Many ngoma contexts
utilize both dimensions, with healers acting both as
diagnostic counsellors (diviners), and therapists, a
distinction that is consciously made (see Janzen
1978a:12; Turner 1975).

A brief elaboration on divination is necessary
here. In the African setting it tends to be a specialized operation in the hands of a specialist. Yet it is
to be thought of as the logical extension of a sufferer's and his family's search for understanding of
affliction and misfortune. Divination's specialties
tend, therefore, at any given time and place, to
reflect the range and degree of common misfortunes,
afflictions, and felt needs for interpretation and
guidance in referral. That divination is often associated with chronic ngoma rituals means that these
problems are often saddled with perplexing cognitive
dilemmas. They need to be interpreted and resolved in
the light of major social values. Therefore it is not
surprising that in some settings, such as the southern
African region, the ngoma complex is often explained as
having entirely to do with divination. On closer
examination, however, the divining diagnostic function
and the therapeutic function have, everywhere, a complementary but varying relationship. Thus, in Turner's
Ndembu studies, divination is commonly handled by the
ngombo basket operator; chronic ailments are directed
into one of twenty ngoma ritual communities. In nineteenth century coastal Kongo society, there were many
types of divination, reflecting a range of influences,
including the ngombo, others for juridical breakdown,
and others for the restoration of chiefly authority.
Some of these were part of the therapeutic process. In
twentieth century Kongo society, the mechanistic
divination methods were abandoned, to be replaced by
inspirational divining, much of it handled by Christian
prophets. In some twentieth century Southern African
settings, the divination with bone throwing has been
supplemented with inspirational diviners who are
mediums of a variety of nature and alien spirits,
including Christian and Islamic spirits. In these settings, each diviner-healer tends to have a number of
apprentices who, together, conduct therapeutic and
purificatory group events to maintain a semblance of
community in the fractious South African setting. The
shape of ngoma in this setting is that of an unending
network-like fabric with events taking the appearance
of temporary nodes on the social fabric. Ngoma, in
South Africa, is not broken up into denominations or
functionally-specific modes, as it is among the Ndembu
as studied by Turner. Rather, all appropriate problems
are channelled into the undifferentiated network of
diviner-healers and their apprentices.

   In a few regions this combined divinatory and
therapeutic network becomes centralized, even bureau-
cratized. On the Swahili coast of Tanzania, the
Sharika la Madawa ya Kiasili (Medical Organization)
with 500 members (healers) in the Dar es Salaam, Tanga,

Dodoma, Morogoro and Bagamoyo districts, operates ngoma
"dispensaries" among cells of healers who conduct the
therapeutic drum-song rites on a strict fee for service
basis. Very few of the "customers" become apprentice
healers. The Sharika is recognized by the government
of Tanzania as a legitimate regional medical organization which may control this kind of medical resource,
and determine its value, as well as the rate of professional recruitment among its practitioners.
     It is apparent then that the ngoma therapeutic
tradition is extremely adaptable to epidemiological,
social and political variables. For this reason it is
not easy to delineate appropriate criteria of health
with which to evaluate efficacy in ngoma organization
and therapeutic practice. A brief listing of some of
the probable areas of effective intervention may be
suggested.
     One area of clear effective intervention would
come under the "positive health" rubric of individuals
entering therapy. There is, in ngoma therapy, an
obvious build up and release of emotional energy;
whether through the taking of drugs, or the commencement of cortical driving (brain wave alteration), and
intensive auto-suggestion, an environment conducive to
psychic relearning is set up. Ngoma therapy is effective psychotherapy.
     The verbal, conscious properties of ngoma therapy
may also be mentioned. The counsel and verbal interpretation of song-dance derived from dreams or peer
prompting, effectively promotes enhanced identity.
Ngoma songs have contributed very widely to the meaningful musical art of the sub-continent.
     It is, however, in the area of social reproduction
that ngoma therapy may be most significant, in the way
it lays the groundwork and builds up bonding between
individuals of a common affliction, and channels
resources into that setting. Throughout Central and
Southern Africa ngoma ritual groups have formed around
sectors of pronounced personal or social disintegration
and perceived threat: in Central African cities such
as Kinshasa and Bukavu, one finds ethnically rooted but
increasingly universalistic communities of the alienat-
ed; women experiencing difficulty, or lineages in
fragmentation; in the Western Cape, in the face of
divided families, crowded difficult living conditions,
labor insecurity, and depressed work conditions, one
has noted the formation of a universalistic support
network around (mostly female) healing networks; in
Swaziland, in the face of rapid industrialization and
the opening up of the social order of a capitalistic
society, the perceived need for diviners' schools to
deal with the extensive cognitive uncertainty, especially prevalent among young adults. In East Africa, the

emergence of ngoma groups is both professional, as
noted above, and entertainment oriented, as practitioners seek to consolidate their work with government
support, and as the general public desires to utilize
the richness of this tradition for the enhancement of
its cultural heritage. The government also is involved
in sponsoring and promoting this outlet of ngoma. In
an indirect way, then, ngoma may even improve the
quality of life and enhance health statistics seen, as
the" absence of disease".

Ngoma has been presented here as a distinct therapeutic tradition that is part of the classic heritage,
millenia old, of Central and Southern Africa; yet it
continues to evolve and find new outlets in the urban,
industrial, post-colonial African setting. Its practitioners are both educated and uneducated; in some
regions it has government support, at least legitimacy,
in other regions not. It is rooted in wider world view
concepts and values; it may be evaluated in terms of
analytic health concepts that make it relevant to
today's national development priorities.

Conclusion

     The historical study of African therapeutic
strategies has barely begun, if one compares the field
with historical studies of Asian and Western health and
healing. Whatever the reason for this delay, there are
several imperatives for beginning immediately to focus
theories and to perfect techniques that are at hand.
The intrinsic interest of the subject and the desire to
carry out good scholarship provide one imperative. A
greater imperative however is the practical concern
grounded in the need to know what therapies of the past
have made a difference on health, what we mean by
health in the African setting, how we define the arena
or scope of study, and how we formulate policies for
the self-conscious promotion of particular strategies,
and then, how we evaluate decisions undertaken or
tendencies allowed to run their course.

     The present paper has introduced several dis-
courses into the discussion. The first has been that
of the health profile of socioeconomic settings, suggesting that demographic, disease, and therapeutic
responses are unique, according to the type of setting.
In Africa, distinct profiles have been recognizable in
hunting and gathering societies, autonomous agrarian
societies, peasantries in the shadow of kingdoms,
empires, and trade routes; colonial societies, industrial and recently urban-industrial societies. The
point was made that the socioeconomic setting in large
part determines the epidemiology of disease, and the
type of recourse to health care available.

A second discourse has to do with <u>definitions and concepts of health</u>, useful both for the reconstruction of a history of ideas as well as for the formulation of health goals in the present, and the evaluation of programmes undertaken.

A third discourse introduced is that of the <u>total context</u> in which therapeutic strategies are undertaken, emphasizing the panoply of strategies entertained and undertaken by real individuals, in real communities, solving real and complex health problems in infinite variety. The context of health-seeking decisions and actions cannot be locked into boxes of custom, ethnicity, the traditional, or native; new options are continually opening. Therefore, our methodological and theoretical perspectives must capture the changing, dynamic relationships between therapeutic alternatives in concrete settings.

A final discourse of great usefulness is that of the <u>therapeutic tradition</u>, which includes values and perspectives from the wider culture applied to the therapeutic function; a focus of affliction types regarded appropriate for the therapeutic tradition-- i.e., a classification of the "epidemiology" of diseases treated; a set of specific therapeutic measures, a kit of techniques; legitimation in terms of an ideology or worldview; and social organization of all these dimensions. The therapeutic tradition, as an analytic notion, permits us to view on-going behavioral-conceptual-historic-adaptive institutional ways of responding to perceived diseases. The particular case studied, an African ritual therapy mode known as the "drum" or "cult of affliction" (<u>ngoma</u>), which utilizes rhythm, song, dance, counselling, therapeutic initiation, network building and exchanges, around stress points in the society, is but one of many therapeutic traditions. However others may be analyzed with the criteria suggested, such as the tradition of Islamic medicine, or of Biomedicine, utilizing this or a related set of comparative criteria.

These discourses emphasize the historical perspective of scholarship. This means that they emphasize conscious, deliberative decisions by actors; changing patterns and structures; the role or ideals and goals in terms of which actions are undertaken, and in terms of which they may be evaluated. Above all, they take into consideration the aspiration to improve health, using several criteria, by sharpening goals and clarifying appropriate options.

References Cited

Berger, Iris. The "Kubandwa" Religious Complex of
    Interlacustrine East Africa: An Historical Study,
    C. 1500-1900. Ph.D. Dissertation, History Depart-
    ment, University of Wisconsin, Madison. 1973.
Boorse, Christopher. Health as a Theoretical Concept.
    Philosophy of Science, Vol. 44: 1977.
Douglas, Mary. Natural Symbols: Explorations in
    Cosmology. New York: Pantheon, Random House.
    1970.
Faris, James. Social Evolution, Population and Produc-
    tion. Steven Polgar (ed.) Population, Ecology and
    Social Evolution. The Hague: Mouton. 1975.
Gregory, Joel W. and Victor Piché. African Popula-
    tion: Reproduction for Whom? Daedalus. Spring
    1982.
Hartwig, G. W. and K. David Patterson (eds.). Disease
    in African History. Durham: University of North
    Carolina Press. 1978
Janzen, John M. The Quest for Therapy in Lower Zaire.
    Berkeley, University of California Press. 1978
    (a) The Comparative Study of Medical Systems as
    Changing Social Systems. Soical Science and
    Medicine, vol. 12. 1978 (6).
_____. Ideologies and Institutions in the
    Precolonial History of Equatorial African
    Therapeutic Systems. Social Science and Medicine,
    vol. 13B, 1979.
_____. The Development of Health. Akron: Mennonite
    Central Committee (Development Monograph Series
    8), 1980.
_____. The Need for a Taxonomy of Health in the
    Study of African Therapeutics. Social Science and
    Medicine 15B (3) 1981.
_____. Lemba 1650-1930: A Drum of Affliction in
    Africa and the New World. New York: Garland
    Publishing, Inc. 1982.
_____. Towards a Historical Perspective on African
    Medicine and Health. In Joachim Sterly (ed.)
    Ethnomedizin und Medizingeschichte. Berlin:
    Verlag Mensch und Leben. 1983.
Janzen, John M. and Steven Feierman, (eds.) The Social
    History of Disease and Medicine in Africa. Social
    Science and Medicine (Special Issue) 13B, (4).190
Janzen, John M. and Gwyn Prins, (eds.) Causality and
    Classification in African Medicine and Health.
    Social Science and Medicine (Special Issue) 15B,
    (3). 1981.
Köhler, Oskar. Die Utopie der absoluten Gesundheit.
    Heinrich Schipperges, Eduard Seidler und Paul U.
    Unschuld, (eds.) Krankheit, Heilkunst, Heilung.
    Freiburg: Verlag Karl Alber. 1978.

MacCormack, Carol P. Health Care and the Concept of
    Legitimacy. Social Science and Medicine, vol.
    15B, (3). 1981.
Patterson, K. David. Health in Urban Ghana: the Case
    of Accra 1900-1940. Social Science and Medicine
    1, (4). 1979.
Polgar, Steven. Population, Evolution and Theoretical
    Paradigms. Steven Polgar (ed.) Population,
    Ecology and Social Evolution. The Hague: Mouton.
    1975.
Ranger, Terence O. Dance and Society in Eastern
    Africa: The Beni Ngoma. London: Heineman.
    1975.
Sautter, Gilles. De l'Atlantique au fleuve Congo: Une
    géographie du sous-peuplement. The Hague:
    Mouton. 1966.
Schipperges, Heinrich. Motivation und Legitimation des
    Ärztlichen Handelns. In Heinrich Schipperges,
    Eduard Seidler und Paul U. Unschuld, (eds.).
    Krankheit, Heilkunst, Heilung. Freiburg: Verlag
    Karl Alber. 1978.
Sibisi, Harriet. The Place of Spirit Possession in
    Zulu Cosmology. In Martin West and Michael
      Whisson (eds.) Religion and Social Change in
      Southern Africa. Cape Town: David Philip.
    1975.
Temkin, Osawi. Health and Disease. Dictionary of the
    History of Ideas. New York: Scribners. 1973.
Turner, Victor W. The Drums of Affliction. Oxford:
    Clarendon. 1968.
_____. Relevation and Divination in Ndembu Ritual.
    Ithaca: Cornell University Press. 1975.
Unschuld, Paul. Medizin in China: Eine Ideengeschite.
    München: Beck 1980.
World Health Organization. W.H.O. Statistical Annual
    1978. Geneva: World Health Organization. 1979.

CHAPTER 6

THE ISANGOMA: AN ADAPTIVE AGENT AMONG URBAN ZULU

Brian M. du Toit

Underlying much of the belief and action of man in every day life is a culturally defined cosmology. By this is understood the theory of the universe which is held by a particular people. While it is correct to state that we cannot really understand action unless we also understand the belief and theory on which it is based, the converse is also true. We cannot fully comprehend belief unless we see it in action. This opens up dimensions of powers and supernatural agents which cannot be learned from an objective statement of the cosmological system. Through an understanding of the universe held by a people we can better comprehend their belief in supernatural agents and the values which underlie social interaction. It is universally true that some person or persons stand between the members of the community and the supernatural agents which are recognized as influencing their lives. These persons may be specialists or occasional agents; they may also perform this role on a fulltime basis or appear only when there is a need for their services. They may appear in ritually designated locations or buildings attired in ceremonial regalia or simply perform their roles as functionaries in the community when the need arises. In every case, they are satisfying a need of the members of the community and performing a function without which discomfort would result.

I.

This paper is concerned with the diviner and the traditional healer in Africa and especially among the Zulu now living in modern urban conditions. I will briefly touch on relevant literature dealing with this subject before discussing my findings in recent urban research.

Speaking of traditional healers in Ghana, Jahoda remarked in general that "one might hazard the guess that in most underdeveloped countries, these (traditional healing agencies) not merely supplement such limited facilities for Western type treatment as are available, but do in fact bear the brunt of the burden" (Jahoda 1961:245). But when speaking of traditional healers we have to recognize that the traditional African generally does not distinguish between or compartmentalize physical treatment as contrasted with psychiatric treatment. The treatment of body and mind go hand in hand. Giving a person assurance and faith facilitates the curing of the body. The cause of disease may be mental or it may originate with agents, such as witches, outside the person. In any case it is believed to be caused supernaturally.

Due to this complex causality we also find a complex method of treatment. Thus the Shona "witch doctor" is simultaneously herbalist, diviner, specialist (Gelfand 1964:12), and his Zulu counterpart performs the same role. The Zulu in fact employ variations of the same noun to denote the person who professes to cure sickness by physical means and the one who claims to detect and counter the activities of witches. Thus, we can distinguish the inyanga yokwelapha (elapha: treat medicinally - the doctor for curing) and the inyanga yokubula (bula: divining with sticks - the doctor for divining) Bryant 1966:13). A person in this latter category may also be denoted as isangoma, when he relies to a large extent on divination to discover the cause of discomfort, or isanusi, when he "smells out" such causes.

The isangoma (and I am including most of the izinyanga here) may perform any of a multitude of roles as a specialty. It seems that when a specialist goes beyond merely treating with herbs, he may be called an isangoma. Thus Krige points out that "the diviners who, though often called by the name inyanga or specialist (in divination), are usually known as isangoma or isanusi" (Krige 1950:299). In the same context of various kinds of specialists the author also refers to a category of izinyanga zisithupha (thupha: thumb), or thumb diviners, who perform their skills by having the people consulting them beat the ground with sticks to indicate agreement or corrections in their divination.

Each category has its own sub-group of specialists. Thus Reader (1966:287-288) discusses the role of the inyanga yezinsizwe, (-zwe: nation tribe, clan), who is the tribal medicine man and strengthens the army, and the inyanga yamagungo (gungo: blood-lust, fit of insanity), who is the specialist that purifies a man who has killed in battle, thereby preserving his sanity. Thus there are izinyanga who specialize in the treatment of boys or girls at puberty, who are approached when a girl recently married does not become pregnant, and who are experts in the treatment of snake

bite and other specialties. These specialists have
usually inherited their knowledge and will pass it on
to a son or daughter.
    A person who is called by the spirits to wander
off into the woods and to become an isangoma has no
control over this. He usually knows or learns a great
deal about herbal treatment since he would then be able
to treat his own patients rather than sending them to
an inyanga. The isangoma also fall into different
categories and while all have supernatural aid, their
special abilities may prescribe their modus operandi.
Thus we find stick diviners, bone diviners, umlozi
(whistling doctors) who listen to the voices of the
spirits, thumb diviners, heaven doctors who cause rain
to fall, ukuvumisa diviners who depend on verbal
responses from those who are consulting to guide their
statements, and others. In short, the continuum from
basic herbalist to divining specialist is not clearly
separated into izinyanga and isangoma, and most persons
in the former category do use dreams and visions to
assist and guide them thus relating closely to the role
of the diviner. Diviners may also, irrespective of the
method employed, make predictions of what is to follow
or perform acts to discover what is not known or to
find things which are lost. Junod (1927:559) shows the
first kind of divination for the Thonga in the prophecy
of a migration. I will discuss, for the urban Zulu,
examples of both prediction divination and discovery
divination.
    For the purpose of this paper, then, I am using
the referent "diviner" to include all persons who attempt to elicit supernatural guidance and information,
whether this is done with the aid of devices (bones,
entrails, scapula), whether the diviner acts as medium
for supernatural communication, or whether the diviner
interprets omens, dreams, voices etc. The person who
diagnoses illness, or learns about treatment in the
above sense, is a diviner whether he personally treats
the client or patient, or whether he sends such a
person to an inyanga.
    Every traditional Zulu community had access to the
services of such agents who could act as intermediaries
between man and the supernatural world. While such
persons were usually women (Bryant 1917:143 and
Köhler 1941:6) they may also have been men who were
called in when ritual impurity or negative forces
resulted in sickness, misfortune, or unnatural events.
These persons were expected to analyze the cause of the
discomfort and to prescribe ways of dealing with it.
They were also, and this is very important for people
such as the Zulu (du Toit 1960), in direct contact with
the ancestors and could relay or interpret messages to
their living descendants. Thus when a child was ill,

an adult troubled by bad dreams, or the cattle infertile, a man would seek the cause of his ancestors' displeasure. But man, being as smart as he is, knows that he can forestall trouble by keeping certain taboos or by performing particular rituals in advance. Such precautions as planting inthelezi or having a specialist perform the ukubethelela ritual were commonly performed as a safeguard rather than cure. While an individual could perform a number of actions to insure safety and health for himself and his family, the person who was especially gifted and called to perform these duties for others was the specialist. Krige points out that "when disease breaks out, when cattle are lost, when omens appear, or a wizard is suspected of having caused things to go wrong, the man who is consulted is the diviner. He will discover the cause and prescribe what steps are to be taken to set things right again" (Krige 1950:299). While a sacrifice is frequently called for, this does not substitute for the payment due the specialist for his services. The doctor may therefore become a fulltime specialist with hereditary abilities, or an agent who has been specially called by the spirits.

The Zulu, then, differentiate between the inyanga, who is an herbalist in the true sense of the word, and the isangoma, who is a diviner combining his special abilities in divination with a thorough knowledge of medicinal herbs, roots, and the like. While much of this paper deals with the inyanga I am including discussion of the isangoma and of powers which are his special domain. The reason for using this latter referent in the title of the paper is due also to the fact that during the research on which this paper is based most persons who called themselves inyanga were in fact more than simple herbalists and combined this specialty with other abilities.

Krige's statement above suggests that the diviner is a person in great demand, yet she was really speaking about the rural and more traditional Zulu. A logical extension of this would be to look at the man in the city, the person who now lives in a square house on a paved street, and who in many cases is a member of a Christian church to which he pays monthly dues. It is with reference to these people that Vilakazi has pointed out that "no Christian may consult a diviner (isangoma) on pain of excommunication; and the calling in of an African medicine man (inyanga) is frowned upon by the church. In fact, no Christian, in a Christian community, would call in an inyanga in broad daylight" (1965:103). Depending on the definition of "Christian community," this statement could suggest that the traditonal Zulu doctor is being replaced to make way for the modern medically trained doctor and the minis

ter or priest.   An examination of this statement is a
major concern of this paper.

II

It is important to note that the diviner is still
very much a part of the urban community and an important figure whose role has been redefined to fit the
urban situation. The diviner is of importance for the
very fact that when man is faced with unknown and unpredictable situations then it is through consultation
with the diviner that he receives the will of the
ancestors and consequently his doubts are removed and
his anxiety reduced. A number of examples and situations will be discussed below in which the diviner
still is the psychological buffer on which people may
rely.

For six months during 1969 I worked on a project
among the urban people, primarily Zulu, who live in Kwa
Mashu just outside Durban.[1]   Kwa Mashu is an African city with a population of at least 100,000 people.
Numerous churches and denominations have buildings or
allocated sites and many more, particularly the Separatist cults, meet in private houses during the week
and on Sundays. Nearly every city block has a house
which is marked by a tall bamboo post holding a flag
which designates it a "Zionist" leader's home while
simultaneously protecting it against lightning.   In
many cases these persons combine their role as religious cult leaders with various forms of healing. Some
use blessed water, others heal by faith, while a large
number of these new religious leaders combine the role
of the old inyanga and even that of the isangoma with
their new position. One such cult group is discussed
in detail elsewhere (du Toit 1970 and 1971). Whether
in fact the Separatist church leader doubles as healer
or not, nearly every city block in Kwa Mashu houses at
least one person who is recognized as an inyanga or
isangoma. Some are more open about their trade than
others since the Medical, Dental, and Pharmacy Act (Act
13) of 1928 endangers the isangoma on certain points of
practice.

It is quite common in Kwa Mashu to find that persons have safeguarded their homes against evil spirits
and against danger by installing some form of inthelezi. Generally this refers to any protective charm or
protective medicine but it usually takes on the form of
a wide leafed plant which is planted outside the front
door. Informants explained that the presence of the
plant, which they simply referred to as inthelezi, kept
dangers at bay. Closely associated with this practice
is the use of some protective charm or medicine which
is buried at the front door, at the gate entrance, or

on the borders of the yard all along the fence. This
is very closely related to the practice of ukubethelela
in which a doctor is called in to fortify the house
against lightning and other dangers. A very complex
concoction of plant and animal products is prepared and
applied to either stones or sticks which are buried at
specified places near the house. This will protect the
house and the inhabitants. One of my informants had
traveled, within a week, as far south as Port Shep-
stone, inland to Estcourt, and north to Empangeni in
addition to performing certain healing ceremonies in
Kwa Mashu.[2]   Relating how he had gone about fortifying a village near Empangeni, he explained: "The
first night when I arrived at Empangeni my grand-
father's spirit (idlozi) appeared and informed me that
the head of this village was no longer visited by his
ancestors. This is why he was sick and unlucky. I
prayed to his ancestors on his behalf and gave him some
medicine to make him vomit. We then sacrificed a white
hen.   Actually the ancestors had called for a white
cock but since we could not find one we placed twenty
cents on the sacrifice to make it acceptable."   This
diviner and his family were living in the city as were
his parents.
     The sacrifice which was mentioned above is a very
common practice. Every Sunday, (during the week people
are too busy and usually too tired), there are ceremonies and feasts at which the meat of sacrifical goats is
eaten with the traditional beer. In most of these the
household head takes the initiative in sacrificing a
goat to his ancestors to assure health, a job, or good
luck. It may also be the ukubuyisa ceremony in which
the spirit of a deceased father is "brought home"--
thus installed to its rightful socio-jural position
within the cult of the ancestors. In traditional Zulu
huts the back part of the hut was set aside as the
umsamo where the ancestors could easily be reached.
This was the place where a boy sat during his puberty
initiation, and this was the place where a sacrifice
was hung in order that the ancestors might take their
share before the meat was removed to be cooked. In the
square house in Kwa Mashu one frequently finds that
there is a particular place where the sacrifice is
always hung. In most cases this turns out to be in the
bedroom where the head of the family sleeps, for it is
the most likely place where his ancestors will visit
him during sleep. This is also the place where the
sacrifice will be hung for the night with a small pot
of beer next to it, only to form part of the feast the
following day.
     In cases where a person has an upsetting dream, or
dreams the same thing repeatedly, he will go to a doctor, usually an isangoma, and ask for an explanation.

While working in Kwa Mashu I learned of the condition
of a Dlamini boy.   It turned out that he had had a
number of important dreams over the past months about
the neighbors who, in his dreams, had repeatedly
threatened him. His father decided that he was gifted
with particular visionary abilities because of these
dreams.   Though only twelve years old this little
fellow was taken out of school and sent to the country
where he could be trained as an isangoma.[3]   But
this does not imply that every thwasa (initiate-- from
ukuthwasa, lit. to come out like the new moon) must go
to the country for training. A number of very powerful
doctors reside in Kwa Mashu and at the time of the
study at least two in the area where I worked had
initiates whom they were training. These initiates can
be seen walking down the streets, their faces smeared
with clay while they carry a small drum as token of
their new state.[4]
     The primary reason for the high esteem in which
these doctors are held is their ability to see into the
unknown.   It is interesting, for instance, that in
BONA, the monthly Bantu magazine, the horoscope is
headed: Isangoma sakho sezinkayezi kulenyanga (Your
prophecy of the stars this month).   The isangoma is
turned to for any dream interpretation and this applies
also to "playing the numbers."   Most South African
Bantu live in pitiful poverty and have to make ends
meet by employing a variety of ingenious means. While
some methods are more constructive, or at least employ
means which are more predictable regarding likely
returns, the Fah Fee is the most popular. This is a
betting game, run by an anonymous "Chinaman", which is
very widespread and in Kwa Mashu this game involves a
few hundred dollars every day in bets of between one
cent and a dollar. The amount which a person is willing to bet depends partially on his financial condition
and partially on the clarity of his conviction regarding the number to bet. When a person dreams he goes to
the isangoma for an interpretation of his nocturnal
visions and this decides the number he should bet and
may also influence the amount he bets.
     It is perhaps in the field of medicinal treatment
that the doctor, be it an isangoma or an inyanga, is
most active and earns the greatest part of his income.[5]   In the research a number of questions were
asked of informants regarding any occasion when they
would turn to a particular kind of specialist for help.
The table was composed in such a way that the horizontal axis went from the categories "ancestors" and
"inyanga" to "medical doctor" and "priest", while the
vertical axis dealt with an increasingly more serious
illness, starting with "colds" and ending with "death."
More than 50% of the informants would go to some kind

of traditional doctor in the case of less serious upsets while in the case of snake bite nearly all would
go to the inyanga for isihlungu, a bitter herbal
extract, which is said to be the most effective treatment. More than half the persons in our sample stated
that they would turn to the isangoma in the case of the
sudden death of a close relative. Repeatedly the answer was given that the doctor would be able to "see"
what had caused the death and would be able to state
what steps should follow. These findings were confirmed by my friend Dr. M.V. Gumede, a Zulu medical doctor,
who did his training at the University of the Witwater-
srand and now practices medicine in Kwa Mashu. He
states:

> The vast majority of Africans still consult the
> diviners and herbalists before they go to
> medical practitioners. Many African beliefs
> and customs have been bundled together and
> classed as banned for all practicing Christians
> as unchristian, heathen and pagan, etc. without
> a careful study to separate the chaff from the
> corn. The African has, therefore, always
> presented two faces, viz, one for himself and
> his own and another for the minister and the
> Church in order to avoid some terrible disaster
> such as excommunication. In the main when he
> is sick, the African, Christian or otherwise,
> often seeks the help of the diviner and the
> herbalist (Gumede 1968).

The diviner has also branched out into new fields
since urban living has become a way of life. A favor-
ite meeting place for the younger men in urban areas is
the all night choir competition. Competitive teams,
each consisting of six to eight members meet on a
Saturday night at a central building where they com-
pete. The men are dressed in their best, most colorful, and most modern clothing and each team has its own
manager who usually acts as musical director. But
before a team leaves its home base they go to an
isangoma who "strengthens" them and after their return
from the choir competition they will report back to
their diviner who either receives their praises and
gratitude or must divine to find the cause for their
lack of success.[6] After such an early Sunday morning meeting in which the isangoma first had to satisfy
the team who had lost the competition and then answer
numerous probing question from this inquisitive anthropologist about his modus operandi, contacts, aims, and
abilities, Mr. Mchunu turned to me and asked the
following questions: "How do your airplanes fly? How
does one make electricity? How does such a large thing
as a rocket go to the moon?" He obviously was not
requesting information nor was he interested in an

answer. He was pointing out to me in a very subtle way
that I had been asking about his secrets and he was
giving me a taste of the same treatment.
    Since the diviner knows and is able to cope with
both worlds, the traditional and the modern, he is also
able to assist others who are experiencing troubles.
The diviner knows what steps to take for a man to get a
job; he knows how a young lady can get her man in a
world of fleeting relationships and mobile workers; he
knows how a young migrant to the city can double-cross
the system of influx controls and retain residence in
the city. Invariably this is initiated by a state of
purification induced by vomiting. Further physical
treatment, such as bleedings, may follow since it lets
out evil powers and brings a balance between the physical and mental state of the patient and the treatment
or ritual action to which he is then subjected. It
also assures an income for the specialist who may do
little physical good (African, Indian, and White medical doctors spoken to in Durban all agree that this
kind of treatment does more harm than good) but is an
essential psychological buffer between the individual
and the new conditions and situations. While treatment
is prescribed or administered, the isangoma gains knowledge about his patient and required prescriptions from
supernatural agents.

                            III

    The questions with which we are confronted are why
this person has retained so much of his status and why
he still forms a functional part of the Zulu community
in the city. I think that the basic reason is that the
isangoma is answering very pertinent questions for his
patients in a way they can understand. Their cosmology
contains spirits and powers which are real, ancestors
who can see and experience what we cannot, and all of
these powers have a direct bearing on the individual.
When he loses his job, when he becomes ill, when his
children are unhappy he turns to the man who is
supremely confident that he can explain the cause and
furthermore, given jurisdiction, can bring about the
desired results provided he is given sufficient time.
Discussing the Shona peoples, Gelfand states: "When a
patient consults him for sickness, his first action is
to diagnose the cause of the illness, not in physical
terms, but in spiritual ones, because Africans believe
that sickness is caused either by the activity of
spirits (usually those of their dead relatives) or by
men and women who are evil and desire to harm others"
(Gelfand 1964:24). This is also the reason that many
sick Africans avoid going to medical doctors, and
especially White medical doctors. Thus the sick Afri-

can "fears that, by consulting a White doctor, he is
provoking--or futher provoking--the spirits of his
ancestors" (Gelfand 1957:15). Given a novel situation
or problem the patient tends to call on the proven
agents and to employ proven means of treatment. And
so, when harmed, the patient views it as the responsibility of the diviner to ascertain who caused the
problem and to prescribe what steps should be taken.
    It is also common to find that Africans believe in
some kind of ecological niche theory. This became
obivious on a number of occasions when informants asked
whether I was not affected by my change in residence.
They would explain that every person, due to his particular make-up, was in balance and at harmony with the
powers in the area where he was living. When a person
changed his residence, and particularly when this
involved major ecological changes, he was susceptible
to natural forces over which he had no control. What
was needed in these cases were the protective activities of the supernatural agents to work out a balance
between man and the forces to which he was now exposed.[7]
    It should also be kept in mind that no person is
able to break completely with his past or disassociate
himself from his cultural values, world view, and
cosmology simply because he has changed his place of
residence (du Toit 1968). The man in the city is still
a Zulu, in spite of the square house and paved streets
where he lives or the pernament job and football game
which occupy his time. The need, of course, is for
education, both in a religious sense and in an academic
sense, in order that the basic premises which are seen
as underlying the world and its existence may be rein-
terpreted. But this education must be sympathetic and
substitutive rather than coming in to sweep away
completely the old values and accepted beliefs. We
need to reinterpret and build on the existing rather
than condemn and sweep away the accepted building
blocks of traditional beliefs. The need is best
described in the words of Gumede, who states:
    Africans today, in all walks of life, urban and
    rural, erudite and illiterate, are everywhere
    swimming in a whirlpool of black and white
    magical conceptions, a characteristic of a
    people that are in search of the truth. They
    will spend thousands of rand[8] annually on
    the herbalist and the diviner and will pay vast
    sums for the "intelezi" which will fortify
    their homes against wizards and witches. They
    will buy armlets to ward off sickness and pain,
    charms to keep away lightning, charms to bring
    them luck and good fortune or carry out sacri-
    ficial rites to appease the ancestral spirits

to look kindly upon them and bless their homes.
Thus it will continue until the African
eventually realizes the true aetiology of
sickness and suffering, that is, until the
spirit and man-made theories are replaced by
scientifically valid arguments (Gumede 1968).

Much of the same thing is true for other parts of
Africa. Jahoda, speaking of Accra in the mid-fifties,
explains that "traditional healers are widely patronized by literates, and the evidence suggests that the
support and reassurance they provide probably often
prevents the occurence of serious breakdowns. A similar need is served by the healing churches..." (Jahoda
1961:268). While a distinction may be made between
European disease and traditional African disease (see
Southall and Gutkind 1957 regarding the Ganda in Kam-
pala), and therefore also the types of treatment which
should be sought, it is possible for the diviner to
straddle both worlds since the spirits are unchanging.
Whites in Africa may in the past have leaned too heavily on their pills and prescriptions while losing sight
of the psychological angle. Thus Lambo (1959) in
Nigeria has served as social psychiatrist to assist the
adaptation of new migrants to the city who are emotion-
ally not able to adjust to the discipline and rigor of
urban living. To a great extent then, Lambo and persons like him are substituting and gradually replacing
the isangoma or his equivalent.

This concept of supernatural forces may be of
significance in modern conditions of migration, urbanization, and culture change in general. Thus there
exists the opportunity for administrators to bring into
use their knowledge about a people with whom they live
and work. In the Preface to his study Shona Religion
(1962) Gelfand states: "I believe that Africa must see
a marriage between medicine and anthropology that will
produce doctors and health officers who combine a knowledge of medicine and an understanding of the African
peoples and their environment." In recent years a
number of cases have been reported in which a "marriage" of sorts has taken place. Thus the Town Council
of Krugersdorp in South Africa hired a Shangaan witch-
doctor Josiah Mangani to exorcise the "evil spirit" of
a former worker at the sewerage pump station who had
been stabbed to death. The spirit of this man was said
to be restless and angry with the other workers because
they could not trace the killer. Mangani performed his
purification rituals and the workers returned to the
pump station which was free of the spirit (STAR, Decem-
ber 3, 1965). Shortly after this it was reported that
the Kenyan Government had officially hired a witch-
doctor to neutralize other witch doctors who were

intimidating the local populace (New York Times, October 16, 1966.[9]   These are cases in which there is a
recognition of differences in world view and also a
recognition of ways to facilitate the adaptation of
people to changed conditions or a change in habitat.
The witch-doctor here and in cases discussed for the
Zulu in Kwa Mashu is performing the role of psychiatrist which later is taken over by a qualified
psychiatrist.   This is the role of Lambo in Nigeria
which was mentioned above.

   Speaking of the Africans in Soweto, Ellen Hellmann
has recently pointed out that "the witchdoctor is frequently the agency whereby people are brought back to a
consciousness of the influence of the ancestors" (Hellmann 1967:8).   This same function is served by the
isangoma in Kwa Mashu.   He stills fears, interprets
unpredictabilities, sanctions certain actions, and
explains novel experiences.   In this role he supports
Wallace's hypothesis (1966:173) regarding the function
of divinatory rituals since he reduces the duration of
individual indecision; he accomplishes a rapid con-
sensus within the group; and through his indefatigable
optimism and self-confidence, he assures persons that
they have made the correct decision.   The diviner may
not be approved by the modern medical specialist or the
Christian minister, but for the common man in Kwa Mashu
he is still of great value and importance.   While Vila-
kaze is partly correct and many practicing Christians
would not openly call upon the diviner, he is nevertheless swamped with work.   Personally I think that in
these kinds of evaluative statements we are making the
cardinal error of attempting to define "urban", Christian", "social class" and many other concepts in terms
of a Western European prototype rather than arriving at
a situational definition which fits the particular
cultural-ecological-historical situation.

NOTES

[1]Research in Kwa Mashu was carried out during
March to September 1969 with financial assistance from
the University of Florida and the U. S. Department of
Education, to whom I would like to express my sincere
appreciation.
[2]This entails a distance of about seven hundred
miles by train and bus.
[3]The quite intensive training ritual of the
diviner (igqira in Xhosa) is discussed in detail by
Hunter (1936:320-18), by Hammond-Tooke (1955) and
Köhler (1941)
[4]Bryant (1966:13) suggests that the term which
refers to the diviner is derived from a root originally
meaning "the drumming one." Thus Mgoma in Swahili

madness." Peter Lienhardt (1968:52) points out that
the medicine man in Swahili is mganga while the
derivitive form uganga refers to magic which is used to
help people.
[5]Both of these specialists earn a relatively
high income as compared to their cost of living.
Figures are given by van Nieuwenhuijsen (1968) for a
rural area and these figures are substantially lower
than my own for Kwa Mashu.
[6]Professor Vilakazi (1965: 92-13) explains
that traditional taboos, e.g., regarding sexual
intercourse before a battle, are applied in modern
times to such situations as a team before playing a
football match.
[7]Mrs. Harriet Sibisi of the Institute for
Social Research at the University of Natal pointed out
during personal communication that this would be the
ideal and perfect context into which health officials
could introduce the germ theory of disease.
[8]The "rand" is the unit of currency in the
Republic of South Africa and equals approximately
$1.40.
[9]This humble palm-tapper called Tsuma Washe
had a "calling" and changed his name to Kajiwe,
translated as "little stone." The implication of this
name was that he was powerful and could not be crushed.
According to lat est repor ts (The Star, November 1 4,
1970) Kajiw e has re tired at the age of 26 to
concentrate on cultivating his large farm with the help
of his seventeen wives.

<h3 style="text-align:center">References Cited</h3>

Bryant, A. T. Zulu cult of the dead. Man 27:140-115,
1917
Zulu medicine and medicine men. Cape Town: C.
Struik, 1966
De Toit, Brian M. Some aspects of the soul concept
among the Bantu-speaking Nguni-tribes of
South Africa. Anthropological Quarterly
33:3:134-142. 1960
Cultural continuity and African urbanization.
Urban anthropology: research perspectives and
strategies. Elizabeth Eddy (ed.) The Southern
Anthropology Society Proceedings 2:58-74. Athens,
Ga.: University of Georgia Press 1968
Emakhehleni-a revivalistic cult, Brian M. du Toit,
(ed.), Communication from the African Studies
(University of Florida) E. T. deJager, (ed.)
Religious revivalism among urban Zulu Man:
anthropological essays presented to O. F. Raum.
1971

Gelfand, Michael. The Sick African. Cape Town: Juta
and Co. (3rd ed.) 1957
_____. Shona religion. Cape Town: Juta and Co.
1962.
_____. Witch doctor. London: Harvill Press. 1964

Gumede, M. V. African Concepts of Sickness and Bodily
Suffering. Paper presented at the Sixth Biennial
Congress of the South African Nursing Association.
Pretoria. 1968

Hammond-Tooke, W. D. The Initiation of a Baca Isangoma
Diviner. African Studies 14:16-22. 1955.

Hellmann, Ellen. Soweto, Johannesburg's African city.
Johannesburg: South African Institute of Race
Relations. 1967.

Hunter, Monica. Reaction to Conquest. London: Oxford
University Press . 1936.

Jahoda, Gustav. Traditional Healers and Other
Institutions Concerned with Mental Illness in
Ghana. The International Journal of Social
Psychiatry 7:4:245-268. 1961.

Junod, Henri A. The Life of a South African Tribe.
Vol. II. London: McMillan and Co. 1927

Köhler, M. The Izangoma Diviners. Ethnological
Publications 9. Pretoria: Government Printers.
1941.

Kriger, E.J. The social system of the Zulus.
Pietermaritzburg: Shuter and Shooter (2nd ed.)
1950.

Lambo, T. A. A Form of Social Psychiatry in Africa.
Bureau Permanent Inter-african pour Tse-Tse et
Trypanosomiase. Publication 2/0. Leopoldville.
1959.

Lienhardt, Peter. The Medicine Man. London: Oxford
University Press. 1968

Reader, D. H. Zulu Tribe in Transition. Manchester:
Manchester University Press. 1966.

Southall, A. and Peter Gutkind. Townsmen in the
Making. London: Kegan Paul, Trench Trubner and
Co. 1957

Van Nieuwenhuijsen, J. W. The Witch-doctor Institution
in a Zulu Tribe. In the Valley Trust annual
report. Botha's Hill. 15-22. 1968

Vilakazi, A. Zulu Transformations. Pietermartizburg:
University of Natal Press. 1965

Wallace, Anthony, F. C. Religion: An Anthropological
View. New York: Random House. 1966.

CHAPTER 7

WITCHES, MERCHANTS AND MIDWIVES: DOMAINS OF POWER AMONG URBAN BARIBA WOMEN

Carolyn Sargent

In 1983, a Bariba woman in northern People's Republic of Benin traveled from the village where she lived to visit her brother, a civil servant in the administrative capital. The woman, who had grown up in town and married a rural chief's son, was nine months pregnant, and intended to purchase baby clothes in town, while spending a few days at her brother's home. She was pregnant for the eighth time, and had delivered the previous seven children at home in the village, unassisted. While at market in the town on this visit, she went into labor and in spite of her reluctance, was compelled by her brother's wife to deliver at the government hospital. The family took her to the hospital, arguing that their social position would be compromised were she to deliver in their household compound. The features of this illustration of a decision to select a particular form of obstetrical care are indicative of the complexities and contradictions inherent in medical decisions, such as choice of obstetrical care, for contemporary Bariba.

The purpose of this paper, then, is to examine concepts and practices associated with obstetrics and to discuss the implications of these for the status of women in two Bariba communities in Benin. In particular, I will focus on Briba concepts of the causation of misfortune and discuss the prevalent Bariba belief that witches are primary agents of evil who must be detected at birth and dealt with efficiently. I suggest that assuring the availability of measures to control witchcraft affects women's choices of obstetrical care in rural areas. However, transformations in both concepts and practices characterize obstetrical care preferences in an urban Bariba population.

The research upon which this discussion is based was conducted in a rural Bariba region in 1976-77 and in an urban center in 1982-83. Both research projects focused on factors influencing Bariba women's utilization of available obstetrical care services. The

96

Bariba are one of the major ethnic groups of the People's Republic of Benin; they have an estimated population of 500,000 and inhabit the area of Guinean savanna ranging from the western border of Benin into western Nigeria. The Bariba, who are patrilineal and patrilocal, have traditionally been agriculturalists with an economy based on staple food crops of yams, millet and sorghum and an increasing dependence on cash-crops of peanuts, cotton and rice. The urban Bariba are primarily engaged in local commerce and long-distance trade.

Rural Maternity Practices.

The rural portion of this study involved research in the village of Pehunko, which was selected as a research site because of its position as a crossroads market center, from which a number of alternative obstetrical services are accessible. These include national health dispensaries and maternity clinics, missionary health services, indigenous midwives, herbalists and diviners. However, even a cursory consideration of birth practices among Bariba women in this region suggests that women are reluctant to use any cosmopolitan health services.

This initial research project led me to conclude that a multiplicity of factors influenced a woman's decision to select a particular option for birth assistance. Among these factors were such constraints as time, distance, money or as James Young who has written on medical choice in Mexico would state, "factors of accessibllity and exclusion." Also significant were cultural factors such as concepts of sickness etiology, expectations regarding the characteristics of competent obstetrical care, and responsibilities associated with attaining adult female status. As elsewhere in Africa, the significance of reproduction to Bariba women lies in the fact that a first pregnancy is indicative of a critical change from the position of young girl to that of mother. An adult woman's reputation and claim to respect is to a large extent derived from her role as mother of many living children, in particular, sons. One primary means for a woman to enhance her status is to produce numerous healthy children; moreover, a woman's reputation among both men and women is increased by a demonstration of courage and stoicism during delivery. Behaving as the "ideal wife," amassing capital through trade, laboring industriously in agricultural operations all accrue to a woman's prestige. The practice of midwifery, healing, membership in a spirit cult, and divining could also enhance a woman's position. However, a necessary route to achieving any

position of respect and influence for every woman is to
be "a mother of children," and professional specialization does not exempt a woman from the obligation to
produce offspring in order to obtain full and meaningful status as as adult woman.
    Perhaps the most fundamental factor to note in
considering birth among the Bariba is that intrinsi-
cally, pregnancy and delivery are not defined as
pathological processes. In general:
    1) Bariba do not define pregnancy and normal
    delivery as a disease in the sense of "an
    undesirable deviation in the way a person
    functions" (Fabrega 19:293);
    2) in the event of a normal birth, the assistance
    of a specialist is not necessary; the Bariba are
    noteworthy in idealizing the solitary delivery,
    which is not a prevalent practice in Subsaharan
    Africa (Ford 1945:55)
    3)in the event of complications, however, birth
    becomes a life-threatening crisis requiring a
    specialist's intervention.
Pregnancy, then, is not considered abnormal or a
disease, but is nonetheless a period of danger, and
delivery carries the risk of death. This assessment of
the risks of birth will be discussed further below.
    According to the Bariba, every woman should learn
how to behave while pregnant; she should also learn
simple medicines to ensure a safe, quick and easy delivery, and ideally, she should deliver alone. Even a
primipara, a woman at her first delivery, is expected
to try to demonstrate courage during delivery without
assistance. Information on primiparas is scant because
of the difficulties encountered in interviewing them
due to their modesty and reluctance to discuss reproduction but in the sample of 120 women who responded to
questioning, approximately 14% of the primiparas
delivered alone whereas about 43% of the 96 multiparous
women interviewed delivered their last child without
any other present. After delivery, the woman called a
female member of the household to cut the cord (cord-
cutters varied from husband's mother to parturient's
own mother, sister, mother's sister, co-wife and as-
sorted others) or sent for a neighbor for that purpose.
    If a pregnant woman is expected to be competent to
deal with a normal delivery, one might wonder under
what conditions did the 60% of the survey sample who
were assisted at their last delivery deliver? Typical
reasons given by Bariba for calling a midwife are:
    1) the woman is fearful
    2) the woman has experienced difficult deliveries
    in the past
    3) the delivery is in progress and is considered
    problematic.

In the latter two instances, the family and the delivering woman initially decide that the birth cannot
be considered "normal." A midwife may then be called.
The midwife's role thereafter is to study the symptoms
and signs, define the situation, try to remedy any
complications and assist the birth to progress.
    A birth always has the potential for being abnor-
mal, in spite of the fact that in the absence of
complications, the intervention of a midwife is not
required. The primary indicator of a delivery which is
"not good" or "not normal" is that the child is born
with the mark of the supernatural, in other words, the
child is believed to be a witch. Due to this possibility, those awaiting a birth always harbor an underlying
anxiety that the child may present itself as a witch
baby (bii yondo) capable of killing its mother during
delivery or of growing up to provoke havok among its
patrilineal relations. An important function for the
midwife, then, is to observe the delivery process and
verify that labor is proceeding predictably; in other
words, nothing unexpected or visibly abnormal is occurring which would lead one to await or fear a witch
child. The midwife tries to prevent the death of the
mother in case a witch child is attacking her; she
observes the actual delivery to proclaim the normality
of the child, or she may call for the appropriate
specialist in the event that a witch child is born.
    The significance of detecting a witch child can be
appreciated by the realization that in Bariba culture,
witches represent one of the major causes of misfortune, together with poisoners, God, and malevolent
spirits of the bush. An adult cannot become a witch;
rather, a person is born with the power of witchcraft.
A Bariba elder, a former Land Chief of Pehunko respected for his knowledge of good and evil, explained that
birth is the moment when a witch arrives on earth and
must be apprehended. According to Bariba informants,
the signs indicating a witch child are:
    1) a breech birth
    2) child which slides on its stomach at birth
    3) child born with teeth
    4) child born with extreme birth defects
    5) child born at 8 months (lunar months)
    6) child whose teeth come in first in the upper
       gums
One popular story told by Bariba midwives illustrates
the features of a birth considered to bear the mark of
the mystical. In this case, a woman died in labor. In
such instances, the parturient and infant are buried in
separate graves, requiring specialists (the gravedig-
ging family) to surgically remove the unborn child.
During the episode in question, an elder, armed with
protective amulets, removed the child, which was still

alive, very large, had all its teeth and was smiling. This, according to informants, is truly a child which killed its mother, the epitome of a witch baby.

These characteristics which signify abnormality to the Bariba might also be considered unusual in western obstetrics in the sense of being statistically less probable to occur. Thus 96% of births are predicted to be vertex presentations and less than 4% predicted to be breech births. Approximately 10% of deliveries are likely to terminate in a presentation where the baby might slide on its stomach, and very few babies are born with teeth. It seems, then, that Bariba have a biomedically accurate perception of what constitutes both the probable course of a delivery and the most frequently occurring types of presentations; births which deviate from these norms are accordingly defined as abnormal and indicative of witchcraft. Customarily a child born with any of the characteristics of witch children is killed shortly after birth. However, Bariba allege that adult witches may be responsible for causing misfortunes. By what means, then, if witch babies are destroyed at birth, do these adult witches remain? The answer seems to lie in the fact that whether a child is defined as a witch and killed is debatable; first, if a woman delivers alone, and, for example, the child slides on its stomach, she might theoretically decide to move it into another position before someone arrived to cut the cord. Bariba questioned on this subject agreed that a woman who could bear the risks and keep a secret forever in her heart might attempt to disguise a possible witch birth. It is not impossible that a midwife might also connive in such a fashion. Moreover, the fact that some breech births, depending on the point of view of the specialists whose opinion is sought, might be defined as acceptable, allows an element of doubt into the situation. One might wonder why a woman would want to allow a suspected witch to live. Discussions with women suggest that one provocation might be a long-desired pregnancy for a woman who had never conceived or who had no living children.

The case of Adama offers one example of an instance where the desire for a child outweighed the risk of witchcraft. Adama, in her fourteenth pregnancy, had no living children. When she commenced labor in the eight month of pregnancy, she expressed concern to the researcher that the premature labor might indicate a dangerous child. However, when the baby was born (the mother retired to her room to be alone for the delivery), and appeared lively and healthy, no further mention was made of the possibility of witchcraft; the child was alive and thriving several years later. To such a woman as Adama, the risk of a potential witch

might be outweighed by the value of a living infant. In
these and similar ways, then, a dangerous child might
slip through the screening mechanisms and live to grow
up and cause harm. The significance of witch children
in affecting decisions regarding obstetrical assistance
should not be underestimated. Delivering alone provides a woman and her family with flexibility of
options--the woman who delivers without assistance may,
as described above, try to alter the situation; a midwife present at an "abnormal" birth may assist the
mother by trying to protect her from the witch child.
If a witch child is delivered, the midwife may then
call another specialist to deal with the situation
without divulging the truth beyond those immediately
involved. Relatives and neighbors might be told that
the woman had delivered a stillborn child. Thus, the
options fall in both directions: flexibility to keep
or to destroy the child.

On the other hand, if a woman delivers at a maternity clinic, her options seem more limited. First, the
delivery is more public than a home delivery. However,
usually the woman delivers in a room with only the
clinic personnel present; the relative or friend who
accompained her is not allowed in the room. Women
often assert that the government midwife, especially
when she is a member of a different ethnic group, is
not aware of the importance of identifying a dangerous
child. Because the mother is obliged to deliver lying
down, rather than in the Bariba style of kneeling, she
herself cannot determine in what position the child is
delivered in order to note if it is a breech or other
presentation, indicating a witch child. Even were she
aware of the presentation, if she delivered a healthy
child, it would be difficult to poison it or not feed
it while at the maternity clinic. Although theoretically it is possible to do so, most people today are
concerned with the likelihood of being reported to the
police or army and sanctioned for destroying a witch
baby.

The effect of this restriction of options is to
cause some rural women to hesitate before delivering at
the maternity clinic. This hesitation was articulated
by women in the district of Kerou, where several young
women were trained as auxiliary midwives by Catholic
nuns of a nursing order to do home deliveries. One
young trained auxiliary said that women were reluctant
to call her to assist them at deliveries because they
feared it was "like going to a maternity clinic."
Eventually it became clear that what the village women
feared was (a) that she would force them to lie down to
deliver, which is disliked for a variety of reasons,
one being the ensuing difficulty in expelling the
child, and further, the restriction of visibility of

the child's position at delivery, and (b) that she
would either spread the news of an abnormal birth or
report it to the authorities. However, the woman
continued, she had tried to reassure them that what she
saw at a delivery would never be divulged, and some
seemed to believe and accept her. To recapitulate,
then, many rural Bariba women prefer an indigenous midwife if they experience obstetrical complications,
because of expectations regarding the type of intervention likely to be necessary at birth. These expectations derive from the definition of birth as a normal
but dangerous state, which signifies the potential for
the manifestation of abnormality and evil and requires
immediate action to protect the family and society from
future misfortunes.

The Urban Setting

One question which remained to be answered following
the initial study of Bariba birth practices was the
relative extent to which factors of accessibility of
cosmopolitan medical services or cultural factors such
as belief in witch babies constrained women from
selecting a clinic delivery. This issue represents a
current theme in the study of health care decisions.
Young has argued, for example, that extrinsic factors
such as accessibility and exclusivity largely explain
health service use. Moreover, his data suggest that
mystical causation is not a factor which significantly
influences medical choice. Contrastingly, much research on the utilization of alternative medical services in Africa suggests that concepts of etiology do
affect treatment choices (cf. Janzen 1978:127; Maclean
1976: 290). The most recent research, then, aimed to
clarify this issue by examining a population with
greater access to hospital assistance. The research
was conducted in the administrative and commercial
center of Parakou, a largely Bariba town with a population of approximately 60,000. Women in Parakou have
the following delivery options.
    1) a 32-bed hospital maternity center, supervised
    by government trained nurse-midwives, offering
    free delivery but charging for a required five-day
    stay and any medications prescribed;
    2) two private clinics, one run by a nurse-
    midwife, the other by a nurse's aide. Both
    clinics provide prenatal consultations and charge
    a fixed price for delivery. The woman is free to
    leave as soon as she chooses following delivery;
    3) home delivery assisted by relatives, friends,
    or indigenous midwives, or unassisted delivery.

Interviews with 58 women attending a prenatal
clinic, 36 pregnant women contacted at home and 50
women employed at a cashew processing plant indicated
that approximately 22% had ever experineced a home
delivery. So, correspondingly, 75% have relied on
hospital assistance at birth. In the sample of 36
women followed throughout their pregnancy, women were
interviewed regarding preferred type of delivery
assistance (hospital or home delivery), reasons for
utilizing the hospital and explanations for not
delivering at the hospital. Responses demonstrated
that 17% of the women had selected a home delivery.
Among the primary reasons offered for not using the
hospital were distance (62.2%), lack of time (12.2%),
being a stranger in town (12.2%). Those women who did
deliver in the hospital gave as explanations a variety
of reasons including greater safety (45.7%), greater
medical assistance (14.3%), influence of relatives
(8.6%), less suffering (5.7%), public influence (2.9%),
habit (2.9%) and facilitating acquisition of birth
certificate (2.(%). All informants discussed the
general attitude of those women who prefer home
deliveries and suggested that women do not choose a
hospital delivery due to lack of money (34.3%),
distance (14.3%),habit (5.7%), embarrassment (5.7%),
shame, habit and embarrassment (5.%), lack of need
(2.9%) and lack of "civilization" (2.9%).
     The responses citing factors of accessibility as
explanations for not choosing a hospital delivery might
suggest that such constraints are the primary determi-
nants of delivery choice. However, more profound
investigation regarding public policy concerning home
delivery and urban perspectives on the cosmological
implications of birth is necessary in order to assess
the influence of beliefs and values on delivery preference. The marked contrast between the prevalence of
hospital delivery in the urban sample and prevailing
birth practice in the village provokes inquiry regarding the ideology of birth, in particular, the fate of
the witch baby in the urban setting. Do Bariba women
who deliver in hospitals maintain a belief in the
possiblity of a witch birth? If so, how is the witch
detected and dealt with and does the belief in witchcraft, a potential cause of affliction, affect delivery
choice? In Bariba tradition, two varieties of children
possessing extraordinary powers may exist: the abiku
child, born only to die and then to be reborn, but to
die again, and the biiyondo, or witch baby, who shows
certain identifying signs at birth and if not promptly
killed, will eventually cause harm to patrilineal kin.
This sample indicated that belief in both abiku and
biiyondo persist in the urban environment. Questioning
on the topic of witch babies proved particularly diffi-

cult; given the delicate nature of the subject. Reluctance to discuss actual experience with witch babies is
evident in the high percentage of evasive responses
indicated.

Table 1
Extraordinary Children

Category	Yes	No	Evasive
Abiku Knowledge	91.4	0	8.6
Abiku in Town	88.6	2.9	8.6
Yondo Knowledge	80.0	2.9	17.2
Yondo in Town	77.1	2.9	20.0

All 56 women interviewed on the subject expressed
belief in witch babies and 77% express the conviction
that such witches are periodically born in town. Predictably, none of the sample claimed any personal
experience with witch births. However, a number of
sources indicated that infanticide was decreasing in
the Parakou area. Rather, those families unfortunate
enough to confront a witch baby were turning to the
option of neutralizing the witch by means of special
medications prepared by elderly Bariba male healers.
Such neutralizing medicines ensured that the infant
would not harm its kin and could be expected to lead a
normal life. Women who delivered in the hospital,
then, would return home with the child and subsequently
consult an appropriate elder either in town or in a
neighboring village. The elder would medicate the
child, subsequent to which the child would return home.
Interestingly, this has always been an option (according to village elders) but never selected due to fear
of the consequences for the child's kin.

It seems, therefore, that belief in witches and
concern for the consequences of a witch birth need not
constrain a woman from selecting a hospital delivery.
On the other hand, the reasons for selecting a hospital
delivery are not difficult to determine. Government
pressure, the possibility of fines and public humiliation in the event of a home delivery, publicity regarding increased safety for mother and child in the
hospital setting, and for civil servants financial gain
in the form of monthly benefits for the properly
registered child (allocation familiale based on the
French social security system), all encourage hospital
births. These pressures may well explain the unexpect-
edly large percentage of women delivering in hospitals.
Moreover, it seems likely that those women who selected
a home delivery might be reluctant to express an actual
preference for home delivery, thus indicating a preferred option counter to government policy. Apparent
"factors of accessibility," then, might disguise other

significant influences affecting selection of delivery
assistance.
     Following this consideration of the relevance of
the belief in witch babies for choice of delivery
assistance, it is illustrative to examine additional
dimensions of the decision not to deliver at home.
Research on rural Bariba women indicated that the
solitary home delivery provided a woman with the opportunity to determine the fate of her child, in other
words, the solitary setting offered a means to control
this aspect of reproduction. Furthermore, women serve
as specialists in complications of pregnancy and
delivery and skill in midwifery has supplied women with
a rare avenue to enhanced prestige. Lombard, a French
ethnographer writing on Bariba social organization in
the 1950's, claimed that midwifery served in fact as
the sole outlet for a woman to achieve regional fame
(Lombard 1965:143). Correspondingly, women who select
a hospital delivery have relinquished the control of
the reproductive domain characteristically held by
rural Bariba women. Moreover, as urban women cease to
rely on midwives for back-up support at home deliveries, the midwives themselves find their position
diminished and interest among potential apprentices
similarly declining. Although urban midwives continue
to practice, some are shifting to specialize in infant
health problems and midwifery is by no means the
optimal route to achieving reknown in the urban area.
     A comparison of status determinants in rural and
urban Bariba communities suggests that for the rural
woman, status is a function primarily of family origin,
status of spouse, and motherhood; position may be
enhanced by behavior such as courage at delivery and
prestige accrued by a specialization in a healing
skill, most probably midwifery (spirit cult members who
are clairvoyants attain particular prestige). The
status of the urban women is also set in part by family
and marital linkages; however, urban women may achieve
an economic independence, unparalleled in the experience of most rural women, by means of which they may
accrue prestige, wealth, and respect. Among women
interviewed at the Parakou cashew processing factory, a
majority stated that the desirable enterprise for a
woman in Benin today was commerce; a small beginning in
petty trade might lead to a more substantial commercial
undertaking and eventually to profitable investments in
long-distance trade. For a minority of women, opportunities may be found in salaried employment with one of
several urban factories or in civil service jobs which
allow time for the mother to return home periodically
throughout the day to breastfeed, as opposed to low-
ranking civil service jobs, which are less flexible.

The following vignettes illustrate some options available to urban women.

Buyon, for example, engaged in trade, selling such
items as cheeses, grain, and old yoghurt containers to
friends and neighbors. In addition, she obtained a job
in the cashew processing plant after passing the entry
exam, (which usually requires an elementary school
education). Having acquired this salaried position as
a low-ranking civil servant, she nevertheless relied on
intermittent commercial enterprise to supplement her
salary. Although she would prefer to enlarge her
commercial investments, her husband disapproves of the
traveling which such work entails, so her long-term
goal is to enter the health civil service, perhaps as a
nurse's aide. Much of her current profits are rein-
vested in trade, or spent on her three children.

Juliette, on the other hand is divorced, in her
late thirties, childless, and devotes herself to her
cloth trade. Periodically, she travels between Niamey,
Niger, and Cotonou, the capital of Benin, to buy and
sell bolts of cloth; she operates in both retail and
wholesale enterprise and has achieved a notable profit
from her commerce. Known throughout her neighborhood
as a shrewd and competent, yet diplomatic woman, she
serves as the only female governmental delegate in
town. Her home is furnished with luxury items such as
electric fans, record player, radio, and imported
knick-knacks.

A final example is that of Barikissou, who left
school to marry a veterinarian, divorced, worked as a
laundress, engaged in petty trade, and studied independently to pass examinations to enable her to enter the
civil service. She has two children, both of which she
has supported through her endeavors, although one now
lives with his father. Initially she obtained a job in
the cashew factory, but eventually passed a higher-
level examination which permitted her to find a
position in the post office, where she now works an a
telegraphist. She does not trade at the present time
and hopes to move further up the civil service hierarchy to become an administrator. These three women,
when discussing reproductive practices, state that the
urban woman is likely to select a hospital delivery to
demonstrate her commitment to the urban mode, or
fashion. In this perpsective, they echo the comments
of those Parakou women cited earlier, who urged their
visiting relative to deliver at the hospital in order
to avoid shaming her urban kin.

Aspirations to achieve success in commerce or
civil service are frequently accompanied by efforts to
adopt behavior perceived as "civilized" (that is wear-
ing European clothing, adopting European food habits,
demonstrating competence in French, displaying famili-

arity with bureacratic procedures. The French term
"civilizé" is a commonly heard reference for such
behavior.) According to women employed in the cashew
factory, hospital delivery is a requisite for the urban
woman. Home delivery, contrastingly, is an indication
of a peasant mentality. However, to date, the urban
environment allows a mix of values and goals, so that
with the exception of the elite few who categorically
oppose home delivery, most women express admiration for
the "virtuous woman" who delivers at home, thus demonstrating her courage in a situation of danger. The
decision by a woman to deliver at home in town represents a personal preference, reflecting certain values
and priorities--but due to fundamental transformations
in the bases of power in Bariba society, the solitary
delivery no longer represents a unique opportunity for
a woman to augment her prestige and midwifery no longer
serves as a rare vehicle for women to transcend the
limitations of sex and achieve power outside the
domestic domain.

REFERENCES CITED

Fabega, Horatio Jr. Disease and Social Behavior.
    Cambridge, Massachusettes: MIT Press. 1974.
Ford, C. S. A comparative Study of Human Reproduction,
    1964 Edition. Yale University Publications in
    Anthropology #32. HRAF Press. 1945.
Janzen, John. The Quest for Therapy in Lower Zaire.
    Berkeley: University of California Press. 1978.
Lombard, Jacques. Structures de Type "Feodal" en
    Afrique Noire. Paris: Mouton and Company. 1975.
Maclean, Catherine M. Una. Traditional Healers and
    Their Female Clients: An Aspect of Nigerian
    Sickness Behavior. Journal of Health and Social
    Behavior 10(3): 172-83. 1969.
Sargent, Carolyn. The Cultural Context of Therapeutic
    Choice. Dordrecht, Holland: Reidel Publishing
    Company. 1982.
Young, James. Medical Choice in a Mexican Village.
    New Brunswick, New Jersey: Rutgers University
    Press. 1981.

CHAPTER 8

HEALING AND CONVERSION IN NEW RELIGIOUS MOVEMENTS IN AFRICA: CHANGE AND CONTINUITY

Lamin Sanneh

And they say that they [the Blacks] were the first to be taught to honour the gods and to hold sacrifices and festivals and processions... and the other rites by which men honour the deity; and that in consequence their piety has been published abroad among all men, and it is generally held that the sacrifices practised among the Ethiopians are those which are the most pleasing to heaven. As witness to this they call upon the poet who is perhaps the oldest and certainly the most venerate among the Greeks; for in the Iliad he represents both Zeus and the rest of the gods with him as absent on a visit to Ethiopia to share in the sacrifices and the banquet which were given annually by the Ethiopians for all the gods together....And they state that by reason of their piety toward the deity, they manifestly enjoy the favour of the gods, inasmuch as they have never experienced the rule of an invader from abroad; for from all time they have enjoyed a state of freedom and of peace one with another, and although many and powerful rulers have made war upon them, not one of these has succeeded in his undertaking [Diodorus of Sicily, Greek historian of first century B.C.E.]

Healing and conversion are two of the most spectacular and persistent traits in the new religious movements in Africa. Their analysis as a genuine aspect of religious history is more than justified in any concern with modern Africa. The voluminous literature in the field should make this a relatively easy task. What is surprising, however, is the comparative reluctance to take this religious theme seriously so that the authentically religious may be conceived as playing an important historical role. A straight causal analysis of the phenomenon is likely to sidestep the religious centre. External factors may help explain the character of

108

change, but the religious basis would require other explanations, including the predisposition of traditional
societies.
   The approach here is to set healing as an indigenous category alongside conversion as a modern permutation. Indigenous criteria would thus be acting upon new
materials. Conversion might be described in lofty revolutionary language, but the experience of healing
which often undergirds it suggests a less radical break
with the past. Jean Comaroff may be right when he calls
for a reconciliation between cultural form and social
transformation and a willigness to reliquish the
epistemological premise that ahistorical, synchronic
models are sufficient for explaining continuity and
change (see his "Healing and Cultural Transformation:
The Tswana of Southern Africa," Soc. Sci. Med. 15B:367-
378.) But in my reckoning Robin Horton may have gone to
the other extreme by throwing away the baby with his
evolutionary bath water (1971:85-108). Others have
joined Comaroff in pointing out the complex variations
that exist in traditional cosmologies (Ifeka-Moller
1974:55-72) which Horton is apt to view in undifferentiated terms as comprising the 'microcosm' of tribal
deities and the 'macrocosm' represented by cults of the
Supreme Being.   In this theory Christianity (or Islam)[1] merely stimulates, rather than originating,
developments in the macrocosm at the expense of the
microcosm. This approach assumes a static, ahistorical
view of cultural form, and its consequence would be to
postulate a wholesale uprooting of social systems by
virtue of external developments. It is much more rea-
sonable to contend that the pressures of modernization
are absored into pre-existing currents of adaptation.
Cultural systems may be profitably viewed as being both
historical and affirmative. Assimilation of new
materials and experiences presupposes active contact
with historival transmission. In this view healing is
an assimilative category, combining ancient reflex with
new experience.   Dreams are another (Charsley,
1973:244-257).   And so is prayer in its prognostic
use.[2]   All these categories rest on the epistemological assumption of change and continuity, allowing
African societies to handle new religious materials
within culturally recognizable forms.
   Dr. Harold W. Turner, who has done much to advance
research and study in this field, has alluded in one
place to the modernizing role of new religious movements. He speaks of

      the contribution of medical care through spiritual
      healing, the discipline of disoriented peoples
      when they gave a new 'place to belong', the new
      trans-tribal unities...the authentic indigeniza-

tion of Christianity in many of the independent
church forms and, in general, the great spiritual
and mental shake-up that breaks through the con-
fines of the old world-view and opens the way for
new incentives, new visions of the future, new
basic assumptions and values. These considerations
[he continues] reveal how the...new religious
movements...may in fact be making a most important
contribution to the development and modernizing of
their societies [1979:12-13

The theoretical model being suggested in this
paper has practical application. The phenomenon of
religious conversion would appear to be most strikingly
represented in societies where people have recourse to
explicit traditional religious materials. Wherever
these religious materials are no longer an important
influence, conversion is correspondingly scarce. Some
other factors may influence this situation. Islam,for
example, may succeed in weakening traditional religions
and thus in suppressing any 'revivalist' potential in
the culture (see O'Fahey 1980:115-130 for Dar Fur as an
example). Consequently areas of Islamic influence may
appear roughly to correspond with the absence of conversion movement. Similarly, the active contact of the
West, to think of a contrasting situation, may trigger
a religious response and lead to the emergence of new
religious movements. From this situation we may be
tempted to conclude that conversion is a reaction to
Western humiliation which Islam averted for its
adherents.
     The absence of significant conversion movements
among, say, the Bambara of Mali or the Temne of Sierra
Leone, areas influenced by Islam before colonialism,
would appear to strengthen the case for Islam as an
inhibiting factor. By contrast, the spectacular growth
of new religious movements in South Africa might lend
credence to the 'reaction' argument. But the defect of
both these appproaches is that they assign a determin-
ist function to external factors and agents. One
eminent writer concedes the case when he writes that
Christianity provides the grammar and syntax, and
traditional customs the lexicon to produce the modern
phenomenon of African Christian independency (Victor
Turner in Foreword to Jules-Rosette 1975:8). Yet it is
clear in most of these movements that innovations were
being made on the basis of pre-existing values and
attitudes--and in this sense Horton is the victor. By
an ironic contrast, those writers who saw most clearly
that the new was in the service of the old were also
those most concerned to view the old in the conspira-
torial sense which in South Africa carries the inevit-

able implications of political suppression (Oosthuizen
1968 and Gray's review 1980;415; also Sundkler
1976:190-92, 204n, 306, 328).
     The resilience of indigenous categories should
help us to minimize the significance of imported standards. It should also help to isolate the Islamic
factor. The dramatic occurrence of new religious movements in a place like Yorubaland, where Islam had made
a significant impression, suggests that the Islamic
factor cannot on its own hold back the tide of religious revivalism. Conversely, the relative absence of
movements of Christian Independency in much of French-
ruled West Africa shows that Western contact alone
cannot account for the phenomenon. Yet the coincidence
of the rise of new religious movements with areas of
Western influence demands an explanation. It would
appear that new religious movements, rising out of
indigenous ferment, responded to Western contact by the
help of the vernacular Bible which that contact made
possible. Thus the impact of the West need not be
denied in order to retain indigenous initiative or to
account for reform and change. Long before the coming
of the West, African societies were subject to drastic
change through climatic and environmental factors,
historical events such as military movements and the
waves of refugees that rose and fell on new shores, and
the shifting fortunes of political states and trading
patterns. All these produced corresponding changes in
the religious traditions, as one detailed study of the
anicient Mbona Cult in Malwai has shown (Schoffeleers
1972). This history of adjusting to new experiences by
marshalling into line the old order acquired a fresh
impetus with the availability of the vernacular Scriptures. The alarm expressed by some writers that many of
these movements are only a diversionary facade for
'nativistic' revival shows a slowness in appreciating
what a revolutionary instrument missionaries had
created with the Scriptures in the vernacular.
     The importance of local factors, both structural
and personal, in stimulating movement in religious
values and attitudes is enhanced by the complementary
role of African materials. In much of the evidence we
possess, we have the impression that the leading per-
sonalities embarked upon their mission with great
reluctance and after a dramatic intervention. Some of
this emphasis is undoubtedly aimed at discouraging
religious adverturism which must have existed to
deserve this wariness in the sources. But it also suggests the outlines of an indigenous critique of the
veracity of religious experience. It is a pervasive
issue in the sources, though we may identify a few
typical examples at this state. One of the guiding
spirits of the 'Aladura' revival movement, which

occurred between 1928 and 1930 in Yorubaland, was
Joseph Babalola. He was employed in the Public Works
Department as a driver of a steam-roller on road construction. It was while he was working that his engine
seized. He then heard a voice calling his name three
times with the command to go and preach the Gospel.
Babalola returned home armed with a bell and the message that prayer and the 'water of life' (omo iye)
would cure all sickness. He enterdd the town naked and
covered with ashes and was appropriately taken to be
mad and promptly put in prison for two weeks (Peel
1968:70).
        In the case of Joseph Babalola it was a seized
engine which overcame his resistance and made him
relent. We should also notice the manner in which his
name was repeated to him three times, an emphasis which
established in his own mind that his fundamental identity was not in doubt where it mattered, whatever his
reduced significance as a replaceable source of casual
labor. Furthermore, the major changes taking place in
his traditional environment must have had their effect
in 'the shaking of the foundations'. The experience of
riding the road-roller and seeing the rough earth
levelled under him must have played a part in awakening
him to a notion of a spiritual power which can level
and bring order to the be-strewn pieces of ancient
religious values. The name as the instrument by which
the objective self exists might become the means of a
subjective enlightenment. This is a well-known religious principle. The intrusion of a modern road into a
traditional village symbolized for Babalola and his
types the irreversible speed with which modernity would
impinge on ancient Africa, and only a correspondingly
swift religious carriage could keep pace. Appearing
naked and covered with ashes before an astonished
people, Babalola symbolized the bewilderment of traditional Africa on the threshold of modernity, and for
remedy he combined the healdic appeal of the bell with
the healing quality of 'the water of life' as signs of
a new religious order. Conversion, and healing as its
efficacious, token were brought together in the person
of the prophet. Babalola claimed that the smallpox
epidemic that afflicted the village people shortly
after their rejection of him was a punishment for his
treatment. The sickly appeareance of his ash-covered
body thus foreshadowed the coming affliction of his
people. What smallpox did to the body modernity would
do to the human spirit. And just as retreat into
hygienic quarantine is impossible before the one, so is
religious disengagement suicidal before the other. The
prophet is the via negativa to the new dispensation.
Babalola's road engine would not trample on the com-

munity's sacred objects and memories. He was now
riding the chariot of a different dispensation.
This theme of approach and retreat is represented
in one story concerning the rout of anicent tradition
by the forces of modernity. The story is told of a
gentle oracular spirit, the widow of a long-deceased
Alaye of the village of Efon, who lived a solitary but
contented life in the forest near the village. In the
early 1920's Christianity and new schools and roads
began opening up the place. The oracle was disturbed.
In 1927 she told the reigning Alaye, Aladejare, that
"her pot of indigo dye had been broken by the new road,
and that she was leaving Efon to return no more" (Peel
1968:94). It was a retreat which neither saved her
sacred pot nor halted the advance of the modern world.
She represents many of those who had confided in sacred
vessels of tradition only to have them smashed by an
aggressive modernity. But she is also typical of the
inability of solitary and marginal people to face major
challenge. The disorientation of refugee groups in
African society is a dramatic recapitulation of the
fate of the widow of Efon.
To return to the subject of reluctance to embark
on the religious vocation we are told of the story of a
Zulu Zionist leader, Ma Mbele (b. 1904). She had a
revelation in 1940 in which she was told to heal the
sick. She ignored the summons for more than ten years.
Then in 1951 she passed through an unconscious state
and had a vision. God told her: "I need you as a
Healer and Helper of many" (Sundkler 1976:83). That
terse message achieved its purpose and her resistance
was overcome. She subsequently founded a community
dedicated to spiritual healing. But she retained her
reputation as a shy and withdrawn person (Sundkler
1976:82). In the concentrated message as she received
it, the gift of healing was clearly the operative context of religious truth. Even faith as a personal
conviction appears missing from the material.
The founder of the Church of the Saints in South
Africa, George Khambule (1884-1949) emerged into prominence after a prolonged period of determined resistance. Only a personal tragedy brought about his
eventual capitulation. In 1918 a great influenza
epidemic engulfed the world. Coming so soon after
Halley's comet of 1911 (another is due in 1986, two
years after the year of the modern pre-millenium) the
epidemic was interpreted as the dawn of the apocalypse.
John Mtanti (1873-1937) was one of those griped by the
fever of expectancy, and in 1919 he saw in a dream what
he must do to build Zion as a spiritual refuge for his
people. In 1931 he went public with his message, which
included a detailed sketch of the architectural sym-
metry of Heaven, something in fact of an enterprising

114 AFRICAN HEALING STRATEGIES

blend of modern cathedral style building and the traditional homestead. His confidence boosted, Mtanti re-
signed his job as school-teacher after he had unsettled
his pupils by appearing in the wild garb of an Old
Testament prophet and exclaiming 'Nakho! Nakho!--'Woe,
woe!' (Sundkler 1976:124). Only the new Jerusalem, he
felt, could now avert the fearful fate that hung over
the world, and at that point a suitable dream admonished him to seek out the man who was to found the Church
of the Saints, George Khambule.
    George Khambule had been a mine captain in Johan-
nesburg. He was barely literate, and in the world in
which he struggled to make a living he would be considered inferior to John Mtanti. But in the upside-down
logic of the spiritual Zion, Mtanti looked up to him as
the greater instrument by which the Heavenly Jerusalem
would take earthly proportions. George demurred. But
shortly after this his woman friend in Johannesburg
died after a brief illness, and George was shaken by
the experience. He fell ill consequently and was taken
to hospital. He lost physical consciousness one
evening, regaining it at four in the morning. In that
time he recounted how he had vision of his woman friend
and his sister, both dead. He saw his sister crying

    and saw the angels of Satan with their forks about
    to push the dead into the fire. The Jesus
    appeared--Khambule was now in heaven, the two of
    them were looking from above down at the earth and
    its central point, Telezini. He saw there his own
    corpse, foul and smelling, and his wife crying
    beside it [Sundkler 1976:125].

By the time the vision ceased, Khambule had been given
a detailed levitical code concerning ritual purity.
When he rose from this experience the question no
longer was whether but how soon he could reach home in
Telezini. Eventually a stone temple was erected, and
Telezini, the obscure spot on maps of the Native Reserves, was now bathed in the elevated light of Zion.
    The use of dreams and visions and other unusual
types of religious experience to rebuke doubt and in-
duce compliance is so widespread that it cannot be
adequately followed in this limited discussion. Another
equally major theme is the matter of physical mobility:
people on the move or travelling away from home may be
particularly prone to religious experience. But the
thematic converse of this may also hold: people making
a habit of retiring to a familiar spot for meditation
or rest may come to a new religious experience.
    Certain other theoretical issues may be introduced
at this stage of the exposition. The concept of healing is a dominant one in the sources. One general view

is that human beings are encircled by a hostile world
which threatens to take them to the margins of existence. Healing is the process of unpossessing the ill
and re-possessing them in an integrated community.
Both the healer and the patient are thus exposed to the
same forces, for the power to cure comes from a related
power to harm. The public seance of healing reinte-
grates the healer in to society from which he would
otherwise remain isolated by his professionalism.
Religious healing takes the social understanding of
illness and places it in the appropriate ritual context. Illness demands social action, and ritual shapes
and articulates that action. It is this understanding
of healing which has fired the new religious movements.
Illness has natural causes, but it has a mystical basis
requiring investigation and demonstration in a public
context. This supplies the common basis for social
experience. The rank and file are made to participate
in a community of equal access. The common experience
of disenchantment and the assumption of the mystical
source of illness draw people into a mass catharsis of
deliverance through the crucible of conversion. In
Soweto, for example, there are Faith Healing 'Foun-
tains' around which people congregate at night. "Nobody
is asked whether he or she is Anglican, Catholic,
Lutheran, 'A.M.E.' OR Zionist. At the Fountain, 'The
Lake of Peace', all are alike: the same anxiety about
health and wholeness; the same trust in the blessed
water which they are given to take home" (Sundkler
1976:291). In this important sense, healing gathers
people from the margins of a diminished existence and
brings them into inter-personal relationship. But it
does not fabricate a non-existent community. Healing
is returning a person to a state of integration which
illness threatens to destroy, and ensuring a public
charter for the healer.
    In some areas this might acquire the significance
of an ecological harmony. Isaiah Shembe (d. 1935), one
of the most remarkable of the leaders of new religious
movements and founder in 1911 of the Church of the
Nazarites in Zululand, taught a deep reverence for
nature and an awesome awareness of her suffering. He
admonished his sons not to cut a branch of a tree:
"How would you feel if I were to cut one of your
fingers from your hand?" (Sundkler 1976:171). He
similarly condemned cruelty to animals (Sundkler
1976:171).
    The practice of healing often allows women to play
a critical role. Two redoubtable women leaders, Ma Nku
(b. 1894) and Ma Mbele, both specialized in healing.
The attend above all to mental disorder (ufufunyane)
and, a particularly serious type, isinyanya, and other
forms of hysterical illness. Before a healing service

an animal is sacrificed to increase the healing power.
Later the bones are burned to produce highly valuable
ashes which are mixed in a tub with consecrated water
and with the sacrifical blood, and then placed in the
vestry. The mixture is held to be particularly effective against demon-possession (Sundkler 1976:84). In a
different example water and ashes are served in a mixture as a prescription for the those suffering from a
hysteric disorder (isipoliyana) (Sundkler 1976:221).
    In one example the diagnostic procedure is used to
reinforce the therapeutic use of healing. Offences
against the sexual code are first deterimind and then
prescribed for. Ashes and Sunlight soap are mixed with
water and then dispensed. The ashes are obtained from
an altar built according to measurements laid down in
the Book of Exodus Chapters 30 and 38. Cattle would be
carefully selected and 'baptized' by the prophet of the
new church (in this instance St. John's Apostolic
Church of Swazilaand). The water which is used is
taken from underneath a rock. The prophet rubs the
head of the client with the mixture while praying at
the same time (Sundkler 1976:221).
    Water and ashes are clearly significant ritual
elements, and in the context of religious healing or
spiritual purification they carry great power.
Babalola had stumbled on a major resource. When the
setting is a flowing stream in the open where numbers
can be multiplied then we have public drama of major
proportions, in fact the stage for a command performance. In this particular story we are also confronted
with a discreet if ubiquitous theme, namely, the
encounter of new religious movement with African traditional religions. On that point, the story affirms the
resilience of old values which may receive renewed
stimulus from contact with new Christian materials.
    At dawn two groups of worshippers arrive at a
stream. The first is a group of traditional religious
worshippers led by Dlakude, a woman. Her followers
dance round her as the entire party runs downhill
towards the stream, chanting old sacred songs. On the
opposite bank is a rival group of worshippers, some
dressed in white with green or yellow sashes. They are
members of the Sabbath Zionist Church led by Prophet
Elliot Butelezi. They are also running and dancing
round the prophet as they move along. They are singing
a Christian hymn.
    The Christian party is preceded at the stream by
the traditional religious party. All the members of
the party have brought their calabashes and when these
have been filled with water some medicine is mixed with
it and then rigorously stirred until it foams. The
leader gives each to drink from it and they begin to
vomit. Meanwhile the Zionists look on silently except

when Elliot Butelezi, perhaps sensing that his passive
role in all of this might be construed as an inadequacy, asks Dlakude a rhetorical question: "When are
you going to finish, preacher?" (Sundkler 1964:239).
The Zionist party, given that formal lead, respond with
amused laughter. Dlakude takes no notice, intent on
completing the ritual vomiting. She then finds some
white clay with which she smears herself and her
followers. A short sacred song follows and the whole
group begins to leave the stream for Dlakude's kraal.
She leads the group in a recessional dance, beating
them with branches as they run home.

It is now the turn of the Zionists. One of the
group complains that the water has been defiled from
Dlakude entering it, a veiled criticism of Butelezi's
allowing Dlakude to steal the show and to push the
Zionists into secondary importance. But Butelezi is
reassuring, saying that the vigorous flow of the stream
has removed any impurity. He intones a hymn which the
assembly of worshippers takes up, and then he blesses
the water. He dips his finger in the stream and stirs
it. He looks up to the sky and says a short prayer to
the Lord of the Living Waters that the stream may be
cleansed of vile things. A sick member of the group is
brought to Butelezi by a prayer-woman. He scoops water
into the patient's mouth, shouting at the same time the
Trinitarian formula. Then he assures the patient:
"This blessed water will take away illnesses from this
sick person. Drink!" (Sundkler 1964:239).

Butelezi then takes the patient into the middle of
the stream and makes the woman stoop until the water
covers her head. He puts his hands over her head and
immediately goes into a possession phase. His body
shakes and he shouts in rising tones. The patient
drinks repeatedly from the water, praying in the inter-
vals for the Spirit to descend like a dove. Soon she
also goes in to possession to the accompaniment of
hymn-singing by the worshippers. The sick woman
emerges from the water and starts to vomit on the
rocks.

Other patients succeed her in the water, going
through an identical process of purification and ending
with vomiting. Following this Butelezi takes some
white ashes which he mixes with water into a paste. He
rubs the paitents' faces and shoulders with the mixture. He then ties green sashes round their shoulders.
In a procession Butelezi leads the Zionists home, all
of them singing and dancing (Sundkler 1964:240).

It is clear that the two groups of worshippers are
remarkable more by similarities in what they think
divides them than in what they feel unites them. Zionist advocates in South Africa and in West Africa would
strenuously deny they have anything is common with

Dlakude and her types. But such denial cannot hide the
deep affinity that exists between the old and new. In
the area of actual practice the bond is much closer and
the lines of demarcation are much harder to draw. The
practice of Dlakude and her party in fact provides the
rule of clarification for what followed in Elliot Butelezi and his group of Zionists. The new religous movement was clearly riding on the back of the old.
Dlakude was the chief broker in the enterprise which
Butelezi is anxious to profit by. Both he and his
Zionist followers are steeeped in the same element as
Dlakude and her acolytes. Consequently the new religious vocabulary of Butelezi is directly influenced by
the earlier material. Religious and social renewal
might thus come to mean the indispensable necessity of
a significant carry-over of pre-existing models.

The Waziri of Sokoto, Alhaji Junaidu, in an
address to a convocation of the Ahmadu Bello University
in Zaria 1971 expressed similar sentiments when he
exhorted the students and the general University community to remember that they could only make a meaningful life for themselves in the modern world if they
previously recognized an indebtedness to the sources of
traditional value in their own communities. He cau-
tioned against an uncritical espousal of change,
saying:

> Wise men know that change is part of the necessary
> processes through which all societies must pass if
> they are to grow and to survive in an improved
> state. Wise men know that change can have other
> faces whose influence might well lead to the
> impoverishment of the very society we wish
> tonourish...It is little wonder that our...modern
> elite...violate they very laws and principles
> which the themselves create. When your own world
> has been put aside, you feel no respect for any
> other [Text of address in Brown and Hiskett
> 1975:467-571].

Research into this question has to proceed much
further before we can predict the final outcome of the
confluence of the old and the new. Yet even at this
stage two things stand out clearly. In the first place
at the confluence of the old and the new a striking
degree of parallelism occurs, and the new prophets
navigate the headwaters of the change with indigenous
charts. Thus they have carried forward the religious
enterprise harnessing old forces. In the second place
there can be little question of the profound influence
of the older religious materials in setting the course
and infusing pace into development in the field. In
watching Dlakude' movements carefully, Elliot Butelezi

might indeed suggest a methodological principle by
which we should ourselves approach the subject. His
own arrival at the stream was almost made to appear as
if it was at Dlakude's prompting. The'stirring of the
waters'[3] of that and other streams may have the
effect of prompting a similar process of scholarly
purfication so that writers may strive to pay greater
heed to the amour propre of African societies.
     "Water Church" is how one leader describes the new
religious movement over which he presides (Sundkler
1964:205). By that name he has highlighted the central
preoccupation with the element. Western contact by
virtue of its religion and politics has placed a pre-
mium on indigenous values. Christianity provided the
access route par excellence with the introduction of
the vernacular Scriptures, though the consequent creation of a Water Chruch was hardly the motive for Scriptural translation even if it is its indisputable result. Those who attend the Water Chruch are convinced
that the pool around which they congregate is inhabited
by snakes, crocodiles and the evil works of Satan. The
world as a hostile environment is thus recalled, with
water serving the role of ritual scapegoat for the
hazards and traumas of existence. The Biblical pool of
Bethesda (John 5) is thus transposed into its numerous
local equivalents into which, like bulging lagoons of
African cities, are discharged the effluents of float-
ing populations. Personal purification reverses this
process of physical deterioration, and in its collective form provides a social bond of rehabilitation and
integrationl. The challenge thus for the new religious
movements is to demonstrate that they possess the
resources to diagnose and prescribe for the African
condition. Many therefore plunge into the newly available Christian materials to take the measure of the
full potential for personal and social well being. The
prophet approaches the evil-infested pool carrying a
bucket of ashes. He is quickly reminded of the grave
risks that lurk in the water. He breaks into a prayer
and waves his staff, symbol of prophetic office, and
with that scatters the imaginary forces that have
established tutelage over the pool. He then prays for
peace in the water, and entreats the Angel of the
Waters to descend with power and cleansing into the
pool and thereby remove all the dangers (Sundkler
1964:204). Meanwhile he is watched and encouraged by a
public audience.
     An indispensable resource is thus regenerated and
made available to fill a correspondingly extensive
need. Bottles are brought to the pool and filled with
the precious element and given to the mothers in the
gathering. Some ninety-six children, aged from one to
seven, are then taken from their mothers and plunged in

the water three times. The symbolic stages of this
ritual, contrasting the separation and reunion of kin,
transmute the painful experience of economic and
political alienation which Zion would transcend. The
children were handled by a woman leader who turned
their frantic crying and gasping into a justification
for upbraiding the mothers, charging that it was because the women had not confessed their sins that their
children were distressed. Adults followed where
children led, going in turn through the purficiation
exercises.

The hazards of which the prophets are warned by
their followers may be proved to exist even if it take
tragedy to secure the point. The bishop of a new
religious movement in Johannesburg in 1943 once chased
Satan into the baptismal pool, leaving his followers to
recount the story subsequently of how he fought
valiantly with the enemy who blocked his exit with an
immovable rock (Sundkler 1964:205-206). His death
confirmed the view that the illness exists on the
margins of existence, and is pursued there at great
peril. The pool as the place of combat is also the
source of healing: that which takes life may also
preserve it. In that limited combat marginality is a
condition of the healer, though in this case it proved
a fatal condition. (I am impressed in these stories by
the notion of the category of divine affliction which
ascribes to treachery or tragedy the not unrecognizable
face of a frowning providence. The sun in some glor-
ious crisis of the dominance of noon or the distress of
nightfall receives the appropriate tribute of sacrifice. The skies in some dark passage of time heave and
convulse with thunder and the forked lightning and thus
elicit a divine compliment. The somebre march of waves
or the reflective stillness of the waters deserve the
obeisance of Neptune. All this proves that humans also
stand under the 'left hand of God' and taste of His
inscrutable doublesidedness. The drowning of a Zionist
prophet is not the solution to the mystery of evil, but
the sign that its reality is undeniable. It deserves
recognition in any sober reckoning, and no setting is
more appropriate than that of a developed ritual
setting.)

Surrounded by a panoply of hostile and evil forces
which threaten isolation, the prophet and prophetesses
of the new religious movements adorn themselves with a
colorful assortment of ritual garments and symbols of
authority in order to blunt the sharpness of the contact with these forces. Sacred pools must similarly be
cautiously approached, with the final contact preceded
by a series of ritual acts to deflect enemy assault.
Prayers of exorcism may shackle the enemy; the ritual
act of circumambulating the pool may pin down the

monsters of the deep; the symbolic staffs may cast a
shadow over the waters and bind Satan.   All this
entails huge demands on existing resources.   Then the
larger society has to be faced, for it represents the
forces of alienation, with the agents of modernization
enthroned in their unapproachable isolation.4 Faced
with these problems an imaginative religious leader
might contrive an enterprising permutation, capitalize
on the situation and adopt a technological device to
mobilize the vintage craft of tradition.   One leader,
Ma Nku, already described, decided to do precisely
that. At the annual meeting of the Church huge quantities of water were dispensed in buckets and bottles for
the pilgrims to take home for future use.   The rising
demand for the element had to be met, and so Ma Nku
installed an electric water pump on the Church premises
(Sundkler 1976:81). When modernity fills the vessels
of need in this uncharacteristic fashion, then it is
possible to turn its power into building community.   In
its characteristic impact modernity is pretty unfeeling
and isolating.
     The interest in the ritual and healing power of
water is raised by some leaders into a major theological subject, as was the case with Pastor J. Ade Aina of
the Church of the Lord (Aladura) in Yorubaland.   He
wrote   a   short   theological   exposition   of   the
significance of water in the 1930's at the height of
the 'Aladura' revival (Harold W. Turner 1979:225-230).
It is not necessary to repeat such theological material
in order to appreciate that an ancient theme has been
released in the propitious setting of the vernacular
Bible. A return to ethnic consolation is not only now
possible but, with Abraham, Moses, Aaron, David and
Daniel goading the ancestors of the rece to attempt
greater things in accents of native dignity, it becomes
unavoidable. This is the aspect I will next attempt to
sketch out.
     The new religious movements have often sought
legitimacy by an authoritative appeal to tradition,
with the important adoption of rules of sartorial
propriety, social etiquette and stands of ethical conduct. Joseph Babalola, for example, is summoned by
ringing tones to affirm the efficacy of tradition in
omo iye. The widow of Efon meets the threat of a dis-
integrative modernity by turning her back on it. Such
fidelity to tradition might create the impression that
no serious change is involved in some of the new
religious movements. But that only assumes a 'stair-
case' view of human progress and social development.
Change might also mean a subterranean alignment from
external impact, occuring as a delayed effect.

Paul Nzuza (1896-1959), leader of a Zionist
church, received his call in May 1916 while he was
visiting the grave of King Shaka, the great Zulu
nationlist hero (Ritter 1955, rep. 1972). The offical
constitution of the church described how Paul Nzuza was
enveloped by the Holy Spirit and chosen along with his
followers to be the 'elected family of Jehova god according to the texture of their skin and hair" (Sundkle
1976:97-98). Another was Timothy Cekwane (1873-1949).
After Halley's comet appeared he and his followers
assembled on the top of a mountain to await the spirit.
Here is a description of what happened:

> They felt the Spirit coming over them like a mighty
> wind. They ran over the mountain; they screamed;
> they sensed an irresistible urge to take off charms
> and amulets from their wrists, and their
> medicines...; they had to confess their sins before
> God and men, in an outpouring of the soul in which
> nothing was to be left hidden. The branches of the
> bushes from the Mountain they gathered and beat
> themselves and one another, driving out the demons.

In that spirit-filled night on the Mountain, Timothy
was gripped by an ecstasy that overpowered him.
Gesticulating and gyrating as if intoxicated by the
Spirit, he prayed and screamed in an unknown tongue.
He opened his hands...he saw blood trickling from the
palms of his hands...Water was brought to him; as he
prayed...it turned into blood. This sacred fluid was
powerful, filled with healing qualities for the sick
[Sundkler 1976:109-110].

The significance of blood was quickly grasped by
Cekwane. Others might see in it a duplicate of the
stigmata and the reference to Christ. He, on the other
hand, derived a much more specific meaning from it.
This was clear when he designated his son as successor
in the symbolic words: "He is my blood. He is I"
(Sundkler 1976:111). A natural interpretation that
reinforce communion with Shaka's spirit as the
primordial kin. It was in that exalted company that
Paul Nzuza arrived at his vision of Zion. Timothy
Cekwane turned for his part to the importance of
investing his kin relatives to carry forward the work
be commenced.
      In one poem the two themes of posterity and the
ancestors are fused and saturated with notes of a harsh
existence. The author is Isaiah Shembe of the
Nazarites.

      You lass of Nazaretha,
      cry like a flowing stream

because of the shame which is yours
in your own country.

You lad of Nazaretha,
cry like a rapid stream
because of the shame which has come over you,
you lad of Shaka [Sundkler 1976:203].

One of the most significant and complex of new
religious movements was that founded by Simon Kimbangu
(1889-1951) in Lower Zaire in 1921 (Martin 1975). The
Kimbanguist Church claims about four million adherents
and was admitted as a member of the World Council of
Churches in 1969/70. As we saw with Elliot Butelezi,
many of the new prophets are inclined to distinguish
themselves sharply from their immediate traditional
religious context. Garrick Braide (1882-1918) of the
Niger Delta was one such (Tasie 1978:166-201; Harold W.
Turner 1979:133-145). Another was Prophet William Wade
Harris, a Liberian who worked along the coast from
western Ghana (Apollonia) to Liberia between 1914 and
1916.[5] All these great religious figures depended
for their effectiveness on the strength of the African
religious tradition, whatever their protestations to
the contrary. Kimbangu was no exception, whatever
major permutations he introduced into Congolese society. He consciously held up the light of the ancestors
to illuminate for his followers the path of renewal.
One contemporary witness observes: "Neither Kimbangu
nor his apostles have ever appealed for ancestor worship to be abandoned; their tombs were kept clean,
paths leading to them were laid out and their return to
life was going to initiate the Golden Age" (Lisembe
1979:153). The culture of ritual veneration of communion with the spirits of the dead and of sacrifice,
which has existed in virutally all African societies
producing new religious movements, explains a great
deal of the attitude of the new religious leaders. One
poem describes this with compelling power:

The dead have never left us. They are among us.
The dead are everywhere:
    They are in the shadow as it clears.
    The dead are not below the ground:
    They are in the rustling tree.
    They are in the moaning forest.
    They are in the running water.
    They are in the still water.
    They are in the huts, they are in the crowds.

    The dead are not dead:
    They are in the woman's breast.

They are in the wailing child
And in the log as it bursts into flames.

The dead are not below the ground:
   They are in the dying fire.
   They are in the dripping shrubs.
   They are in the whining rocks.
   They are in the forest, they are in the home.
   The dead are everywhere [Lisembe 1979:150].

Those verses bring together several major concerns: the notion of the self and its integration with
larger social units, the unbroken bond of kinship
between child, mother and father as well as between the
dead and the living; the link between social well being
and the state of the natural environment; the strong
sense of ecological balance between the just demands of
living through consuming the fruits of nature ('the log
as it bursts into flames') and replenishing the stock
(nature is alive with the spirits of the dead: 'the
dead are everywhere'), and the wider concept of community as past, present and future. In this scheme the
whole is at stake in the parts and the parts encapus-
late the life of the whole. Community solidarity and
individual fulfillment are thus complementary aspects
of the same theme, so that social and historical events
are the consequences of the mutal interplay of individual enterprise and community legitimacy. This
strenghtens the bonds of personal and social solidarity
and acts as a supportive network in illness and healing.
   The Kimbanguist Church has similarly preserved the
tradition of kin responsibility by officially observing
the birthdays of Kimbangu's three sons. As one
present-day leader puts it: "The sons of the prophet
are for us the vanguard of Christ. They are concerned
with our spiritual and material problems. In them, the
prophet still ives for us..." (Ndofunsu 1978:580). It
would seem here and elsewhere that the route along
which the new message is transmitted, i.e., Kimbangu
and his successor-sons, has become inseparable from the
ultimate destination. Here also the modern permutation
of conversion takes place within the revived setting of
the older heritage. In the successful combination of
this heritage and religious conversion new ideas and
styles of living emerge which carry foward individual
and communal well being. The role of the natural
environment and the healing process should not be lost
sight of, for an integrated environment is a prerequisite of healing.
   One example must suffice to show the important
place that nature occupies in African traditional religions. The great missionary explorer, Dr. David Living-

stone, unbowed by the strange unfamiliarity of the dark
continent, decided to engage a Tswana speaker in a
theological duel. He asked the local man what he
understood by the word for 'holiness', biotsepho. Then
came this refreshing answer:

When copious showers have descended during the
night, and all the earth and leaves and cattle are
washed and clean, and the sun rising shows a drop
of dew on every blade of grass, and the air
breathes fresh, that is holiness [Livingstone
1865:64].

Such an aesthetic appreciation of holiness, a logical
extension of traditional reverence for nature, should
be relevant for projects of modernization in Africa. A
pleasant and life-imparting environment is indispensable to the quality of life, and, in its traditional
understanding, it transcended artifical barriers of
class and rank. Stewardship of nature is a concomitant
of a sense of fidelity to kin.

The final theme must be the urban-rural dichotomy.
Here the missionary part of the story is of critical
importance, for by paying close attention to the
sources and modes of African religious values, missionaries were within the range of affecting the foundation
of African perception. Since traditional religions
constituted the most developed intellectual resources,
their modification would have reverberations throughout
the culture. It is a vast subject, but we may content
ourselves with two brief examples.

Dr. Livingstone's challenge to his Tswana compan-
ion had assumed that theological reflection would be
unknown or rudimentary among Africans, which would
justify him in his wish to bring Africans to a sense of
realism about the right division between myth and
science. In other words to clear the way by which
secularism might enter indigenous consciousness. His
assumption did not remain unstated forlong. He encountered a traditional rainmaker whose profession he
tried to expose to the corrective light of reason. He
accused the rainmaker of charlatanry, saying the diviner waited for rain clouds before using his medicine so
as to claim the credit for having brought rain. The
rainmaker rose to his challenge, saying:

We are both doctors and not deceivers. You give a
patient medicine. Sometimes God is pleased to
heal him by means of your medicine. Sometimes
not--he dies. When he is cured, you take the
credit for what God does. I do the same.
Sometimes God grants us rain, sometimes not. When
he does, we take the credit of the charm. When a

126   AFRICAN HEALING STRATEGIES

patient dies you don't give up trust in your
medicine. Neither do I when no rain falls
[Livingstone cited in Lienhardt 1966:142].

Logical exposition is obviously a slippery instrument
which the adversary might skillfully seize against us.
The rainmaker's claim of a professional solidarity with
his missionary visitior (a similar solidarity is claimed by another enterprising local man with an early
seventeeth century traveler, Jobson 1623) closes the
distance implied in Dr. Livingstone's whole approach
and creates a logical scenario which the missionary is
challenged to repudiate at the cost of his faith in a
Supreme Being. Few would willingly grasp that nettle.
     Our second example concerns a missionary who
decided to take the law into his own hands. The missionary in question was resident in the village of
Hastings near Freetown, Sierra Leone. Hastings was
highly regarded in missionary circles as a showcase of
Christian piety and locally was given the epithet, 'the
Bethlehem of West Africa' (Fyfe 1962:526). Consequently when the Engungun masquerade secret society began
asserting its authority over the place in a public
procession, the missionary went out to meet it head on.
The story of that dramatic encounter is relished--and
probably embellished--in the local accounts. The
missionary fell on the masked figure and began physi-
cally to attack it. Obviously he had to accept that he
was fighting a real not a mythological enemy. But

     he only flogged a mass of empty Egugu clothes.
     The bodies inside the clothes had mysteriously...
     vanished. The missionary marched back to the
     Parsonage; his whip had dropped, but a broom
     belonging to one of the...Egugu escorts followed
     him to the Parsonage, gyrating, in fact executing
     a little dance of its own behind the worthy
     Cleric's back [Peterson 1969:266].

     Standard interpretations of this story settle
squarely on missionary intolerance or, equally misleading, on the penchant of Africans for Pagan rites. The
real signficance of such stories, however, can only be
uncovered by submitting them to indigenous rules of
understanding.
     It is clear that in the story the missionary was
being challenged to do spiritual combat on a ground not
of his choosing. However we define his role, whether
as the disguised front of Western secularism or the
lofty representative of a Scriptural religion, the
missionary was compelled to acquit himself in the language and style recognized by the local people. He
produced the Bible, much as a cult object, and flour-

ished it in the face of the pursuing broom which consequently fled from the scene, leaving the missionary unharmed. Convinced that he had demonstrated the superiority of Christianity, the missionary had missed the clear implication that Christianity could engage indigenous traditions only by itself being transformed into familiar epistemological categories. The Bible as a symbol of spirit power was drawn alongside the gyrating broom infused with similar power. At his place of residence, the missionary was within the proper limits of the spirit power of the Bible, with the retreating broom conceding the point. Thus <u>Engungun</u> and Christianity, at least in local perception, were debating and competing within a common epiostemological discourse, rather than about whether such a discourse existed at all. The real conquest was on ground prepared by <u>Engungun</u>. As Christianity moved into the territory it was embodied in the Parsonage which rested on the double margins of physical isolation and symbolic alienation. Dr. Livingstone got off comparatively lightly considering where he started.

The phenomenon of the <u>Engungun</u> broom may be related to the claim of Zionist worshipper, Aaron Mjwara, who once declared in a worship context: "Elijah was given a broom on the mountains. My calling is to be the besom of God. The House of Africa has been perfected through the Broom. It is perfected" (Sundkler 1976:115). In the accomplished hands of domestic servants and field laborers, both prey to the forces inherent in the isolation of urban-rural dislocation, the broom stands for the affliction of a new class of people. For them, too, it may be transformed into a healing symbol.

The rural factor is an important structural issue in the rise and development of new religious movements. The rural exodus into towns creates a class of disenchanted Africans who may constitute a captive audience for the movements. The movements themselves become a line of defence against ultimate wretchedness. Inadequate or inappropriate education, the economics of low wages and seasonal labor, the elitist basis of modern medicine, the slide into the synthetic culture of drugs, alcoholism, prostitution, and gambling that afflict the urban poor, all this creates fertile ground for religious initiative. When rural migrants find themselves adrift in decaying inner-cities, their only form of relief might come from such religious initiative being taken for them and by them. Religion is often quite simply the last foothold before the precipice of final hopelessness.

Urban life, even for those who succeed in finding jobs, may engender wrong attitudes. Two may be identified. First, an antagonistic attitude may develop

towards village life and values. Second, the money
economy which fuels town life rewards individual
performance and so places no value on community goals.
Such an atomized view of life throws the individual on
his own resources, thus leaving him with no meaningful
context. Because economic rewards can never offset the
loss of many other advantages associated with the older
life-style, the rural migrant compensates for this
often in negative terms.

The new religious movements are acutely aware of
the nature of the challenge they face with regard to
the impoverishment of rural areas. The parasitic
dependence of town dwellers on the rural populations
for food and raw materials has resulted in fact in the
candle being consumed at both ends. Rural wealth is
sucked away into the towns where rural labor is attracted and exploited without any corresponding compen-
sation. The loss to the rural sector is obvious. But
the towns themselvse are not immune. Without a replen-
ished source of food supply, raw materials and a
productive workforce, growth and development are stunt-
ed. The loss to the urban sector is equally clear.

It is partly for this reason that some new religious movements have proceeded to place great value on
the rural roots of the people. Many of the early pre-
cursors in fact began by retracing their rural roots.
For example, in 1900 one Shadrach Mogun arose from
Ekiti country in Yorubaland. He had been baptized by
the Church Missionary Society agent, Rev. Hinderer. A
contemporary report described him thus: "He lives
alone with Jesus Christ—to use his own expression...He
preaches to the farmers, and now and again visits the
town to preach. He looks like an Old Testament prophet, and is a veritable John the Baptist preparing the
way for Christ's second advent" (John Peel 1968:58).

A second example is Egunjobi, a hunter also from
Ekiti country. He came to Ibadan after 1900 and was
baptized at the local Baptist church in 1907. About
1912 while he was hunting north of Ibadan he said he
had a vision of an angel shining in the dark. The
charms which were hung about him (for he is described
as being 'powerful in juju') began to jangle terribly,
and fell off. The angel told him of God's anger and
prophesied coming war and epidemic. Egunjobi turned
his gun upside down and water poured out, a sign of
rebuke, he belived, at his obstinacy. The angel made
him preach and then disappeared, leaving a footmark in
the rock. After a year of hestitation, Egunjobi was
troubled in his sleep by dreams until he was eventually
driven to start preaching. His message was apocalyptic
and emphasized the power of prayer. He practised healing by mixing herbs with water and adding a Psalm to be
recited, saying it was the power of Jesus that healed.

He went to Lagos in 1918 to preach and thereafter disappeared from public notice. He probably died in the
1920's (Peel 1968:58-59).

A third example of a charismatic figure to appear
in this style is Moses Orimolade. He was born in the
1870's at Ikare, also in Yoruba country, where Christianity was introduced in the late 1890's. Orimolade
was an early convert. He fell seriously ill for seven
years, but after a vision and taking the waters of a
nearby stream he made a partial recovery though he
remained lame for the rest of his life. He became a
wandering preacher in spite of that handicap. In 1916
he arrived at the C.M.S. church in Owo, and later
travelled as far as Kano and Jos. At the Yoruba Muslim
town of Ilorin further south he built a prayer-house
and was known locally as Alhaaji-n-yisa (Yisa being the
local name of Jesus). Later a leading Lagos Muslim
trader took him in because he was "a holy man." "The
power of prayer was his constant theme" (Peel 1968:59-
60).

In the origins of the extremely successful new
religious movement, the Church of the Lord (Aladura),
the rural factor is again to the fore. The founder,
Josiah Olunowo Oshitelu (d. 1966), had his base in the
small village of Ogere where he began his public
religious career in June, 1929. Ogere was to emerge
into international prominence as the headquarters of
the movement which began to spread to other parts of
West Africa, Britain and the United States. It was
made accessible to a far larger audience by a twovolume
study published by the Oxford University Press (Harold
W. Turner 1967). In Oshitelu's case he explicitly
combined a role in the world of traditional culture
with a strong sense of vocation in the new. In 1941 he
had conferred on him the title, Doctor of the Psychi-
cal, by the National Union of Spiritualists of Nigeria.
Traditional healers had obviously discovered a kindred
soul. Such recognition need not be that explicit to be
acknowledged as an influence with other religious
leaders.

A major conceptual innovation still waits to be
made in the area of the rural factor in historical and
cultural change. In the most significant examples of
movements of reform and renewal in Africa and elsewhere
we are dealing with the critical impact of rural ideas
of society on urban styles of living. Alongside the
comparative boundary of the convergence of Western
influence and traditional cultures an important related
corridor has opened up in the urban-rural nexus. It
would be necessary to shake down the category of the
'millenium' in order to grasp the ideological seriousness implicit in rural critique of town life. It is a
phenomenon that can be traced back into the mists of

antiquity. Its dramatic manifestation in the new religious movements of today provides a unique opportunity
for learning about motives for change and renewal and
their sources in rural life. The great Ibn Khaldun
(1332-1406), writing in the fourteenth century, confi-
dently called attention to this question. He wrote:

> Thus, the group feeling (asabiyah) that goes with
> (common descent) likewise is (stronger). It draws
> those who have it to desert life and the avoidance
> of cities, which do away with bravery and make
> people dependent upon others. This should be
> understood and the proper conclusion be drawn form
> it [Ibn Khaldun, tran. and ed. Rosenthal
> 1967(2):267].

Yet new religious movements may also represent
significant changes in society. Polygamy is one
example. Yet both George Khambule and Simon Kimbangu
developed a stern anti-polygamy code, and in Khambule's
case he went to the uncharacteristic extreme of espousing celibacy (Sundkler 1976:127). Most of the movements in fact rivet on their followers the heavy chains
of discipline and self-denial, requiring sometimes
superhuman feats of personal endurance as a prerequisite for full membership. In this connection the work
ethic may be rescued from its inferior associations and
promoted as a necessary principle of salvation. In the
church founded by Isaiah Shembe, for example, the
morning liturgy "contains the most uncompromising,
unrelenting and persevering exhortation to work, and
against laziness" (Sundkler 1976:197). The muscular
religion was addressed to an agricultural community
following the Natives Land Act of 1913. The address
called on the worshippers not to be lazy,

> for laziness is a sin. A lazy person is like a
> dog begging for food from people. At the
> conclusion of this Prayer take your hoe and dig
> with it. Thus you shall live and not need to go
> and beg for food from people...If the sun is
> shining-- dig...If it is raining--dig and weed and
> be on guard (against birds eating the crops)...
> All the lazy ones will be cast away. Their blood
> will be exacted out of their hands because with
> their laziness they pour shame on God. God gave
> them hands for work...they pour shame on God
> [Sundkler 1976:179].

It echoes the Wolof saying, 'Yalla, Yalla! Bei sa tol!'
('Instead of shouting, God, God! till your land')[6]
Neither the murmur of magic nor of the millenium
stirs in the otherwise clear tones of that stern admon-

ishment. Man shall not live by the Spirit at all if he
neglects the provisions of nature.

It is consistent with the nature of the indigenous
understanding that a 'practical theory' of life be
developed. With its introduction at this stage of our
exposition we may consider the paper completed. However a brief recapitulation of the significance of new
religious movements for the reform and modernization of
African societies should be attempted in conclusion.
The theoretical issue of professional specialization in
religion has practical consequences of modernization.
The existence of a specialized religious sphere has
pointed to a contrasting sphere for politics and world-
ly affairs. This encourages secularization, but it
also inhibits the notion of an omnicompetent state. It
brings into being a pluralist world where diversity of
life-style and vocation may exist simultaneously. It
is, of course, not new to Africa for historical chron-
icles concerned with medieval Africa to describe the
tradition as full-fledged in those times. But the
reassertion of this tradition in an era that has
witnessed the growth of statism in Africa should have
new significance. The widow of Efron, even in her
enfeebled corner, is right to protest at the disinte-
grative intrusiveness of modernity, for much harm comes
from its introduction to Africa. The eminent Bishop
Samuel Ajayi Crowther (1807-1891) expressed this senti-
ment in one of its earliest forms, and he should have
the final word. He reminded people that Christianity
had not come to destroy national assimilation and,
having in mind the colonial government of the time, he
went on: "while we render unto all their dues, we may
regard it our bounden duty to stand firm in rendering
to God the things that are God's" (Ajayi 1965 and
1969:224). Crowther, the agent of new forces entering
the continent, given his great accomplishments in the
field, would understand the 'things of God' to include
indigenous resources as factors of continuity in an era
of rapid change.

NOTES

[1]Humphrey Fisher called attention to the
Muslim dimension in response to Horton's article.
Fisher: "Conversion Reconsidered: Some Historical
Aspects of Religious Conversion in Black Africa,"
Africa 43(1):27-40. Horton replied at some length and
in strident fashion in: "On the Rationality of Conver-
sion, " Part I, Africa 45(3):219-235; Part II,
45(4):373-399.

[2]Monica Wilson , Communal Rituals of the
Nyakusa (Oxford, 1959), pp. 134-139, and E.E. Evans-
Pritchard, Neur Religion (Oxford, 1956), rep. 1974),
pp. 22-27. See also Lamin Sanneh, The Jakhanke: The

History of an Islamic Clerical People of Senegambia
(London, 1979), pp. 185-213 for examples from the
Muslim tradition.
    [3]The concept of the 'stirring of the water's
(see John 5) was widely used in theological circles in
the 1960's to refer to the confidence with which modern
man was proceeding to bring down the Ptolemaic scaf-
folding with the help of the Copernican revolution, a
step that would, it was believed, sweep away the rem-
nants of traditional authority. I use the phrase here
to indicate a kind of unsettling which comes about from
the impact of modernity on traditional societies without implying that change has to involve a radical
rupture. In his influential book, From the Stone Age
to Christianity: Monotheism and the Historical Process
(New York: Doubleday, 1957, first published 1940),
William F. Albright expounds the thesis of epochal
shifts as characteristic of the general history of
culture. He says: "When one culture yields to another
there is nearly always (probably always under simple
conditions) an abrupt change, a true mutation of
culture, in which a generation may suffice for changes
which might otherwise take a millenium to effect...a
culture may last for centuries with only the slightest
modification, after which there is a sudden
interruption in its continuity, accompanied by changes
so rapid that it is often hard...to distinguish the
successive steps" (123-124). It is debatable whether
as a general theory historical change obliterates so
sucessfully all traces of earlier epochs.
    [4]One Zulu public leader declared in 1958: "As
from 1913 we knew one thing--there is no God with the
White man" (Sundkler 1976:311).
    [5]G.M. Haliburton, The Prophet Harris (London,
1971); John D. Hargreaves, France and West Africa: An
Anthology of Historical documents (London, 1969),
pp.247-252. A three-volume study of Harris was
completed recently, though still unpublished: David A.
Shank, "A Prophet of Modern Times: The thought of
Willliam Wade Harris" (Aberdeen, 1980).
    [6]Reference is intended to the well known book,
Magic and the Millenium by Bryan R. Wilson. The sub-
title of this book reveals the author's methodology: A
Sociological Study of Religious Movements of Protest
among Tribal and Third-World Peoples. Published in the
United States by Harper and Row, New York, 1973.

REFERENCES CITED

Ajayi, J.F.A. Christian Mission in Nigeria: 1841-1891:
     The Making of a New and 1969 Elite. London and
     Evanston. 1965.
Brown, Godfrey N. and Mervyn Hiskett, eds. Conflict
     and Harmony in Education Tropical Africa. London:
     1975.
Charsley, S.R. Dreams in an Independent African Church.
     Africa 43(3):244-257. 1973.
Fyfe, Christopher. A History of Sierra Leone. London.
     1962.
Gray, Richard. Review of C.G. Oosthuizen's Post-
     Christianity in African. Bulletin of the School of
     Oriental and African Studies, 43, Part 2. 1980.
Horton, Robin. African Conversion. Africa
     41(2):85-108. 1971.
Ibn Khaldun. al Muquaddimah. Translated and edited by
     Franz Rosenthal. Princeton: 1967.
Ifeka-Moller, Caroline. White Power: Social
     Structural Factors in Conversion to Christianity,
     Eastern Nigeria: 1921-1966. Canadian Journal of
     African Studies 8(1):55-72. 1974.
Jobson, Richard. The Golden Trade of a Discovery of
     the River Gambia, 1620-21. London: 1623.
Jules-Rosette, Bennetta. African Apostles: Ritual and
     Conversion. The Church of John Marankjea. Ithaca.
     1975.
Lienhardt, Godfrey. Social Anthropology. Oxford:
     Oxford University Press. 1966.
Lisembe, Phillippe Elebe. The Role of Kimbanguism in
     the Development of the Self-awareness of the Zaire
     Nation. Christian and Islamic Contributions Toward
     Establishing Indenpendent States in Africa South
     of the Sahara (Africa Colloquium Bon-Bad
     Godesberg). Stuttgart: Institute for Foreign
     Cultural Relations of the Federal Republic of
     Germany. 1979.
Livingstone, David. Expedition to the Zambezi.
     London: John Murray. 1865.
Martin, Marie-Louise. Kimbangu: An African Prophet
     and His Church. Oxford: Blackwell. 1975.
Ndofunsu, Diakanua. The Role of Prayer in the
     Kimbanguist Church. In Christianity in Indepen-
     dent Africa. E. Fashole-Luke, Richard Gray et
     al., eds. London and Bloomington: 1978.
O'Fahey, R.S. State and Society in Dar Fur. London:
     1980.
Oosthuizen, C.G. Post-Christianity in Africa. London:
     1968.
Peel, John D.Y. Aladura: A Religious Movement Among
     the Yoruba. London: 1968.

Peterson, John. The Province of Freedom. Evanston and
     London: 1969.
Ritter, E.A. Shaka Zulu. London. (Reprint 1972).
     1955.
Schoffeleers, Matthew. The History and Political Role
     of the M'bona Cult among the Mang'anja. Terence
     O. Ranger and I.N. Kimambo, (eds.) The Historical
     Study of African Religion. Berkeley: University
     of California Press, 1972.
Sundkler, Bengt. Bantu Prophets in South Africa.
     London: 1964.
Tasie, Godwin. Christian Missionary Enterprise in the
     Niger Delta: 1864-1918. Leiden. 1978.
Turner, Harold H. History of an Independent African
     Church: Church of the Lord (Aladura). Oxford.
     1967.
_____. Religious Innovation in Africa. Boston.
     1979.

CHAPTER 9

HEALTH CARE SYSTEMS IN NORTHWEST ZAMBIA

Anita Spring

In the religious and medical spheres in many societies, the acquistion of specialized knowledge may be
predicated upon long apprenticeships and shared experiences. The construction of the total or "big picture"
concerning of the cosmological, religious, and medical
belief systems as it is knowable to the individual
comes with increasing age and maturity. This knowledge
may be differential in terms of the individual's sex,
access to information, interest, and life experience.
In some kinship based societies, to become a religious
leader or curer requires personnel experience. One
must have been a participant in a ritual to train as a
ritual expert; one must have been ill and recovered to
be a candidate to learn curing. Those desiring to
attain the status of curer, midwife, or diviner must
serve an appenticeship to the expert and build up the
knowledge and experience. By contrast, the biomedical
tradition involves a coordinated curriculum for study,
but its practice is not predicated on personally experiencing its cures. By comparison to kinship based
societies, few people become trained as biomedical
experts, although many experience its practice. This
paper focuses on women's access and knowledge of a
system as it is practiced indigenously in an area in
Zambia and as it incorporates the biomedical tradition.
Major topics include the apprenticeship system, the
transmission of the healing repertoire, and the method
of incorporating aspects of the biomedical system into
indigenous healing strategies.

Janzen has written about the ngoma mode (ngoma
means drum) providing a therapy strategy that is
critical to healing in Central and Southern Africa.
The ngoma mode is associated with the "therapeutic
features of song, dance, rhythm, divining, counselling,
sacrifices, feasts, social exchanges, and the construction and maintenance of permanent support gourps"
(Janzen, 1982:1). It is argued here that the ngoma

mode also functions as a mneumonic device, locking into
place certain sequences of events, putting certain
aspects of curing in the public domain which in turn
help to structure private therapies that might otherwise be unregulated.   In the pluralistic medical
situation, people use "all available traditions and
resources" (Janzen 1983:2).   Janzen asks what variable
account for the selection of the ngoma therapy when
other modes are available, and what variables account
for the

> "organizational relations of divination and
> therapeutic support communities...in the face
> of a series of other therapeutic modes
> including biomedicine, psychotherapy,
> herbalism, and a variety of other medical
> traditions' (Janzen 1983:4).

It is argued here that when therapies other than the
ngoma mode are employed, the absence of structure
provided by the ngoma sets the stage for unregulated
combinations or therapies in which combinations of
therapies, and alternative usage of treatments and
practitioners occur.

THE STUDY AREA

     The research for this paper was carried out from
1970 to 1972 and in 1977 in Northwest Zambia (Spring
1976a, 1976b, 1978a, 1978b, 1980a, 1980b).   (Although
the Luval people are the primary focus, the traditions
of the surrounding Lunda, Chokwe, and Luchazi are similar.)   The biomedical tradition brought by non-Africans
also is important in the area.   The Luvale are a matrilineal group who have descended from the chieftancy of
Mwanta Yavwa in Zaire and who have resided in this part
of Zambia since the last century (Hansen and Papstein
1979).   Influxes of Luvale people from Angola and Zaire
have been occuring regularly throughout this century.
The Luvale people share similar life styles with other
peoples in the area being shifting hoe agriculturalists
who cultivate cassava or millet depending on the ter-
rain, fish in the rivers and streams, and trade in
surplus foodstuffs, fish, and locally and imported
manufactured items.   In the current scene, people are
linked with Zambian towns and cities through a network
of relatives, through their job and travel experiences,
and through radio broadcasts in ChiLuvale, one of eight
national languages.   The Luvale and other northwest
peoples are known in Zambia and environs for their
medicines and ensorcelling capabilities.   Renewal of
indigenous techniques has been facilitated by the
influx of Angolan refugees during the 1970s.   These

people had little or no access to biomedicine in Angola and therefore were not pluralistic in their health system. Their presence in Zambian border villages stimulated a resurgence of ngoma therapies as well as other indigenous rituals (Spring 1978b, 1982).

THE APPRENTICESHIP SYSTEM

The apprenticeship system is best viewed as forming a regular program that may have disparate or noncontiguous steps, but which ultimately forms a coherent pattern. The Luvale ritual and curative system for men and women produces pupils and teachers, midwives and doctors. The various apprenticeships and the knowledge imparted enables individuals to understand the system and indoctrinate others. It also serves as a bonding mechanism creating mutual aid networks that cross-cut kinship ties. In addition, participation in the healing system strengthens ties between matrilineally related women. By contrast, carriers of the biomedical tradition tend to come from outside the area, although a few local people have been sent for training and some local women have received some instruction in midwifery.
I shall discuss two types of indigenous ritual learners and leaders--the non-specialist leader which all women may fulfill and the specialist leader which few women attain. It should be noted that women participate in a strong "single sex tradition" (in which the transfer of knowledge and the performance of certain rituals and treatments usually is carried out by women for women or by men for men). A corresponding system exists for men and is, in fact, more widely described (Just 1972; Turner 1967, 1968; White 1961).

Non-specialist roles

The girl's puberty ritual functions in the widest sense to integrate each female into the community of women, to provide the initial learning experience of self-medication, and to formally induct a woman into her matrilineage. Most public rituals require the participation of women to participate in singing and dancing in the ngoma mode. All life crises whether physiological or social serve as ritual modes where the subject, ritual expert, and community of women come together. Girls are initiated alone at menarche, while Luvale boys are initiated in groups. Most writers have remarked upon comradeship and solidarity that the boy's rituals promote and the solitariness of girls (Just 1972; Richards 1956; Turner 1967; White 1953a 1953b, 1961). From an outsider and male point of view, the young woman seems alone. In fact, there are young

girls who are apprenticed to her, and she herself is
appenticed to an older woman. Solidarity is then with
younger and older women and not simply age mates.
During the girl's puberty ritual (mwali), the young
woman will be taught certain medicinal treatments for
sexual enhancement, menstrual problems, and "female"
illnesses. She learns that other women and her teacher
(chilombola) in particular are entrusted with her
health care and fertility by their participation in
this ritual and in any future rituals and health care
that she may need. She learns that certain illnesses
may be self-medicated, others require the assistance of
more knowledgeable (and usually older women), and still
others are under control of specialists (men and woman
who are experts on various treatments).

The teacher herself gains expertise in carrying
out a ngoma ritual and in providing the herbal medications. Each chilombola may have one or more vamwale,
or puberty girls. The teacher's understanding of the
sequence of events and the medications involved may or
may not be perfect. The ritual's telic or purposive
structure (Turner 1967) is guided by other women
especially in the public phases. Public phases, usually those events where ngoma is present, help to remind
all concerned that certain private aspects (such as
labial elongation and medicines for menstrual problems)
must be carried out (Spring 1976b).

Many women in the society fill the role of chilombola, and some do so repeatedly. In addition to the
traditional girl's puberty ritual (that is multiphasic
and may last as long as one year) there are a variety
of alternative rituals that may be used depending on
the financial situation of the family, and whether or
not the girl is schooling and/or the family is Christian (Spring 1976a). Also, a woman will have a chilombola at other time in her lifetime such as at marriage.

Specialist Roles

The most well-known specialist types among women
are the midwife (chifunguji), herbal doctor (singular
is nganga, plural is wanganga), and spirit possession
doctor (nganga wamahamba). Men fill roles as diviner
(ngombo), herbal doctor and spirit possession doctor.
It is possible for men and women to combine all three
specialties in the healer-medium role. Among women,
usually both midwives and possession doctors know
herbal remedies. One needs to have been a patient to
become one of the doctors. Christians who comprise
about 20% of the population are forbidden by their
Protestant church to be possession doctors and diviners, but Christian women may be midwives, and Christians of both sexese may be herbalists.

Relatively few women are midwives; those who become midwives learn from female relatives (mother, grandmother, mother's sister or sister).or from a friend who has the necessary skills. A woman who desires to learn midwifery has observed many births, usually in the company of her relative of friend, and may act as a helper to the expert in terms of the collection and preparation of medicines of the administration of certain techniques. Unlike the apprenticeship route for doctors and diviners, and similar to most biomedical specialists, to become a midwife one does not need to go through the sequence of illness, recovery and apprenticeship. Midwives need not have been parturients. In fact, some of the most famous midwives are' themselves barren (Spring 1976a). Informants stress the lengthy apprenticeship as well as the skill required. A midwife makes her reputation by successful deliveries, especially those with no maternal mortalities. People's greatest fear and concern is the successful removal of the placenta, and midwives who "know the medicine" for removing the placenta enjoy the best reputations. Midwives have techniques for turning the baby and doing episiotomies. The midwife's job requires long time periods expended on each case commencing with the onset of labor and continuing for a week post-partum. Most midwives are without young children and are between the ages of 40 and 60 years. A cultural rule is that women attending the birth must be older than the parturient (Spring 1976a, 1976b). Midwives are usually heralists and the non-Christian ones may be possession doctors specializing in women's and children's illnesses.

Spirit possession doctors are herbalists by definition because all ngoma performances have herbal medications as well. Spirit possession ritual (mahamba) have been described at length by Turner (1968, 1969) for the neighboring Ndembu where male doctors are concerned with hunting cults, female doctors are concerned with women's reproductive troubles, and both sexes treat general illness. The same pattern exists for the Luvale. The prerequisites for learning doctoring are to have been a patient and to have recovered. The method is to contact the doctor who treated and offer payment for teaching. Mutondo tambu, keshi monako ("tree paid for, not just seen") is the Luvale proverb expressing that an apprenticeship has been served and the expert has been compensated, It is easy to see medicines being prepared, but it is believed that one should learn proper usage from an expert for such treatments to be efficacious. A person should not attempt to prepare or offer treatments to others without being properly instructed and declared competent by an expert. Experts should not dispense knowledge

freely, and the final transferrance requires payment.
Access to spirit possession doctoring is a result of
being sick or having problems in child bearing and
child rearing. Ability to "take up the calling is
based on initial illness, diagnosis that names the
spirit cult involved, followed by the enactment of the
possession ritual, and confirmation of the cult and the
cure. Then the person participates as an adept in the
cult as manifested by attending and helping at the
ngoma therapies of others. She then must express the
desire to learn, pay the token fee of interest, formally apprentice herself to the doctor, and pay the final
fee. It may be said that illness outlines and channels
careers, for generally one may become an adept only in
those spirit cults and for those illnesses one has
personally experienced. (By the term "illness", I mean
the socially defined categories of sickness, that is,
how individuals perceive and interpret changes in
bodily states as contrasted with "diseases" that are
defined by biological criteria [Lewis 1976]).
     Herbalists know materia medica (herbals and other
medicines) used in curing a variety of illnesses,
either as part of possession or other rituals for minor
illnesses. Generally, a similar training procedure as
outlined for spirit possession is followed. The
patient is given medicines by the doctors and recovers.
She subsequently desires to learn the treatment(s) and
asks the expert. One differnece is that the doctor may
mention that she also knows treatments for other illnesses and may offer to teach her pupil these as well.
In the case of these other illnesses, the apprentice
does not go through the illness and recovery sequence.

MATRILINEAL CONTINUITY

     For general illness and herbal treatments, doctors
treat patients of either sex and apprentices may be of
either sex. Although the legend is that the first
diviner was a woman, currently all diviners are men.
(However, custom did not prevent the author of this
paper from being accepted as an apprentice for one and
a half years by two diviners.) A divination is required to diagnose the illness and specify the spirit that
is afflicting the patient. Only then can the relatives
(whom Janzen (1978) calls the therapy-management group)
engage a possession doctor and start the process of
enactment, recovery and apprenticeship. Diagnosis is
generally limited to those spirit cults in which the
patient's female ancestors were participants and had
ngoma performances. After death, a woman's mother,
mother's mother, and these women's sisters may be said
to afflict their descendents with illnesses concerned
with child bearing and rearing. Structuralists would

argue that the purpose of ancestral affliction is twofold: to remind the woman to honor and remember her own
martrilineage, necessary because she is living viriloc-
ally (with her husband's relatives), and to confer cult
membership, a way to participate in the mainstream of
the healing tradition (Turner 1968, 1969; Hoch-Smith
and Spring 1978).   I have argued elsewhere that the
disease   vectors   themselves   are   significant,   that
obstetrical and gynecological ailments are many, and
that women turn to the community of women for cause and
treatment (Spring 1976a, 1976b 1978).   Women who lack
matrilineal cult antecedents often are diagnosed as
requiring herbal treatments of spirit possession cults
that come from the "air", i.e., they do not require
ancestral participation.   Some of these   so-called air
spirits   (mahamba   wapeho)   are   animal   spirits   (e.g.,
Nguvu--hippo), others are believed to be a result of
contact with Europeans or modern society. (e.g., Tupelo
-- Angels and Ndeke -- Airplane).
     The   relationship   between   doctor   and   apprentice
(adept) may be close or distant.   Many women learn doctoring or midwifery from female relatives.   Often as a
doctor becomes old she requests that a young kinswoman
help her and learn her knowledge.   Since ancestral
intervention and affliction is believed to stay within
lineages,   this   action   makes   sense.   Matrilineally
related women, dead and alive, tend to be members and
doctors for the same cults concerned with reproduction.
The fees for the apprenticeship are much lower for
relatives, and the apprenticeship more easily carried
out since the junior has already helped her senior
relative.
     The healing system in the ngoma mode with its
divinations, medications, and possessions enable each
woman to be in the mainstream of the curing tradition
and to have a place in the matrilineage as curer,
patient, and ancestral afflictor.   Illness provides the
continuation of matrilineal cult paticipation.   Certain
matrilineages have a preponderance of ritual experts,
but there are other mechanisms to transfer expertise.
Women of different lineages who are in close residen-
tial proximity, who are affinally linked, and who
belong to the same Christian church may help each other
with cures and apprenticeships.   Because of the mechanism of women assisting during puberty or ngoma rituals,
women feel it is their obligation to help each other
during illness.   Even where social interactions may be
less than harmonious, women will rally to aid other
women and offer their healing knowledge -- double
protection where sickness is common and where it is
necessary to dispell the notion of wishing others evil.
Rather than seeing women in "special situation which
regularly give rise to conflict, tension, rivalry, or

jealousy between members of the same sex" (Wilson
1967:366), the apprenticeship system for women (as for
men) may be viewed as one of the bonding mechanisms
that enables women to form ritual groups and enter
arenas other than domestic ones.

Ngoma therapies do not occur randomly, nor do they
occur without a consideration of an individual's medical and reproductive history. Profiles of women's
fertility and ritual performances show that certain
medicines and rituals are performed at specific times
in the life cycle for particular categories of women.
The onset of menarche sets the stage for rituals ensuring fertility; the type of puberty ritual performed
influences the commencement of sexual life. Pregnancy
and parturition require a series of public and private
rituals and medications. Difficulties during this time
require special medicines, recourse to divination, and
appropriate ngoma or other therapies. Illnesses later
in life may be treated with ngoma performances for
nonreproductive cults or treated by herbals only. The
choice of therapy is affected by such extraneous
factors as wealth, marriage, and modernity. There is a
tendency to repeat the ngoma therapies performed for
other women within the matrilineage who were successful
in bearing and rearing children.

The ngoma and other therapies in a person's life
serve as indicators of illness and misfortune. The
performances are public statements about private
individual problems. Although informants may not
recall all their past illnesses, they do remember all
of their ritual performances and treatments. Ritual
performances including the ngoma mode are clues to
illness, curing therapies, and specific medicines that
a person has experienced. As Rappaport points out,
"the occurrence of the ritual may be a simple quantitative representation of complex qualitative information"
(1968:235). Rituals not only provide a record of the
medicinal treatments that a person receives in life,but
also directly affect the therapeutic style. The performance of a ritual in the ngoma mode or of a variant
that does not require ngoma provides a mechanism that
regulates and sanctions use of herbals and other treatments. Usually specific medicines accompany each
therapy, although substitutions are possible. However,
variations are inhibited by the proscribed and purposive structure of the curing sequence. The public
ngoma ritual sets in motion the private phases during
which certain treatments and medicines are utilized.
The public performance thus becomes a marker of private
events. Ngoma and other rituals "lock in" the medicinal treatments assuring their application and continuity. They also may limit the patient to one type of
treatment at a time.

COMBINING THE INDIGENOUS AND THE BIOMEDICAL SYSTEMS

I have written elsewhere (Spring 1980a, 1980b) that African consumers of health care, like consumers everywhere, pick and chose medicines and curative treatments that are available to them. In a pluralistic system, sometimes the choices are consistent with the "traditional" or the indigenous belief systems, other times they are not. For analytical purposes, I utilized a conceptual framework (Harrison and Ulin n.d.) that categorized the indigenous and the biomedical systems. The former was divided into 1) Taboos: Prescriptive and Preventative, 2) Ritual Manipulations, 3) Herbalism, and 4) Traditional Midwifery. The cosmopolitan or biomedical system was divided into analogous categories of 1) Preventive Medicine, 2) Surgery, 3) Pharmaceutical Services, and 4) Maternal and Child Health Services. The component of each system had its counterpart in the other.

"Herbalism finds its counterpart in pharmaceutical services, and traditional midwifery corresponds to the area of maternal and child health. The surgical aspects of cosmopolitan medicine find their correlates in manipulative rituals... Finally, traditional taboos with their aim of prescribing appropriate health behavior... and prohibiting actions which may threaten health...correspond to preventative health measure (Spring 1980b:58).

The paradigm is helpful in explaining usage in the pluralistic environment. People in Northwest Zambia attribute most illnesses to causative agents, but they recognize natural causes as well. The choice of treatment for an illness is influenced by the defintion of a sickness as being natural or unnatural, as being curable by Luvale medicines and rituals or by biomedical treatments, as well as the patient's and therapy management group's belief in each system. The model of choosing among alternative treatments stems from a variety of sources, the first being the indigenous system itself. Alternative treatment paths are always available, whether or not they are for the girl's puberty ritual or to medicate an earache or diarrhea (Spring 1976b). A variety of medicines, curing techniques and divination modes are available. Substitutions of standard treatments are a result of expediency, reduced circumstances, availability of materia medica, etc. Such things as the financial situation of the family or individual, as well as the amount of concern that the therapy management group has for a particular patient affect treatment styles.

144 AFRICAN HEALING STRATEGIES

People choose from the indigenous system, but also
may utilize the biomedical one. In Northwest Zambia,
the biomedical was introduced by Americans of the
Plymouth Brethren (Christian Missions in Many Lands) in
the 1920s. Currently the Brethren run several hospitals that specialize in maternity services. In addition, the Zambian government introduced a clinic and
medical personnel in the area starting in the 1950s.
People conceptualize and utilize biomedical facilities
in a variety of ways. Christians are forbidden by
church edict to participate in the ngoma mode, for this
will involve the singing and dancing connected with the
ancestral-based religion. Rituals and taboos therefore
are excluded from their repertoire, but herbalism and
some aspects of women's medicines for child bearing and
rearing are not. These become part of Luvale "home
remedies" that Christians utilize in addition to the
biomedical system. Non-Christians utilize any or all
of the biomedical repertoire depending on proximity to
facilities and perceived usefulness of the treatments.
Biomedical care does not require payment because of
socialized medicine, but transportation becomes an
issue. People must go or be brought to the hospital or
clinic and out-patients must return daily to receive
medicine and treatments. Often medications are given
on a daily basis rather than dispensing the entire
prescription at once in fear that people will take too
much or too little at a time or stop medicating once
they feel better. Sometimes the course of treatment is
never completed because outpatients only attend clinic
sporadically.

Many people have access to the biomedical treatments, but the majority have no idea that they are
dealing with a system. Rather, the biomedical system
is thought of as discrete medicines and treatments.
For example, people have rank-ordered the types of
medicines they perceived were offered. Injections are
believed to the best medicine, pills and tablets, are
next, and liquids to drink are perceived as the least
efficacious and least desirable medicine. People do
not know which medicine they will receive for an ailment, and sometimes ask for another method or type. In
terms of Luvale people becoming biomedical specialists,
a few persons in the area have taken short courses to
be able to work as clinic personnel and several women
have received some basic instruction in midwifery.
However, there is nothing analogous to the apprenticeship system, and of course, one does not have to have
experienced illness to be a practitioner.

Because the biomedical system is perceived as providing materia medica that may help, there were many
cases in which people were treated by both systems or,
within each system, utilized multiple medications and

treatments. Many treatments are efficacious but some
produced disastrous results especially when people
overmedicated. In one case, a child received herbal
treatments in the village and was taken also to the
clinic and to the hospital where she was given injections of chloroquinine and penicillin. She went into a
coma after the second injection. Another type of
situation is when Christians or those who consider
themselves "too modern" to engage in an indigenous
treatment, in fact participate in a minor ritual or
utilize the herbal medications. As a result, a variety
of "non-ngoma" type treatments are being employed.
Although these combinations may be thought of as harm-
less, or as not causing more harm than indigenous
treatments, healing for some people now consists of
utilizing parts of each type of medical system somewhat
haphazardly. The consequences are social as well as
physical. Patients no longer have the prerequisties
they need to paticipate in the apprenticeship system
and people utilize pharmaceuticals carelessly.

   Elsewhere I have discussed a variety of patterns
that people employ in seeking cure (Spring 1980a,
1980b). Table I sums up utilization patterns of traditional (non-Christian) and Christian Luvale in terms of
their expected and actual use of the "traditional"
indigenous medical and the biomedical systems in the
area. The "classic" pattern of using all aspects of
the traditional system and none of the biomedical would
hold for those opposed to or disinterested in the biomedical, or for those living where biomedical services
are unavailable. Similarly, Christians would disavow
all aspects of the traditional, although many retain
beliefs in some of the herbals and this would be their
"classic" pattern. Most non-Christians commonly use
the biomedical maternal-child care services that may
include pharmaceuticals and immunizations. Some people
use all aspects of both systems. Christians may have
to rely on traditional midwifery if labor commences
before the parturient can go to the hospital. If
difficulties arise, traditional rituals might have to
be enacted. Finally, another pattern is the enactment
of a minor ritual that does not involve ngoma. Oc-
casionally, even Christians will participate in a ngoma
ritual (carried out away from the family's Christian
residence) for a sick child or woman with repeated
problems in child bearing. Ideally, this should not
occur, but in reality Christian families sometimes turn
to these methods.

   What do the specialists who have been trained
through the apprenticeship method think of the biomedical system and how do they utilize it? Some midwives
send their patients to pre-natal clinics for confirmation of pregnancy. At least half of the attenders at

AFRICAN HEALING STRATEGIES

Table 1

Utilization Patterns in Traditional and Biomedical Systems

INDIGENOUS MEDICAL

		Midwifery	Rituals	Herbals	Taboos
TRADITIONAL LUVALE	A	x	x	x	x
	B	x	x	x	x
	C	(*)	x	x	x
CHRISTIAN LUVALE	C	0	(*)	x	0
	B	(*)	0	x	0
	A	0	0	0	0

BIOMEDICAL

		Maternal-Child	Surgery	Pharma-ceuticals	Preventa-tives
TRADITIONAL LUVALE	A	0	0	0	0
	B	x	0	(*)	(*)
	C	x	x	x	x
CHRISTIAN LUVALE	C	x	(*)	x	x
	B	x	(*)	x	x
	A	x	x	x	x

A = classic   x = full participation

B = most common   0 = no participation

C = alternate   (*) = partial participation

the pre-natal clinics at the Christian Mission Hospital
(where I have data) have village deliveries using
indigenous midwives. Midwives will be employed to give
herbal medicines during pregnancy and the "washing the
baby ritual" (Mitchell 1962; Spring 1976a) in which all
non-Christian hospital parturients engage. Spirit
possession doctors and herbalists will claim cure and
demand payment from a patient who recovers, even if the
patient's cure may be as a result of biomedical treatment.
     In the pluralistic environment sometimes even
ritual experts incorporate aspects of biomedical treatments into curative patterns for themselves and their
families in the same way as other villagers do.
Midwives have utilized some breathing and massage techniques they have seen the hospital staff use. The
wanganga in the area may parody the methods of biomedical techniques during the ngoma mode and other rituals.
Unlike some areas in urban Zambia, herbalists are not
seen in markets in this rural area selling packaged
drugs (that are often outdated or countraband pharmaceuticals). Ritual specialists and others believe that
cosmopolitan medicine cannot cure everything, and that
there are some illnesses that are immune to biomedical
treatment. Thus far there has been no overlap of
ritual specialists and biomedical specialists except
for the Christian midwives.
     It has been proposed in other places in Africa
such as Nigeria that traditional curers be retrained
and utilized to carry biomedical health care, as they
know the local culture and have recognized status.
Many of the Luvale indigenous women health care experts
such as midwives or traditional birth attendants would
be ideal in this role, and some of the wanganga would
be involved in "barefoot doctor" type activities. However, even though the biomedical system is actively
utilized, it is conceputally different from the indigenous. The apprenticeship system differs radically from
the biomedical system in that it is not experiential
and sick people are not preferred as curers.

CONCLUSION

     Turner (1968) has written that women form a "com-
munity of sufferers" as they participate in the ngoma
therapy mode. The community of apprentices and experts
comes together in an individual's adult life with the
girl's puberty ritual. Here the public phases include
ngoma which provides the tempo, pace and structure of
the ritual sequences that lock in the private phases
where the materia medica are administered. Women
continue to participate in curing in the public and
private spheres during pregnancy and parturition, and

private spheres during pregnancy and parturition, and
for their own illnesses and those of their children.
All the while women are being learners and leaders,
apprentices and experts. Women's illnesses are central
to the mainstream of the healing system just as boy's
puberty, men's illnesses, and the male concern with
misfortune has its practitioners and rituals. The
girl's puberty ritual and the apprenticeship system for
midwives, spirit possession doctors, and herbalists
function as the training curriculum whereby women learn
the religious and medical system. All women participate to some extent. The experts are those who have
the experience in terms of being ill and recovering, or
those having the interest or inclination.
       By contrast, the biomedical tradition is utilized
by people in the area, but is not perceived as a system
by them although its components have been systematized
here. Very few Luvale have undertaken the study of the
new curriculum or understood the principles. The basis
for being an expert is different from the indigenous
system and the long study periods are not perceived as
apprenticeships, probably because individual experience
with illness is not a prerequisite. The Luvale and
other ethnic groups in the area add all or some of the
parts of the biomedical system into their healing
strategies, even though they do not understand the system. Utilization often depends on various factors such
as distance to facilities, volition of the individual
or of the therapy management group, finances, modernity
and Christianity. Sometimes the biomedical treatments
will be efficacious especially when an entire course of
treatment is completed; other times the efficacy of the
treatments in reduced when a haphazard course of treatment is followed. Christians disavow the traditional
medical system, but are sometimes forced to use it. At
times Christians go against their religious tenants and
employ ngoma and other therapy modes when they feel
that the biomedical treatments are not working.
       People in Northwest Zambia, as elswhere in Africa,
are in the process of syncretizing and integrating
indigenous healing strategies with biomedical strategies just as they have been incorporating ideas about
curing from neighboring peoples for centuries. Indigenous medicine gives women a significant place in the
religious and healing tradition and people see it as a
system. The biomedical system dispenses medicine to
people who do not perceive it as a system and who cannot yet perceive their participation as practitioners
within the new tradition. Whether or not women will be
able to play equally important roles as men in biomedicine in the area becomes a question for future
consideration.

REFERENCES CITED

Hansen, Art and R.J. Papstein (eds.) The History of the
Luvale People and Their Chieftanship. Los
Angeles: African Institute for Applied Research,
1979.
Harrison, Ira and Priscilla Ulin, "Traditional Healing:
Continuity, Discontinuity and Consequence", MS.
4pp. n.d.
Hoch-Smith, Judith and Anita Spring, (eds.), Women in
Ritual and Symbolic Roles. New York: Plenum
Press, 1978.
Janzen John, The Quest for Therapy in Lower Zaire.
Berkely: University of California Pess, 1978.
_____, "Indicators and Concepts of Health in
Anthropology: The Case for a Social Reproduction"
"Analyses of Health", MS. 22pp, 1982.
_____, "On the Comparative Study of Medical
Systems: Ngoma, A Collective Therapy Mode in
Central and Southern Africa", MS. 36pp, 1983.
Just, Peter, "Men, Women and Mukanda": Transforma-
tional Analysis of Circumcision Among Two West
Central Africa Tribes", African Social Research
13: 187-206, 1972.
Lewis, Gilbert, "A View of Sickness in New Guinea, in
J. Loudon, ed., Social Antrhropology and Medicine.
London: Academic Press, pp 49-103, 1976.
Mitchell, Clyde, "Marriage, Matriliny, and Social
Structure among the Yao of Southern Nyasaland",
International Journal of Comparative Sociology 3:
29-40, 1962.
Rappaport, Roy, Pigs for the Ancestors. New Haven:
Yale University Press.
Richards, Audrey, Chisungu: A Girl's Initiation
Ceremony Among the Bemba of Northern Rhodesia.
London: Faber and Faber.
Spring, Anita, "An Indigenous Therapeutic Style and its
Consequences for Natality", in J. Marshall and S.
Polgar, eds., Culture, Natality and Family Plan-
ning. Chapel Hill: Carolina Population Center,
pp. 99-125, 1976a.
_____, Women's Rituals and Natality Among the
Luvale of Zambia, Ph.D. Dissertation, Cornell
University, 1976b.
_____, "Epidemiology of Spirit Possession Among
the Luvale of Zambia", in J. Hoch-Smith and A.
Spring, eds., Women in Ritual and Symbolic Roles.
New York: Plenum, pp. 165-190, 1978a.
_____, "Women and Men as Refugees: Differential
Assimilation of Angolans in Zambia", Disasters: 3:
4: 423-38, 1978b. (Revised and expanded in A.
Hansen and A. Oliver-Smith, eds., Involuntary

Migration and Resettlement: The Problems and Responses of Dislocated Peoples. Boulder: Westview Press, pp. 37-47, 1982.

_____, "Faith and Participation in Traditional Versus Cosmopolitan Medicine in Northwest Zambia", Anthropological Quarterly 53: 2: 130-41, 1980a.

_____, "Traditional and Biomedical Health Care Systems in Northwest Zambia", in P. Ulin and M. Segal, eds. Traditional Health Care Delivery in Contemporary Africa. Syracuse: Maxwell School African Series, No. 35, pp 57-80, 1980b.

Turner, Victor, The Forest of Symbols: Aspects of Ndembu Ritual. Ithaca: Cornell University Press, 1967.

_____, The Drums of Affliction. Oxford: Claredon Press, 1968.

_____, The Ritual Process: Structure and Anti-Structure. Chicago: Aldine, 1969.

White, C.M.N. "Conservation and Modern Adaptation in Luvale Female Puberty Ritual, Africa, 23: 1: 1-23, 1953b.

_____, "Notes on the Circumcision Rites of the Balovale Tribes", African Studies, 12 2: 41056, 1953a.

_____, "Elements in Luvale Beliefs and Rituals", Rhodes-Livingstone Papers, 32, 1961.

Wilson, Peter, "Status Ambiguity and Spirit Possession", Man 3: 266-378, 1967.

CHAPTER 10

RELIGION, RITUAL, AND HEALING AMONG URBAN BLACK SOUTH AFRICANS

Brian M. du Toit

Introduction

Anthropologists are socialized, intellectually at least, with the concept of cultural relativity. Every society must be seen against its own background and setting while behaviors and institutions should be viewed within this nexus. To this philosophy we all pay lip service but whether we truly believe it and practice it is a different matter.

Few social scientists who have had heterogeneous cultural experiences would expect the educated Pakistani to mold his family life on the American model, or the modern New Guinea village leaders to insist on an American experimental school. Yet when it comes to individual behavior in the areas of politics, religion, medicine, or science we tend to forget about cultural relativity. In many cases we expect developing countries to follow closely on the Westminster parliamentary model, Christian converts to somehow forget their traditional religions, and newly educated persons to place all their faith in medical science while turning from practices that proved beneficial for their mothers and fathers. We forget that a person cannot be "born again" in toto where a new basis for belief is accepted or when faith is placed in new curing properties. This is based on two basic principles. First, change in one behavioral sphere does not necessarily effect every other sphere of thought and action, and second, the motivation for change in one sphere might not apply to other spheres of belief and behavior.

The subject of this paper is religion, ritual, and healing. In particular I will focus on urban blacks in Durban, South Africa.[1] Most of the subjects under discussion have had a few years of schooling,[2] most have lived in the city for at least a decade, most visit a modern medical clinic and are served by medical doctors, and most are active members of Christian churches. This might suggest that our research subjects would compare well with other educated, Christian, urban dwellers outside southern Africa, or that

151

they would compare well with persons of other ethnic
groups in Durban. Neither of these, of course, is the
case relative to the topics under discussion. The
reason for this is that these people are members of a
southern Bantu linguistic and cultural stock (83.8% of
them are Zulu-speaking) who have long traditions in
this particular regional and ecological setting. While
they might go to the clinic or pharmacy for certain
preparations, this will not necessarily replace the
traditional pharmacopoeia; while they might be active
members of Christian churches, there will be certain
realms in which the shades continue to be important;
and while new rituals might be accepted or required,
these will not necessarily replace traditional rituals.
In no aspect of life is this more true than that of
healing. A primary reason for this is that healing
has very clear religious bases and overtones, and that
these are enhanced by rituals.

It is frequently suggested that women are "more
religious" than men and that they are more regular
attendants at religious services. If this is true, its
effect will be neutralized in this sample[3] in which
260 men and 172 women responded, and also due to the
importance of men in the traditional religion and
ritual.

The remainder of this paper will focus successive-
ly on religion, ritual, and healing. The conclusion
will suggest an integrative approach.

Religion

The Traditional Picture: The southern Bantu-speaking
peoples traditionally were characterized by a very
strong belief in and reverence for their deceased
ancestors. Since the latter in the form of shades,
maintained contact and either communicated or actively
influenced the living there was a need for praises,
thanksgiving, libations, and sacrifices. Such beliefs
and rituals resulted in a particular form of religion
and assured a conservative retention of traditional
values.

In addition to the ancestors there were other
supernatural agents that had to be recognized by all
people but that could be manipulated by diviners and
sorcers. Within this supernatural context most diseases had their origin. Cure for a disease was based
on treatment but also on the restoration of a balance
in supernatural relations, and this was best achieved
by a sacrifice. Rituals, usually accompanied by sacrifices, marked all critical periods in a person's life.
This concept of "critical" involved facing the unknown
or being confronted by a new set of life forces. Such
confrontation involved movement in space and through

time. Thus, a sacrifice might be made before a person
went on a journey or migrated to the city, before he
entered a new phase in interpersonal relations, or
before he entered a new stage of the life cycle.
Inherent in the rituals, the sacrifices, and the
accompanying prayers was always thanksgiving for what
lay behind as well as a request to the shades for continued protection or support.

Religion, then, was a part of everyday life as the
shades were always in attendance. It was also a very
meaningful experience because it gave continuity,
though at a different plane, to parental and familial
bonds. Vertical relationships that were of prime
importance in childhood were carried into adult life,
and so into the afterlife. As parents warned, protected, gave advice, educated, and healed so the shades
would continue to do, provided the avenues of communication were kept open by regular ritual and sacrifice.

The Coming of the Missionaries: For the past century
and a half Christian missionaries of various denominations have worked in the region covered by this study.
The result is that most of the blacks are Christians,
though this does not mean that they have broken completely with the traditional family religion. South
Africa, perhaps more so than most other countries, has
also been marked by a phenomenal growth in the area of
religious independence resulting in churches, cults,
sects, offshoots, and offshoots of offshoots. Today we
better understand some of the motivating forces that
lead to religious independence, but earlier anthropologists saw it differently. In fact, Eiselen (who later
was professor of anthropology at the University of
Pretoria) stated: "One can hardly condemn the malady
of separatism too strongly. Besides making a laughing
stock of both the Bantu people and of Protestantism it
has the most injurious effects on the development of a
Christian way of living within the well-established old
mission churches" (1932:76).

During this research in 1973 the majority of persons in our sample were still members of the official
mission-derived churches, but the "malady" had not been
eradicated. Table 1 shows the churches to which
respondents belonged, but the right-hand column shows
the churches they belonged to previously if they were
converted to their present church affiliation. It is
perhaps this second column that is of primary importance. Of the 30.7% who have changed from a specifically mentioned church or belief system, 22.8% changed
from formal "mission" churches.

TABLE 1. Current and Past Church Affiliation of
Respondents

Name of church	1973 membership		Converted from	
Roman Catholic	66	(15.3)	19	(4.4)
Methodist	65	(15.0)	20	(4.6)
Zionist	56	(13.0)	4	(.9)
Anglican	41	(9.5)	16	(3.7)
Traditionalist	34	(7.9)	15	(3.5)
Lutheran	30	(6.9)	14	(3.2)
American Board	28	(6.5)	17	(3.9)
Presbyterian	11	(2.5)	9	(2.1)
Full Gospel	10	(2.3)	1	(.2)
Baptist	9	(2.1)	0	0
African Congregational	8	(1.9)	5	(1.2)
Apostolic	5	(1.2)	0	0
Zulu Congregational	5	(1.2)	3	(.7)
United Congregational	5	(1.2)	0	0
Dutch Reformed	4	(.9)	2	(.5)
Apostolic Faith Mission	4	(.9)	0	0
Swedish Mission	4	(.9)	1	(.2)
Shembe	3	(.7)	3	(.7)
Jehovah's Witnesses	3	(.7)	0	0
Church of Christ	3	(.7)	0	0
Assemblies of God	2	(.5)	0	0
United Apostolic	2	(.5)	0	0
Free Methodist	2	(.5)	0	0
Twelve Apostles	2	(.5)	0	0
Apostolic Church of God	2	(.5)	0	0
African Methodist Episcopal	2	(.5)	1	(.2)
Old Apostles	2	(.5)	0	0
Ethiopian	1	(.2)	3	(.7)
Other (one member each)	21	(4.4)	11	(2.5)
NR	2	(.5)	29	(6.7)
NA			259	(60.0)
	432	(99.9)	432	(99.9)

One reason for the growth and popularity of independent churches particularly those of the Zionist type
(see Sundkler 1948), is the aspect of healing. While
some persons incorporate herbal remedies, most of this
healing is in the form of laying on of hands, faith
healing, use of holy water, and similar nonempirical
aspects. A growing literature deals with this phenomenon of separatism and religious expression.

One of the most thorough compendia on the subject
of African religious movements is that of David Barrett
(1968), who not only offers a survey but also treats
the underlying factors. He suggests that healing

abilities are not sufficient cause for independence in
the absence of other factors and refers to Josue Edjro,
a Methodist healer in Ivory Coast, and Mrs. Samuel
Nwahune, an Anglican in Eastern Nigeria. In both cases
these persons practiced healing without establishing
independent movements. Others, such as John Maranke
with his message of miraculous healing (Jules-Rosette
1979), Grace Tani (Breidenbach 1979), and numerous
others, employed preparations, holy water, and the Holy
Spirit to cure and restore health. Speaking in general
of traditional African religions, John Mbiti states
that African "prayers are chiefly requests for material
welfare such as health..." (1969:65). Jahoda surveyed
17 independent churches in Ghana, "most of which have
healing as one of their primary objects" (1961:255).
This includes healing that is spiritual as well as
patently magical, and treats barrenness, sickness,
difficulties in life, and worry caused by witches.
Rather than catering only to a traditional clientele,
traditional healers are patronized by literates, and
Jahoda found that the support and reassurances they
provide probably prevents serious breakdowns in many
cases.   "A similar need is served by the healing
churches" (Jahoda 1961:268).
     We should keep in mind that the church family, the
communitas (Turner 1969), functions in much the same
way as the family does in the traditional social setting. Its members support, assist, and act much as the
family members do in cases of illness and witchcraft
(Hautvast and Hautvast-Mertens 1972). This concern for
health is carried over into independent movements and
frequently is the reason a person first contacts or
joins such a movement. While deep commitment and
involvement may follow, practical considerations are
frequently the initial stimulus for association.
     The religious background and family context of
respondents in our sample are represented in Table 2.
One notices that a relatively smaller percentage of
parents were Christians, while the "don't know"
category increases. This is particularly true in the
cases of the spouse. A familiar response was, "I don't
know, you'll have to ask him/her."

TABLE 2 Religious Affiliation of Respondents and
Family

Person	Traditionalist	Christian	N/A, N/R, D/K	Total
Ego	34 (7.9)	394 (91.2)	4 (.9)	432
Father	30 (6.9)	359 (83.1)	43 (10.0)	432
Mother	25 (5.8)	366 (84.7)	41 (9.5)	432
Spouse	5 (1.2)	2 (65.7)	143 (33.1)	432

Syncretism in Action: Out of our total number of
respondents only 34 (7.9%) indicated that they did not
belong to a Christian church or sect, while another 2
(.5%) did not respond.   That means that 396 persons, or
91.5% of all the respondents, are formal members of
churches, pay their dues, and attend regularly.   In
fact, 181 (41.8%) of all those persons interviewed had
been to church at least once during the 2 weeks that
preceded the interview, and 203 (47.0%) planned to
attend at least once during the next 2 weeks.   The reasons for using 2 weeks as a unit is that many blacks
work either in industry or as domestics and might have
to work alternate Sundays.   We should, however, note
also that most separatist churches have midweek services and Thursdays are particularly important for
women who belong to a manyano[4] group.   Table 3
contrasts real patterns of religious participation with
ideal and planned.
        Later in the interview these same persons were
asked about contact with their ancestral spirits.   This
included contact initiated by them as well as visions
of or messsges from the ancestors.   When asked, "Have

TABLE 3.   Religious Group Attendance: Real, Ideal, and
Planned

Frequency of attendance	When last attended	Ideal attendance	Planned attendance
Within 2 weeks	143 (33.1)	158 (36.5)	196(45.5)
1 to 2 weeks	38 (8.7)	28 (6.5)	7(1.6)
Monthly	38 (8.7)	23 (5.3)	3(.7)
Within the year	70 (16.2)	59 (13.7)	24(5.6)
Less than once a year	87 (20.6)	0	0
Only on holy days	0	21 (4.9)	0
Never	34 (7.8)	98 (22.7)	7(3.9)
DK/NR	22 (5.0)	45 (10.4)	185(42.9)
Total	432 (100.1)	432(100.0)	432(100.1)

you received messages from an idlozi?"[5] almost as
many answered in the affirmative as answered negatively.   In fact, 211 (48.8%) answered yes, 215 (49.8%)
answered no, while 6 persons (1.4%) did not respond.
When asked about one occasion when they saw an ancestral spirit, most explained that this had been in the
form of a vision.   The most frequent expression was as
a snake (106 persons, 24.5%), while others saw a mantis
(36 persons, 8.3%), a lizard (4 person, .9%), some
other animal (14 persons, 3.2%), or some other form (4
persons, .9%).   The rest of the respondents either had
not seen such a vision or did not respond.

Such visions, either during the waking hours or in dreams, naturally result in action on the part of the living. This may take the form of consulting a diviner or of independently communicating with the ancestral spirits. Table 4 contains the responses to our question concerning the respondents' approaching the shades.

Can a person hold two seemingly antithetical views in which Christian dogma is accepted and Christian church rituals supported while simultaneously recognizing the shades and sacrificing to them? It is obvious that this goes on every day. It is also obvious that the antithesis exists in the Western scientific mind not in the philosophy and world view of persons not so trained. Religion, says Howells, is "a diplomatic conspiracy against the invisible" (1948:22) and the allies employed in this conspiracy would obviously differ from person to person and from group to group. Syncretism represents one set of allies as selected by these people.

Ritual

This is not the place to attempt a definition of ritual but it is sufficient to point out that rituals may occur in either secular or sacred contexts. Ritual refers to the sequence of events that are performed; their context and connotation gives them meaning and purpose.

TABLE 4. When Was the Last Time You Approached the Amadlozi?

Frequency	Persons	Percentage
Last week	29	6.7
Last month	12	2.8
Within the last 3 months	25	5.8
Within the last year	104	24.1
Over a year ago	112	25.9
Never	141	32.6
NR	9	2.1
Total	432	100.0

Life Cycle Rituals: Following van Gennip, social scientists recognize the individual's life cycle as consisting of various phases. Transition from one to the other is fraught with potential danger, and one generally finds protective or strengthening rituals for the individuals and frequently also for the closest relatives.

Traditional African societies, like most people the world over, marked transitions in the life cycle with ceremonies and even sacrifices. These occurred at

birth, at puberty, at marriage, and at death. While
birth and marriage are of critical importance, the
significance of puberty among males has been downgraded
among the Zulu, first, because Chaka discontinued circumcision, and second, because of Christian teachings
and urbanization. While a protracted ritual can be
performed, the cattle are not always present for the
old time ritual or for the sacrifice. Yet the rituals
are still performed. Table 5 contains responses to
three questions concerning rituals. One could argue
that people do not know what happened when they were
born, and there is in fact a fairly high percentage who
stated that. Yet when asked about sacrifices made to
accompany the above-mentioned rituals, a fairly large
number of persons were very specific. Table 6 presents
the information on sacrifices, though the totals do not
quite agree with the positive response in the previous
table. It is entirely possible that urban residence,
education, and Christian church membership have influenced this response pattern. To remove the issue from
the personal level, each of our respondents was asked:
"Do you feel that your sister's child should have a
traditional puberty initiation with ritual and sacrifice?" Here we find 269 (62.3%) answering in the affirmative while only 140 (32.4%) responded negatively.
The rest would leave it up to the sister or did not
know. The reason for selecting sister's child is based
on the strong avuncular-nepotic relation and the institutionalized role of the malume or mother's brother

TABLE 5. Rituals and the Life Cycle

Question: Were rituals performed at your ...

	Yes	No	Don't know	No response
1. birth	236(54.6)	151(35.)	42(9.7)	3(.7)
2. puberty	104(24.1)	320(74.1)	2(.5)	6(1.4)
3. marriage	404(93.5)	28(6.5)	0	0

among the Zulu and closely related Nguni peoples.
       We should keep in mind that two factors converge
in this protective ritual for a child. First, accidents do not occur randomly. Africans see them "in
direct and personal terms" (Mitchell 1965:194), and for
that reason the individual needs to be protected.
Second, newborn children have a tendency toward death,
and for this reason existential powers must be balanced
by human action. Barker says that "health and sickness
depend upon how we resolve the equation of the spirit,

TABLE 6. Sacrifices and the Life Cycle

QUESTION: Were sacrifices made to mark the rituals at your...

	Yes-NFI	Yes-cow	Yes-goat	Yes-chicken	No	Don't know No response
1. birth?	9(2.1)	4(.9)	213(49.3)	0	4(.9)	202(46.8)
2. puberty?	6(1.4)	17(3.9)	42(9.7)	1(.2)	15(3.5)	351(81.3)
3. marriage?	9(2.1)	208(48.1)	81(18.8)	0	63(14.6)	71(16.5)

the balance which is forever to be maintained by propi-
tiation and ritual" (1973:81). This twofold coping
action results in act and attitude that converge in a
lifelong series of sacrifices, libations, offerings,
and a variety of rituals.

A significant part of life cycle ceremonies are
related to strengthening the individual and protecting
him/her for the new life phase. Part of these rituals
may include prayers to the ancestors or to God, anoint-
ing or treating the body, as well as eating or drinking
medicines or special foods. But there are also rituals
specifically earmarked as protective rituals.

Protective Rituals: People are constantly moving. In
the previous section we identified one form of movement, biological changes that inexorably accompany
people from birth to death. But there are other kinds
of movement. In southern Africa these include migrant
labor, changing to a new house (both rural and urban),
and changing jobs (or finding the first one). On all
these occasions as well as in attempting to assure
continued success or safety, rituals will be performed.
Obviously, all of these rituals would also contain an
element of thanksgiving and some are basically a way of
saying, "Thank you, but keep it up!" Table 7 refers to
rituals at the family level. Included here are two
rituals that are basically of a thanksgiving nature
either for birth or for the health of the children. We
find a fairly high incidence of ego performing the
ritual, and this is entirely in keeping with the traditional religion that is basically a family religion.
Once again the goat is the most frequently used sacri-
ficial animal except where people are extremely poor.
In the latter case chickens may be substituted.

Healing and Health: In a recent study Ngubane pointed
out that "the environment progressively becomes riddled
with changes. In order to survive despite these
changes, everyone must be frequently strengthened to
develop and maintain resistance. In other words
everyone must establish and maintain a form of balance
with his surroundings" (1977:6). This balance is best
achieved and maintained by regular protective rituals
and frequent rituals to strengthen the individual. The
parent does it for the child, and later on adults
perform these for themselves and for each other. But a
lack of health can also be caused by sorcery or by the
shades. In the former case, protection is required; in
the latter, the maintenance of harmonious relations
with the ancestors. Both require rituals.

Anything that comes between a person and the other
world, or anything that upsets the balance, is pollution. This is a mystical force that "diminishes resis-

TABLE 7. Rituals and Sacrifices at Family Level
QUESTION: Have you performed or had others perform rituals...

	Yes-no further information	Yes-by ego	Yes-by a relative	Yes-by a specialist	Yes-by a Christian specialist	No	Don't know No response	Totals
To assure success?	52(12.0)	50(11.6)	52(12.0)	5(1.2)	8(1.9)	235(58.6)	12(2.7)	432(100.0)
Giving thanks for safe return from a journey?	65(15.0)	65(15.0)	39(9.0)	0	1(.2)	248(57.4)	14(3.2)	432(99.8)
For wife during childbirth?	156(36.1)	12(2.8)	7(1.6)	16(3.7)	1(.2)	219(50.7)	13(3.0)	432(100.0)
For dedication of your home after moving?	2(.5)	9(2.1)	0	69(16.0)	10(2.1)	342(79.2)	0	432(99.9)

161

tance to disease and creates conditions of poor luck,
misfortune..." and other negative conditions (Ngubane
1977:78). The southern Bantu-speaker, and in particular the Zulu, is thus constantly involved in an effort
to maintain this balance with reference to nature,
spirits, and the shades. Part of this effort involves
rituals, normally performed by the household head at
the family level but in more serious cases by a specialist, to protect, guide, strengthen, and purify the
patient. Such rituals may be as simple as a sacrifice
and address to the shades or as elaborate as vomiting
or drinking strengthening medicines coupled with blood

TABLE 8. Health and Protective Rituals for Subjects,
         Their Children, or Their House

Question	Yes	No	N/A or NR	Total

Were rituals performed for your health?
        222 (51.4)   205 (47.5)   5 (1.1)   432 (100.0)
Were rituals performed for the health of your children?
        322 (74.6)   108 (24.9)   2 (.5)   432 (100.0)

letting. They may protect the patient, his/her family,
or the house. It is very common to find a plant, inthe-a
lezi, growing outside a house in town or to learn that
specialist was brought in to perform the ukubethelela[6] ritual at the four corners of the house.   In
both cases the ritual serves as a safeguard.   When
subjects were asked whether such protective rituals had
been performed, a majority answered in the affirmative.
Table 8 presents the results of these questions.   But
we were also interested in who performs the rituals.
Table 9 indicates that the majority of rituals are
performed by traditional specialists.   These may be
either those who are predominantly diviners or those
who are herbalists. The need would designate the type
of specialist employed and the remuneration required.
It will be noticed that some persons employed a Christian specialist to perform the ritual.   This refers
specifically to Zionist church membership and will be
discussed below.

Healing

The Belief System: The concept of healing has different implications, depending on one's belief about
existential forces, the nature of disease, and disease
causation.   Treatment must affect both the cause and
the disease itself and frequently involves rituals to
strengthen or protect the individual.
        In a series of very valuable discussions, Robin
Horton offers an analysis of African traditional

TABLE 9. Who Performs Rituals for Healing and Protection?

QUESTION: Who performed the rituals for...

	Yes-NFI	Yes-by ego	Yes-by relative	Yes-by traditional specialists	Yes-by Christian specialists	No	DK NR	Total
your health?	42 (9.7)	4 (.9)	4 (.9)	145 (33.6)	27 (6.3)	205 (47.5)	5 (1.1)	432 (100.0)
the safety of your house?	47 (10.9)	14 (3.2)	9 (2.1)	75 (17.4)	11 (2.5)	272 (63.0)	4 (.9)	432 (100.0)

163

164 AFRICAN HEALING STRATEGIES

thought as it relates to scientific thinking. Drawing
on Kalabari ethnography, he points out that certain on
Kalabari ethnography, he points out that certain kinds
of diseases do not respond to herbal treatment and the
conclusion reached is that "there is something else in
this sickness." The diviner or diagnostician, as I
have referred to him, will now be called and the
disease located in a wider context of causation. "What
we are describing here is generally referred to as a
jump from common sense to mystical thinking. But...it
is also more significantly a jump from common sense to
theory" (Horton 1967a:60). As a theoretical system
this body of explanations absorbs cause and simultaneously reduces anxiety, for it is a coping mechanism.
When the system fails to offer explanations, anxiety
rises and chaos looms. For this very reason coincidence and chance cannot be accommodated. In the first
place, events cannot occur haphazardly. Therefore,
witchcraft enters as part explanation not of the how
but of the why of any occurrence (Gluckman 1944:64-65).
Such an explanation also opens avenues for action.
Disease and related misfortune may be the personal
result of other people's witchcraft or the displeasure
of the ancestors. Thus, Mitchell (1965:202) found that
misfortune caused by the angered spirit of a deceased
kinsman was very common among the Yao. Almost the
opposite was true for the southern Nguni, where
Hammond-Tooke (1970:33) established that a small number
of misfortunes were diagnosed as having been caused by
the ancestral shades. These two explanations of causation of misfortune open specific avenues for effective
action; they also form part of the theoretical system
within which cause and effect can be understood and
explained. Without such a logical causal explanation
there would be chaos. Horton explains: "The idea that
the whole thing could have come about through the
accidental conveyance of two independent chains of
events is inconceivable because it is psychologically
intolerable. To entertain it would be to admit that
the episode was inexplicable and unpredictable: a
glaring confession of ignorance" (1976:174). Ignorance
of cause and effect leaves a person ineffective and
once again increases anxiety. Knowing, on the other
hand, what causes or threatens misfortune leads to a
range of actions, some prophylactic, some precaution-
ary, and some positive. This is part of the theoretical system and is the action component.
    It is also within this context that the "tradi-
tional African psychiatrist" (Edgerton 1966, 1971)
functions so effectively. The illness, physical or
mental, is seen "in the broad psychosocial-religious
context" (Foster and Anderson 1978:119) and this
facilitates treatment by the healer and belief and

trust by the patient. When many of these elements are incorporated in the formal structure of a new religion healing and success become components of the system. While many persons first associate with a religious group for healing and therapeutic reasons, they remain and become active members because of the continuous support and reinforcement.

Among the Zulu, and other southern Bantu, healing has two basic foci--curing the ailment and restoring the balance of patient to ecology. But in order to learn what action is required, the patient must visit a diagnostician. Such a diagnostician, the diviner (isa-ngoma), may either diagnose ritual or social causes or refer the patient to the herbalist (inyanga) for treatment. This is true for a large percentage of rural and city folk alike. Dr. Gumede, a Zulu M. D., explains: "When he (the African) falls ill in town, he leaves all the doctors and hospitals in town and goes home to his kin so that they may consult a diviner, an isangoma, to find out the cause of his illness; whether it is amad-lozi (ancestors), izipoki (ghosts), abathakati (sorcer-ers) or simply umkuhlane (fever), and in particular to find out what would be the prescription required to restore health and mental ease" (1968:3). The treat-ment or prescription may call for sacrifices, but will almost certainly call for certain forms of treatment such as purification (enema or vomiting) or herbal medicines. Such medicines may consist of bark, root, or leaves, or may be composed of a complicated concoc-tion. Many of these concoctions contain herbs that are medically sound. Many others contain herbs that are irritating or toxic when used in the wrong proportions or in overdose.

Within this general region of southern Africa a number of extremely thorough anthropological studies have been made. One of these deals with the Venda peoples in northern Transvaal. Stayt (1968:262-308) begins his discussion of magic and medicine among the Bavenda with the premise that these two terms represent two ways of viewing the same phenomenon. Saying that all herbal and medicinal treatments, even those we would consider therapeutic in and of themselves, depend upon magic for their efficacy, he claims that every object, animate or inanimate, has an inherent kinetic power of good and evil. As an example of how this power manifests itself, he mentions the story of a tree branch that extended over a particularly treacherous section of a foot path and was grasped by everyone who passed by as a support in negotiating the path. The branch became associated with a good force by everyone in the area and small pieces of it were used as charms for travelers. This is contrasted by a root that was in such a position as to cause everyone who passed by

it to stub their toe or trip. Pieces of the root were
cut off fromtime to time by people preparing charms to
use against their enemies. Thus, the art in the magic-
medical profession consists of the ability to control
and channel these forces that exist in all objects.

It is the individual skill of the practitioner in
his use and interpretation of this force, combined
with his knowledge of the specific effects of
certain herbs and concoctions, that make or mar
his reputation. When once a practitioner proved
his powers and established his reputation he can
perform his rites and work his cures with the
utmost confidence, believed and trusted implicitly
by the credulous people. While the magical element in the treatment is scientifically useless,
the personality of the practitioner, often
combined with undoubted hypnotic power, and the
stimulus and excitement caused by the divinatory
rituals, fortified by the implicit faith of the
sick person and his relations in the practitioners
powers, so work on the mind of a patient that a
cure is affected. The native is immensely
susceptible to auto-suggestion, and examples of
natives who suffer from supposed illnesses and
pine away for no physiological reason, or who
simply die through fear of death superimposed upon
them by a more powerful personality, are common
knowledge (Stayt 1968:262-263).

The above quotation is illustrative for two reasons. First, it demonstrates the interrelatedness of
medicine and magic in bringing about a cure --an interrelatedness so strong in the traditional context that
most Bantu languages make no distinction between what
for us are two highly contrastive concepts. Second,
Stayt bears witness to a tendency that has been regret-
tably common among those who would study medical practices in Africa, on the one hand labeling the magical
element as "scientifically useless" and on the other,
after couching the same phenomenon in terms more amenable to Western science, informing us that it does
indeed play an extremely important role in bringing
about a cure. This is indicative of our failure to
understand the problem we are facing and of the smug-
ness of Western science in the face of a so-called
nonempirical way of dealing with nature. The dismissal
of the role of magic in curing is made increasingly
difficult for one interested in making a serious study
of indigenous medicine by A. Winifred Hoernle's reminder: "The very same beliefs and practices --same in
principle if not in detail --were an integral part of
the European civilization of our own ancestors. Right

down into modern times, the belief in witchcraft was
not felt to be in conflict with Christianity. It was
shared, and acted on, by learned and unlearned alike--
by priest and doctor, by judge and magistrate, no less
than by the private burgher in towns or the peasant of
the countryside" (1953:221).   Further, J.D. Krige
(1954) asserts that the Bantu do indeed base their
healing art on empirical observation. According to
Krige, the Bantu are empiricists within their own
culture and they make a much more effective use of
vegetation than do Europeans (see also various chapters
in Ackerknecht 1971). He sees a ready-made body of
knowledge onto which we can graft our scientific
conceptions if only we are able to adequately come to
terms with it. Finally, H. J. Simmons (1957) offers
additional insight into the world view that helps to
shape the role of the healer in the traditional
societies of southern Africa and that is in turn in a
very real sense shaped by that world view. He explains
that their

>   ...notion of the universe may be described
>   as a belief that is both natural and
>   supernatural, or to be more precise,
>   preternatural, if we understand by this
>   term an extension of the natural into the
>   metaphysical and nonmaterial sphere. All
>   forms of life and substance are regarded
>   as being charged with or subject to a
>   supernatural force. This is not defined,
>   indeed there is no word for it in Southern
>   Bantu languages. Its existence is assumed
>   as self-evident and beyond dispute, and as
>   much a part of reality as any material thing.
>   It may operate directly or through matter, at
>   the instance of people or spirits, and for
>   good or evil, and its actual or potential
>   effects has to be taken into account in any
>   situation or enterprise.
>   In keeping with the basic concept, the tribal
>   theory of causality draws no distinction
>   between materialistic and supernaturalistic
>   explanation. There are no equivalent terms
>   in the language for natural and supernatural,
>   corporeal and incorporeal, empirical and
>   transcendental. Natural and preternatural
>   ideas are complementary, not distinct, they
>   form a single, consistent body of knowledge.
>   Natural substance and causes are recognized,
>   but always as operating in conjunction with
>   the supernatural (1957:89).

As one might expect, there is no sharp dividing
line between so-called natural causes of disease and
those diseases that are sent either by an enemy through
witchcraft or sorcery, or by ancestor spirits who are
angry about an occurrence that constitutes a departure
from custom or a departure from traditional norms.
Among the Pondo, a southern Nguni people, Hunter
(1936:272-275) found that certain "natural phenomena"
are associated with causing disease. For example, the
people would avoid eating certain foods that they found
to have made them sick in the past. They would not
kill an animal for meat during the summer and most
would refuse to eat the meat of any animal that had
died of anthrax. Those who would for whatever reason
eat such meat would invariably take medicine in advance
to protect themselves from infection. No importance
was given to the illness that accompanies the intake of
large quantities of beer. Death from old age was
regarded as stemming from natural causes, as were the
slight illnesses that all people contract from time to
time. It was noted, however, that a minor illness can
weaken a person and thus make one more susceptible to
sorcery. Hunter found a difference of opinion among
individuals regarding the origins of specific infectious diseases. Sitting on the damp ground was not
thought of as likely to cause sickness. Accidents were
often regarded as "just accidents" and were also at
times regarded as resulting from socery. Thus, while
many would think of a snakebite or a fall from a horse
as an accident, many others would automatically assume
sorcery. With regard to animals, Hunter noted that
while oxen dying in yoke during the summer would generally be regarded as an accident, the eating of poison-
ous plants was not recognized as a cause of sickness
among cattle, and ticks were not regarded as dangerous.
According to Hunter:

> The dividing line between illnesses believed
> to have been sent (by an enemy or by the
> ancestors) and those which are recognized as
> being due to natural causes is affective,
> not rational. Some people attribute more
> to natural causes than others. If once a
> diviner is consulted the sickness is always
> diagnosed as due to an enemy or to the
> ancestors. No informant could cite a case
> where a diviner had diagnosed natural causes
> for a disease. All agreed that such a thing
> had never happened. A diviner knows that if
> people feel strongly enough about anything to
> consult him, they will not be satisfied with
> the explanation that it is due to natural
> causes (1936: 272).

Hunter has here identified one of the major conceptual stumbling blocks that have plagued those who
would study medicine and healing in traditional Africa.
As scientific Westerners, we separate illnesses into
those for which a cause can be empirically decided upon
and those that seem to be caused by phenomena that are
not empirically detectable. The first are made to seem
more real on the basis of our seeming ability to measure them, and it is this variety that is deemed worthy
of receiving professional attention. The latter are
not measurable; they are therefore less real and less
important, and we tend to expect that the person should
take care of these problems on his own. In societies
such as the one being described by Hunter, however, the
categories of natural and supernatural causes for
diseases tend to merge, and they are certainly equally
real, and perhaps because both types of dysfunction
manifest themselves so concretely in an individual's
behavior, social channels are provided for the allevia-
tion of both types of suffering.

The Herbalist: Up to this point we have only briefly
taken note of the herbalist who in traditional Zulu
society usually was a man. In most cases patients are
referred to him by the diagnostician or diviner, and in
most cases he knows a great deal about plants and their
properties. The herbalist learns from his father (if
the latter was an herbalist) and acquires some knowledge by experimentation; the rest is communicated from
the ancestors. He will prescribe a variety of common
herbs but usually uses some that are peculiar to his
treatment and that he collects on regular visits to the
country.
But pharmacy and dispensary may be no more than a
suitcase filed with packages, or may be as elaborate as
large stores. In most large cities there are "wholesale stores" where people can buy anything from barks
and roots to mixtures containing lion fat or baboon
semen. In Johannesburg's Albert Street there is the
famous old Mai Mai Bazaar with an interethnic clientele
(Longmore 1958). Salisbury (Zimbabwe) has its herbal
markets and practitioners (Editorial 1958) and a Lusaka
(Zambia) suburb has both markets and herbalists (Leeson
and Frankenberg 1973).
Jahoda, discussing research findings from Ghana,
points out that the modern healer has "adapted some of
the trappings of the Western medical man and pharma-
cist" (1961:254). In Durban the urban African could
visit the beer hall, where herbalists display their
wares in suitcases and make diagnoses regarding one
patient's sexual impotence while selling bark to cure
another's runny nose. Patients and herbalists alike

can also visit Kwa David, Ikimisi LaBantu (The Place of
David, the Bantu Pharmacy) in Leopold Street.
    The concern for fertility that brings many women
to membership in separatist churches is simply a carry-
over from the traditional lineage setting.   In the
latter, children were valued and required and many a
woman who did not have children (not always due to her
inabilities) lost the interest of her husband.   John
Watt did an extensive survey of plant use and finds
Ficus capensis and Adansonia digitata widely used as
aphrodisiacs and in treating infertility.   He also
refers to Bena women who drink an infusion of the leaf
of Ximenia americana as an aid to fertility. Since the
active principles are tannin and resin, there can be no
pharmacological effects (1972:80).
    The point to be made in this brief statement is
that the herbalist, though of extreme psychological and
to a lesser extent medical importance, caters at the
individual level.   A patient may visit any number of
healers, first those who deal with the diagnosis and
cure of psychological or spiritual causes, and later
those who concentrate on physiological and bodily
discomforts. This does not guarantee proper diagnosis
or effective medical treatment.   While many plants in
the South African pharmacopoeia have decided medical
value, these plants have in many cases been misused.
This is due in part to a major conception of how to
deal with an illness, namely, the expelling from the
body of the supposed causal agent. This is in contra-
distinction to the view that the illness might be due
to some homeopathic dysfunction.   As a result of this
pervading view, there is extensive use of strong purgative, cathartic, and emetic agents. This often results
in deleterious effects.
    Mokhobo recently reported 12 cases of herb-induced
hepatitis in Africans from the Maseru district in
Lesotho (Mokhobo 1976).   The pathological condition was
brought about by the ingestion of herbs containing
hepatotoxic alkaloids, particularly from the Senecio
species. Of the list supplied by Mokhobo of the herbs
implicated in these cases (which he was able to develop
by interviewing the patients), at least five of the
herbs are mentioned in use in the ethnopharmacopoeia of
the Sotho, the Zulu, and the Xhosa.   He notes that
children are especially susceptible, and malnutrition
confers specific susceptibility on the liver (Mokhobo
1976:1098).   In a related example of a survey of cases
among Xhosa patients, the traditional medicines are
again cited as possibly playing a part in the etiology
of the illnesses (Solleder 1974).   In these cases the
morbidity rate was high.   Of the 50 patients in the
survey, 29 suffered from diarrhea and vomiting due to
the use of a native purgative.   In several cases this

resulted in severe dehydration. In addition, in several other cases the use of the Xhosa medicine apparently brought about a fatal effect from the original illness for which the native medicine was ingested. Unfortunately, no mention is made of the specific herbals that might have been implicated.

Buchanan and Cane report eight cases of poisoning due to treatment by a local herbalist in Johannesburg. Of these, six died. Hypotension was present in seven of the cases and acute renal failure in five. No mention is made of the herbal medicines involved. They do remark, though, that attention should be paid to this problem in that proper therapy would, of necessity, have to be based on the type of toxin(s) involved in the poisoning (Buchanan and Cane 1976:1140). Acute renal failure is also cited in six cases from Zambia (Lowenthal et al. 1974). The patients, six Zambian women, used the traditional herbal medicines for the treatment of gynecological complaints. Dukes et al. mention three species - Securidaca longipenuculata, Euphorbia matebelensis, and Crotalaria laburnifolia - as causing renal damage (1969). Of these three species, Teichler notes that juices from Euphorbia species is in use in Botswana pharmacopoeia for maternity cases and for illness of the eye in children, while it is also used in Zambia and Malawi for eye complaints, he also notes that it seemed that the medicine, often as not, caused blindness as much as it cured the illness (Teichler 1972). Watt and Breyer-Brandwijk and others report the use of two of the above genus groups throughout South Africa. Euphorbia ingens is used in small amounts by the Zulu as a drastic purgative, while the Sotho administer the latex to patients suffering from dipsomania (Watt and Breyer-Brandwijk 1962). There are many different members of Euphorbia species found throughout the world. All contain a highly irritating latex, which can be fatal in certain doses.

Despite the foregoing, there are many plants utilized in the native pharmacopoeias that have definite medicinal use. The Albizia anthelminthica tree has been shown to be a "good worm medicine" (Teichler 1971). Watt and Breyer-Brandwijk report its use throughout southwest Africa, also as an anthelmintic. The baobab tree (Adansonia digitata) has been shown to have extremely high levels of ascorbic acid in the pulp, and it accounts for the low level of scurvy among the low veld Africans who consume the fruit in a variety of manners (Carr 1958). In addition, there are other plants in the native pharmacopoeias also with an antiscorbutic principle. An analysis of "kaffir beer", the native homemade brew, showed significant amounts of vitamins B and C (Fox 1939).

But not all healing, of either a psychological or
a physiological nature, is conducted at the level of
traditional specialists. Increasingly two other levels
of treatment have become accepted, namely, the Western
medical specialist and the faith healer.

Western Medical Specialist: The past century and a
half has made Western medical facilities, specialists,
and cures available throughout southern Africa, and a
growing number of blacks are training and specializing
in various fields of preventative and curative medicine.   Children in towns and cities grow up with the
neighborhood clinic, the Indawoka-Dokotella, the mobile
clinic, and the city hospital. Which of these or the
traditional healers will be selected will vary from one
case to another.   Ngubane states: "There is no
definite pattern followed at this stage, as the behavior depends on the seriousness of the disease, the
availability of particular health agencies, the financial position and the person who makes decisions"
(1977:101).

Urban and rural residents alike might select
traditional health agents in less serious cases and
finally turn to Western health agencies. They may also
try the latter and, if a cure is not forthcoming soon
enough, turn to their traditional healers.   Still
others play it safe by consulting both at the same
time.

Faith Healing: Obviously, the traditional isangoma was
the basis for a great deal of trust and faith, resulting in healing. What I have in mind here, however, is
the role of independent or separatist churches.

With the increase in the number of separatist
churches, some have emphasized their healing roles. It
should be remarked immediately that some Zionist
churches shun medicine and therefore do not allow herbs
or other medications, while others employ the healing
properties of plants but activate them by religious
ritual and faith.
    Discussing independent churches in the Johannes-
burg area, West has stated: "Healing in church services can be both direct or indirect, the latter being
more common. Perhaps the most common form of healing
is through prayer and laying on of hands, and this
usually takes place in one of two ways: either the
patients are called up in front of the congregation,
kneel and are prayed for, or else they are placed in
the center of a circle and prayed for while members of
the congregation dance round the perimeter" (1975:92).
A similar case employing sacrifices, blessed water, and

ritual has been discussed by du Toit (1971). It should
be emphasized here that once a person becomes a member
of a separatist church, much of the decision making
about the choice of a healer is removed. Zionists are
expected to behave alike, to follow the guiding precepts of their leaders, and to submit to the unconscious pressures from the "communitas," as discussed by
Turner (1969).
     To a great extent, I would suggest, the inyanga or
herbalist is being replaced, both by Western health
agents and agencies and by faith healing. While the
herbalist cannot adapt in any major way to the changes,
the isangoma does. As diviners, diagnosticians, and
psychiatrists they are gaining in importance as urbanization and alienation are producing new stresses and
strains (see du Toit 1971). The herbalist will not
disappear but his role and function will decrease and
become increasingly more specialized.

Discussion of Results

     Having discussed various dimensions of belief and
action relative to assuring health, the question arises
concerning their importance. If one selects a sample
of persons who are urban residents, how will they react
to certain choices and certain situations? Are there
in fact certain spheres in which they recognize the
traditional religious agencies over those of alien
derivation? Does the traditional healer in fact have a
realm of undisputed specialization? Does the ethnic
group membership and color of the specialist play a
role?
     In order to answer these questions, we constructed
and administered a series of questions to the sample of
432 urban blacks discussed in the introduction. The
table was composed in such a way that the horizontal
axis went from the categories dealing with traditonal
religious and healing agents progressively toward Western healing and religious agents, while the vertical
axis dealt with a series of questions presuming an
increase in the seriousness of the case - starting with
a headache and ending with death. The question was
then posed: "If you suffered from a headache, would
you approach the amadloze (ancestors), consult an
isangoma, etc., etc.?" and later for males the questions on childbirth pertained to their wives. Table 10
presents the results of these questions.
     A number of very interesting figures appear in the
table. The shades, it seems, are called on both in
times of great stress and (especially) in gratitude.
One does not bother them with such minor ailments as
headaches and flu, but in complicated childbirth and
serious illness about half the respondents would call

TABLE 10. Actions to be Taken in Case of Ill Health.

Forms of ill-health		Amadlozi		Isangoma		Inyanga		Chemist		Clinic		Medical doctor				Minister of religion			
												African		White		African		White	
		#	%	#	%	#	%	#	%	#	%	#	%	#	%	#	%	#	%
Headache	Yes	116	27.2	75	17.5	169	39.7	400	94.8	401	94.6	404	95.3	404	95.7	188	44.2	186	43.8
	No	311	72.8	353	82.5	257	60.3	22	5.2	23	5.4	20	4.7	18	4.3	237	55.8	239	56.2
Flu	Yes	98	23.1	55	12.9	113	26.6	397	94.3	401	94.6	407	96.0	407	96.0	177	41.9	177	41.9
	No	327	76.9	372	87.1	312	73.4	24	5.7	23	5.4	17	4.0	17	4.0	245	58.1	246	58.2
Snakebite	Yes	98	23.2	62	14.6	261	61.7	232	56.6	410	96.9	415	98.1	414	97.9	134	31.8	134	31.8
	No	325	76.8	362	85.4	162	38.3	178	43.4	13	3.1	8	1.9	9	2.1	288	68.2	288	68.2
Serious accident	Yes	173	41.8	74	17.8	93	22.6	168	41.8	403	98.5	401	98.0	400	97.8	175	43.2	174	43.0
	No	241	58.2	342	82.2	319	77.4	234	58.2	6	1.5	8	2.0	9	2.2	230	56.8	231	57.0
Normal childbirth	Yes	247	59.4	8	1.9	98	23.7	320	77.9	382	91.6	375	89.9	375	89.9	347	84.2	346	84.0
	No	169	40.6	408	98.1	316	76.3	91	22.1	35	8.4	42	10.1	42	10.1	65	15.8	66	16.0
Complicated childbirth	Yes	204	48.3	69	16.3	92	22.0	116	28.3	415	99.0	413	98.6	413	98.6	141	34.0	140	33.7
	No	218	51.7	355	83.7	326	78.0	294	71.7	4	1.0	6	1.4	6	1.4	274	66.0	275	66.3
Serious illness near death	Yes	223	53.1	122	29.3	154	37.1	244	59.5	411	98.1	411	98.1	411	98.1	297	71.2	296	71.0
	No	197	46.9	295	70.7	261	62.9	166	40.5	8	1.9	8	1.9	8	1.9	120	28.8	121	29.0
Death	Yes	110	26.1	96	22.7	16	3.8	9	2.2	212	51.7	242	59.6	243	59.6	375	91.2	369	90.7
	No	311	73.9	327	77.3	402	96.2	403	97.8	198	48.3	164	40.4	165	40.4	36	8.8	38	9.3

174

on them. At the conclusion of a normal childbirth
almost 60% of the sample (and keep in mind that only
7.9% of the total sample indicated that they were traditionalists by religion!) would contact the ancestors,
mostly in thanksgiving, quite possibly accompanied by
an animal sacrifice.

The isangoma or diviner receives recognition by
about 15-20% of the respondents, but when serious illness confronts them, a much larger number of persons
would consult the diviner to learn of any taboos trans-
gressed, restitutions to be made, or actions to be
performed.

The inyanga or herbalist currently receives greater support than the diviner, particularly because his
actions are health-related. Whether it is the administration of a purgative, the letting of blood, or the
prescription of herbal medicines these actions all aim
very specifically at relieving pain and curing the
disease. This is particularly true in the case of
headache, where the chewing of a certain kind of bark
may be prescribed, and again in the case of serious
illness, when anything is tried. The most interesting
response in the whole table is under "snakebite." Time
and again, respondents would point out that there is
nothing to match the isihlungu (species of Crabbeanana
Nees and Blepharis Capensis) snakebite antidote used by
their ancestors. Almost 62% of the people would
attempt to get to an herbalist if bitten by a snake.

The chemist (drug store) and clinic are of equal
importance when dealing with medication, but since the
latter has beds and operating theaters, its importance
increases in cases that obviously would imply an
incapacitated patient. The familiarity of respondents
with the clinic is clear from the consistently high
positive responses in selecting clinical treatment.
The same holds true for the role of the Western health
agent, here represented by either a black or a white
doctor.

The minister of religion receives token recognition all the way through the questions. But when all
the other negative responses increase, in the case of
death, the minister's positive responses increase. A
number of persons were asked about their answers, and
their replies made sense: "Well, we have tried everything to keep the patient alive, now the minister must
come and bury them!"

Conclusion

Among urban black South Africans religion and
healing are integrally related. One does not have
success and health without assuring it continuously by
ritual acts and religious behavior. Performing the

correct rituals and acting in accordance with the
religious group requirements should assure health.   But
people need all the help they can get and there seems
to be no contradiction in attending a Christian church
service while a sacrifice to the ancestors is waiting
at home.   The contradiction is in the Western
scientific mind, which attempts to deduce cause and
effect and to relegate each to different spheres of
existence. Disease is caused by an imbalance in nature
resulting in pollution and/or evil spirits and/or
purification and/or God and/or the ancestors. It all
comes down to multiple treatments for multiple causes.
Ritual becomes the enhancing ceremony.

NOTES

1The research on which this analysis is based
was conducted as a prestudy for an extensive project on
drug use in Africa supported in whole by grant number
DA 00387 from the National Institute on Drug Abuse,
United States Department of Health, Education and
Welfare. This support is gratefully acknowledged. All
statements made and conclusions reached are those of
the author and do not imply agreement from granting
agency personnel. This article originally apppeared in
Urban Anthropology, 9(1), 21-49, 1980.
    2Responses from this same sample of persons
have been analyzed from a different perspective in du
Toit (1978). Since this latter publication contains
detailed quantitative analyses, the reader will excuse
my use here of the vague "most".
    3Kwa Mashu, a black satellite city north of
Durban, is divided into 11 neighborhood units. This
sample consists of a 3% random sample of each of the
neighborhoods. The male/female ratio was a product of
this sampling rather than the aim.
    4Manyano societies are voluntary associations
based on religious group memebership in which women,
distinguished by distinctive uniforms, gather on
Thursdays to pray and dance. This weekly meeting is
also used to organize the activities of the group.
    5Idloze (plural amadlozi) refers to the spirit
or soul of a living person and hence the departed
spirit. Normally this is used to refer to the shades.
    6Ukubethelela is the verb that refers to
setting up a charm, protective magic, or medicated
stakes to protect a house against accidents or
lightning.

REFERENCES CITED

Ackerknecht, E. H. Medicine and Ethology. Baltimore:
     Johns Hopkins Press. 1971.
Barker, E. A. Traditional African Views on Health and
     Disease. Central African Journal of Medicine
     19(4):80-82, 1973.
Barrett, David B. Schism and Renewal in Africa.
     Nairobi: Oxford University Press, 1968.
Breidenback, Paul. The Woman on the Beach and Man in
     the Bush: Leadership and Adepthood in the Twelve
     Apostles Movement of Ghana. IN The New Religions
     of Africa. Bennetta Jules-Rosette (ed.).
     Norwood: Ablex, pp. 99-115, 1979.
Buchanan, N., and R. D. Cane. Poisoning Associated
     with Witchdoctor Attendance. South African
     Medical Journal 60:1138-1140. 1976.
Carr, W. R. The Baobab Tree: A Good Source of
     Ascorbic Acid. Central African Journal of Medi-
     cine 4:372-374. 1958.
Dukes, D. C., H. M. Dukes, J. A. Gordon, et al. Acute
     Renal Failure in Central Africa: The Toxic
     Effects of Traditional African Medicine. Central
     African Medical Journal 15:51-56 1969.
du Toit, Brian M. The Isangoma: An Adaptive Agent
     Among Urban Zulu. Anthropological Quarterly 44:
     51-65, 1971.
_____. Ethnicity, Neighborliness, and Friendship
     Among Urban Africans in South Africa. IN Ethnic-
     ity in Modern Africa. Brian M. du Toit (ed.).
     Boulder: Westview Press, pp. 143-174 1978.
Edgerton, Robert B. Conceptions of Psychosis in Four
     East African Societies. American Anthropologist
     68: 408-425, 1966. A Traditional African Psychia-
     trist. Southwestern Journal of Anthropology
     27:259-278, 1971.
Editorial. Mushroom Poisoning. Central African Jour-
     nal of Medicine 4:347-348. 1958.
Eiselen, W. M. Christianity and the Religious Life of
     the Bantu. IN Western Civilization and the Na-
     tives of South Africa. I. Schapera (ed.) London:
     George Routledge, pp. 65-82, 1934.
Foster, George M. and Barbara G. Anderson. Medical
     Anthropology. New York: Wiley, 1978.
Fox, F. W. Some Nutritional Problems Amongst the
     Bantu in South Africa. South African Medical
     Journal 13(3):87-95, 1939.
Gluckman, Max. The Logic of African Science in
     Witchcraft. Rhodes-Livingston Institute Journal
     6:61-71, 1944.
Gumede, M. V. African Concepts of Sickness and Bodily
     Suffering. Lecture to South African Nursing
     Congress. 1968.

Gar_ _nd-Tooke, M. D. _rbanization and the
    Interpret- _on of Misfortune. A Quantitative
    _n_lys_. Africa 40(1): 25-38, 1970.
Hautvast, J. G. A. J., and M. L. J. Hautvast-Mertens.
    Analysis of a Bantu Medical System. Tropical and
    Geographical Medicine 24:406-414, 1972.
Hoernie, A. Winifred. Magic and Medicine, IN The
    Bantu-speaking Tribes of South Africa. I.
    Schapera (ed.) Cape Town: Maskew Miller, pp
    221-45, 1953.
Horton, Robin. African Traditional Thought and Western
    Science. Part 1. Africa 37(1):50-71, 1967.
_____. African Traditional Thought and Western
    Science. Part II. Africa 37(2):155-187, 1967.
Howells, William. The Heathens. New York: Doubleday
    1948.
Hunter, Monica. Reaction to Conquest. London: Oxford
    University Press, 1936.
Jahoda, Gustav. Traditional Healers and Other Institu-
    tions Concerned with Mental Illness in Ghana.
    International Journal of Social Psychiatry 7(4):
    245-268, 1961.
Jules-Rosette, Bennetta. Women as Ceremonical Leaders
    in an African Church: The Apostles of John
    Maranke. IN The New Religions of Africa.
    Bennetta Jules-Rosette (ed.). Norwood: Ablex,
    127-144, 1979.
Krige, J. D. Bantu Medical Conceptions. Theoria, pp.
    505, 1954.
Leeson, Joyce and Ronald Frankenberg. Traditional
    Healers in a Lusaka Suburb. Prepared for distri-
    bution in advance of the Ninth International
    Congress of Anthropological and Ethnological
    Sciences. Chicago. 1973.
Longmore, L. Medicine, Magic and Witchcraft Among
    Urban Africans on the Witwatersrand. Central
    African Journal of Medicine 4:242-249, 1958.
Lonthal, M. N., I. G. Jones, and V. Mohelsky Acute
    Renal Failure in Zambian Women Using Traditional
    Herbal Remedies. Journal of Tropical Medicine and
    Hygiene 77:190-92, 1974.
Mbiti, John S. African Religions and Philosophy. New
    York: Praeger. 1969.
Mitchell, J. Clyde. The Meaning in Misfortune for
    Urban Africans. IN African Systems of Thought, M.
    Fortes and G. Dieterien (eds.). London: Oxford
    University Press, pp. 12-202. 1965.
Mokhobo, K. P. Herb Use and Necrodegenerative
    Hepatitis. South African Medical Journal:
    1096-1099, 1976.
Ngubane, Harriet. Body and Mind in Zulu Medicine. New
    York: Academic Press. 1977

Simmons, J. H. Tribal Medicines: Diviners and
    Herbalists. African Studies 16:84-92, 1957.
Solleder, G. Clinical Observations on Toxic Effects of
    Xhosa Medicine. South African Medical Journal
    48:2365-28, 1974.
Stayt, Hugh A. The Bavenda. London: Oxford
    University Press. (Originally published, 1931.),
    1968.
Sundkler, Bengt. Bantu Prophets in South Africa.
    London: Oxford University Press, 1948.
Teichler, G. H. Notes on the Botswana Pharmacopoeia.
    _____. Notes and Records Botswana 3:8-11,
1971.

    _____. Notes on Eye Diseases in Botswana.
    _____. Botswana Notes and Records 4:237-240,
1972.
Turner, Victor W. The Ritual Process. Chicago:
    Aldine, 1969.
Watt, John M. Magic and Witchcraft in Relation to
    Plants and Folk Medicine. IN Plants in the
    Development of Modern Medicine. Tony Swain (ed.).
    Cambridge: Harvard University Press, pp. 67-102,
    1972.
Watt, J. M., and M. G. Breyer-Brandwijk. The Medicinal
    and Poisonous Plants of Southern and Eastern
    Africa (2nd ed.). Edinburgh: Livingstone, 1952.
West, Martin. Bishops and Prophets in a Black City.
    Cape Town: David Philip, 1975.

PART II
HEALING AND SCIENCE

One of the earliest aims of agents in accultura-
tion was to influence and alter the basic existential
premises of traditonal Africans. However, the question
remains to what degree ill-health caused by Allah or
God was different from that caused by the ancestors or
other supernatural beings. In time scientific bases
were introduced as the medical sciences made progress
in diagnosis and treament.

The papers in this section all deal with the scientific basis of healing strategies. Fako discusses
the history of culture contact and change among the
Tswana by paralelling the growth of traditional healing
strategies. It is interesting finds "the emergent
Tswana bourgeoisee" as espousing most consistently "the
value of allopathic medicine in and of itself" (1981:
374). This includes being a "true believing" Christian. Modern rural Tswana, accoridng to Comaroff,
still recognize the ngaka as diagnotician and employ
traditional medicine while Zionists form a third
category of support especially constitute of urban
proletariate.

Beck looks at the development of the national
health system in Rhodesia and its modern expression in
Zimbabwe as this country emerges from years of warfare.
This introduces the theme of national health schemes.

The last three contributions are by medical doctors. Rosenbloom reports on the Third Annual Disease
Surveillance Conference which was heal in Sierra Leone;
the Smalls deal with the transfer of medical technology
to Africa and especially possibilities to eliminate
tetanus, polio, and measles through immunization techniques; and the Reumans discuss health planning and
problems related to poor decision-making frameworks in
African nations.

It was fortunate that a conference of this nature could bring the medical and the social sciences into the same forum. Each gained in perspective by listening to and discussing with the other.

REFERENCES CITED

Comaroff, John L. Healing and Cultural Transformation: The Tswana of Southern Africa. Social Science and Medicine (B). 15(3B)367-78. 1981.

CHAPTER 11

OLD AND NEW APPROACHES TO MEDICINE IN RHODESIA AND ZIMBABWE

Ann Beck

After independence in the 1960s many African
states were determined to preserve the quality and the
character of the medical systems which they had taken
over from their colonial predecessors. The problem at
this time was not whether scientific medicine and traditional medicine should coexist but whether the financial basis of modern stern medicine could be maintained
in the developing countries of Africa. By 1979, however, after many African countries had experienced
difficulties in coping with an ever-increasing number
of infant deaths and infectuous diseases, while their
plans to bring medical relief to the rural areas did
not progress as fast as they had anticipated, new principles for medical care were discussed at an international conference held at Alma Ata, Union of Soviet
Socialist Republics, which was convened by the United
Nations. The ultimate medical goals presented at this
conference remained the same. The perspectives on
health care, however, changed. It was proposed to make
primary health care the means by which the masses of
the rural populations could be reached. "Primary
Health Care," as stated by the United Nations resolu-
tion, "is essential health care made universally accessible to individuals and families in the community by
means acceptable to them, through their full participation and at a cost that the community and country can
afford." (W.H.O. 1978:2) To make this dream come true,
health professionals would have to be assisted by non-
professional medical helpers such as medical aids,
rural health workers, and village health workers. The
doctrine of primary health care was not a declaration
of war against modern medicine and the professional
practitioner. It was the recourse to a remedy born out
of frustration. It was a firm commitment to bring
medical relief to the millions who needed it. (Beck
1981: 46)

It is against this background that we must now try
to understand what happened to Rhodesia, and its successor Zimbabwe. In 1965 Ian Smith became Prime Minister after he had unilaterally broken Rhodesia's ties
with Britain. His regime lasted until 1979 when the
African civil war came to an end and the republic of
Zimbabwe was established. Between 1965 and 1972 the
Rhodesian medical services continued as before along
the traditional pattern established in most British
colonies. The system was characterized by a central
department in the capital (Salisbury, now Harare) and
several provincial departments headed by a commissioner. Hospitals in the capital and in the provinces had
facilities to deal with surgical, clinical, and infectuous cases even though they were always chronically
understaffed. Rural small hospitals and dispensaries
were available in some rural areas. In many cases the
needs of the outlying areas were not met. (Secretary
of Health: 1980) Generally, curative medicine was
given priority over preventive medicine as can be seen
by the number of positions established for curative
medicine (8,924 in 1978) compared to 638 positions for
preventive medicine. An extensive network of eighty-
three mission hospitals supplemented the medical network in the rural and outlying areas. The medical
school in Rhodesia trained sixty students annually
throughout the period until the end of the civil war.
The Provincial Health Commissioner of Matabaleland
revealed some of the misery when he referred to the
frightening "misery-go-round" of malnutrition-infec-
tion-worse malnutrition in 1979. (Secretary of Health
1979:2)

In spite of the grim statistics during the civil
war between 1972 and 1979, the western institutional
medical services remained the basis of the healing
system in Rhodesia. Planning for a more comprehensive
and inclusive health network began during the civil war
and by 1980 several blueprints for change were ready.
One of them was the health program presented to the
parliament by Dr. Ushewokunze, the first Minister of
Health of Zimbabwe in 1980. His plan presented a blend
of the old and the new. The metropolitan and provincial medical centers were to continue while primary
health care was to be expanded with the greatest
expediency. Primary health care was to serve as the
major weapon against what the British Minister Beve-
ridge had once called the five giants threatening
modern society, namely: want, disease, squalor, ignorance, idleness. (Ushewokunze 1981: 1-4) Primary
health care became, therefore, Zimbabwe's top objective
but it was listed in conjunction with the modern approach to health. This is true even though primary
health care emphasized the strengthening of rural and

village clinics and the use of first aid stations in
the bush, but it would still be modern medicine which
the regular and auxiliary personnel were expected to
practice. On the other hand, Dr. Ushewokunze did not
reject a pluralistic approach to health as long as
certain social and political concepts were preserved.
Mentioned among them during the parliamentary debate on
the new health bill in 1981 was the statement on the
"conscious political" decision to emphasize primary
health care and to end discrimination in health
facilities by having "open" and "closed" hospitals.
(Parliamentary Debates 1980-1981: 1773) Medical
leaders in Zimbabwe have continued the structure of the
health pyramid, with its center in Harare, supported by
provincial centers and reaching out into the vast
hinterland of small villages and isolated settlements,
the latter under the direction of the Provincial Medical Department in Harare. The traditional healers,
however, have been included in this system as part of
the medical establishment in rural areas. The same is
true for mission hospitals.
      In spite of Zimbabwe's ideological orientation to
medicine and its acceptance of western concepts of
science, a reexamination of concepts of healing has
taken place. The writings of Gelfand, Chavunduka and
Sanders, among others, indicate that adjustments are
contemplated while the discussion continues. Most of
the writers agree that the health services must "harmo-
nize the principles of health by the people with health
to the people," i.e., primary health care. (Gilmurray
1979: 47) This involves the creation of a totally new
concept, the village health worker (VHW), who does not
have to have academic training, who may come from the
ranks of midwives, or be an ordinary village resident
interested in keeping the community alert and forming a
link between it and the health cadre above him or her,
referring a sick person to a health center. The value
of such a person, a village health worker, lies in his
or her ability to translate the complaints, health
needs, sanitary shortcomings, and lack of funds to
those directly in contact with him or her, such as the
health assistant or an auxiliary nurse. The most
important thing, however, according to the planners, is
that the VHW has the confidence of the community and a
feeling for the nature of its complaints or wishes.
Ideally, the VHW would be able to cut across bureaucratic layers and perform some of the roles implied in the
approach to disease by traditional healers. He or she
would be aware of the social and psychological problems
in a family group. It is argued that even the health
worker sent from the provincial department might not be
able to understand the type of therapy most congenial
to a particular environment. The VHW is only one link

between the modern medical treatment centers in the
cities and the isolated rural homes. The Provincial
Medical Department in Harare sends regular vaccination
teams traveling many hundreds of miles over unpaved and
dusty roads to reach the remote communities. (Beck
1983) They serve as vaccinators, check up on medical
and family problems, advise on birth control and
nutrition without intimidating the women surrounded by
numerous children. They teach them how to keep their
medical records up to date between visits.

These visits are an effective way to bring the
reality of a remote central government medical establishment to several hundreds of women and children.
The visits should no be compared with clinical ses-
sions. Acute cases of illness requiring professional
treatment in dispensaries or small hospitals must be
taken care of separately.

How does the traditional healer fit into the medical establishment in Zimbabwe today? Before the end of
the civil war in 1979, several studies on traditional
healing were published. In his book, A Service to the
Sick, Michael Gelfand described the work of the traditional healer during the earlier days in Rodesia, prior
to the civil war. (Gelfand 1979) Chavunduka's sociological study of the Traditional Healer and the Shona
Patient is based on more recent field studies supported
by statistics. Both authors shed light on the essential differences between western and traditional
approaches to diseasee. (Chavunduka 1978)

The expansion of scientific medicine introduced by
the colonial medical departments in Africa toward the
end of the nineteenth century followed basically a
similar pattern. It started as a service to protect
the personnel of the colonizing power and expanded
gradually to include the white settlers and the Africans employed by the administration. The expansion of
western medicine in Rhodesia was slightly different.
It took several decades after the arrival of Cecil
Rhodes' "pioneer column" in southern Rhodesia in 1890
before colonial administrations made a serious effort
to deal with the health of the native Africans. By
1920, medical administrators debated the relative
advantages of encouraging the Africans to visit the
urban areas for medical treatment. Fear was expressed
that such contacts might "spoil and undermine sanctions
of tribal life." In 1930, medical director Askins
stressed "the positive advantage of checking infectuous
disease in the native" whom he described as a potential
reservoir of infectuous disease. (Gelfand 1976:122)

The first serious attempt to establish rural
clinics was made in 1931. By 1948 preventive medical
services were more clearly defined. By 1952, eighty-
eight government clinics were popular and accepted by

the African population. (Gelfand 1976: 128) The
medical administration concluded that the time was ripe
to bring the "principles of health" to those who lived
in tribal lands. Throughout these years, however,
traditional doctors continued to treat their patients
as they had done before the arrival of the settlers.
The official medical reports of the Smith government
between 1974 and 1979 indicate the continuation of the
curative and preventive medical services, though on a
very limited scale, while the traditional healers in
rural areas went about their business as usual.

For our discussion here only a few examples will
be given to illustrate the differences between the
western and the traditional concepts of disease and its
treatment. Those who were brought up in the western
tradition of confidence in science and scientific medicine expect to be reasonably free from suffering and
pain through illness. In case of illness, a properly
licensed doctor will be consulted to relieve the cause
of the complaint. The Shona patient's reaction, however, is different, as Chavunduka shows. He considers
a certain amount of pain and suffering as the normal
condition of life. To protect himself he wears brace-
lets or other charms from early childhood on. (Chavunduka 1978:35-37) In this way, feeling safer and more
confident, he does not have to consult a doctor after
the onset of pain unless it continues inspite of his
magic protection. Therefore, the traditional healer
will not ask his patient for the cause of the physical
pain but will try to establish the violation of established rules of behavior, whether in relation to his
ancestors or in his actions toward his community. The
disease process and its treatment, therefore, starts
from a different perspective. The traditional healer
will seek information on social tensions in the community, will want to know about success in a patient's
work which may have caused his opponent's envy, will
probe into his patient's relationship with his co-
wives. This type of inquiry should not be compared
with modern psychoanalysis, although it may fulfill a
similar function. These examples do not refer to the
herbalist healer who fulfills functions more comparable
to western practices. The methods and practices among
the Shona healers and other traditional healers in
Zimbabwe may differ according to region and local custom. But their approach to disease is the same.

Traditional healers do not qualify for their work
through a course of formal studies. They either
inherit their career from a deceased family healer's
spirit or they claim to have been chosen by a non-
family spirit (mudzimu). Some healers learn their art
from an apprenticeship with an established healer.
Their position is the same, whether they learn their

work from experience or from contact with a spirit.
Chavunduka sampled 195 healers to find out what determined them to become a healer. He found that 145
claimed to have been possessed by a spirit, whereas
only twenty-five gave apprenticeship as the beginning
of their profession. (Chavunduka 1978:19-21) The
major departure from the procedure of western medicine
begins with the traditional practice of healing. It is
the approach to disease rather than the methods by
which the traditional healer probes into his patient's
emotional and social problems which establishes the
decisive dividing line between western and traditional
medicine. (Chavundaka 1978: 12-18)

The use of both medical systems by the Shona patient does not seem to have caused serious problems. In
some cases, however, it might be dangerous for hospital
patients to leave their clinical treatment in hopes to
get faster relief from a traditional healer. It seems
that the Shona patient has established his own criteria
for the type of medical system he prefers in each case.
For illness amenable to western treatment, the scientific doctor is accepted. Illnesses, however, suspected
to have been caused by spirits, are referred to the
traditional healer. (Chavunduka 1978:93) One may
question the competence of the patient to make the distinction between psychological and physical causation.
In the interest of the health of the patient some
cooperation between the western doctor and the traditional healer will be beneficial.

From what has been said so far, it appears that
the differences between western and traditional medicine are fundamental. Up to the 1960s, colonial
medical departments did not seriously consider arrange-
ments for recognition or cooperation. But with the
extension of medical systems to the rural areas in all
African countries, a change of attitude has occurred.
The future strategy of medical policy, however, depends
largely on the decisions made by the central government
in Zimbabwe.

There are two conflicting trends. The expansion
of the metropolitan and provincial medical departments
and the increased use of smaller outpatient stations
with auxiliary personnel has brought western medicine
closer to the rural population that formerly was without trained help. Even though dispensaries and nursing
stations expanded very slowly, medical help began to be
available by rotating the personnel. Africans in
remoter areas who formerly consulted the traditional
doctor had now an opportunity to become acquainted with
modern medicine. The expansion of the dispensaries,
first aid stations, and visiting teams from provincial
headquarters had an impact on the rural population. In
spite of the advance of western medicine, the tradi-

tional healer continued to play a role even under the
changing circumstances of the 1970s. This impression
was confirmed when, in 1981, the Zimbabwe National
Traditional Healers Association (Zinatha) was set up
with a membership of 11,000. (Africa Now 1983: 20-21)
Apparently this was an attempt to integrate the traditional healers into Zimbabwe's major medical care
scheme. The council was the brainchild of Dr. Herbert
Ushewokunze, Zimbabwe's first Secretary of Health. His
nickname, "Herbert, the herbalist," indicates his sympathy with some of their practices. Zinatha embraced
more than 11,000 traditional healers by the end of 1981
and became the mouthpiece for medical traditionalism.
The organizational changes made healers respectable and
also permitted the government to have some influence
over them. It is significant that a scholar like Dr.
G. L. Chavunduka was named president of Zinatha in
1981. In his earlier examination of traditional
healing in the Harare area he had found that Africans
sought medical relief from both western and traditional
doctors. In a sample group examined by Dr. Chavunduka,
55.2 percent consulted a western doctor first and then
returned to a traditional healer, whereas 22 percent
consulted a traditional healer first before seeing a
western practitioner. (Chavunduka 1978:41-43) It is
likely that Zimbabwean leaders, at least at this early
stage, found it practical to give legitimacy to
traditional healing. Since it was accepted in many
rural areas, it might just as well be officially
practiced and, if necessary, regulated.

But as it happens with every new organization,
Zinatha has been attacked by another group of healers,
the "Spirit Mediums' and True N'angas Association," or
SMTNACA, a group that traces its existence to the
earliest times of the British colonial administration
in 1896. The n'anga claim to have among their clients
81 percent of customers previously treated by western
doctors, 38 percent traditional cases, 15 percent
gynecological patients, and only 13 percent mental
cases. This would indicate that they attracted some
western-oriented customers and had a percentage of
herbalist healers who were more readily accepted by
modern Africans. (Africa Now 1983: 20-21)

Yet it appears that traditional healers do not
quite fit into the new scheme of rural medicine which
relies on the introduction of the village health workers. To the more socially-oriented planners among
doctors and political leaders, the VHW represents a
better solution. He would represent the government
effectively in the villages however far from the
center. He would cost less and would be a good source
of information to assess reaction to government policy
in remoter areas. He would also be a visable reminder

of the existence of the national government which might
lose contact with the remoter parts of the country.
Apparently, to the leadership in Harare, the VHW
represents a political as well as a medical solution to
the restructuring and reintegration of the new medical
services into a new rurally-oriented society. In 1983,
a writer in Africa Now stated it this way, "The crucial
health worker is not the doctor, western or traditional, but the village health worker---a part-time
non-professional, democratically elected by the village." (Africa Now 1983:21) The view that the doctor,
western or traditional, cannot replace non-professional
medical practitioners does not seem to be borne out by
the great effort which Zimbabwe is making to improve
its medical department and the delivery of its medical
services throughout the country. It has subscribed to
primary health care and it attempts to uphold professionalism in medicine.

REFERENCES CITED

Africa Now, 1983, Harare, pp. 20-21, 1983.
Beck, Ann. Medicine, Tradition and Development in
    Kenya and Tanzania, 1920-1970. Crossroads Press.
    1981.
_____. Personal observations on a trip to Rhneme,
    Mashonaland sponsored by Provincial Medical
    Director P. V. Sang. 1983.
Chavunduka, G. L. Traditional Healers and the Shona
    Patient. Gwelo: Mambo Press. 1978.
Gelfand, Michael. A Service to the Sick. Gwelo:
    Mambo Press 1976.
Gilmurray, John, et al. The Struggle for Health.
    Gwelo: Mambo Press. 1979.
Parliament, Zimbabwe.
    Report of the Secretary of Health for 1979
    Report of the Secretary of Health for 1980
    Debates, p. 1573. 1981.
Ushewokunze, Herbert. Equity in Health.
    Harare. 1981.
World Health Organization. Primary Health Care:
    Report of the International Conference on Primary
    Health Care, Alma Ata, USSR 1978.

CHAPTER 12

THE DILEMMA OF AFRICAN TRADITIONAL MEDICINE: THE CASE OF BOTSWANA

Thabo T. Fako

Introduction

While the growth of Western medical knowledge and technology has had a pervasive influence in shaping the
character of health care delivery systems in many parts
of the world, Western medicine has not intruded upon
any population that had no previous experience with
medicine. In all societies there have always been
individuals who had the responsibility of providing
mental and physical relief from illness, trauma, and
other disturbances. With such people in each community, health and help services were made available, and
close by. Consumers were not faced with a maldistribu-
tion problem which exists in the modern health delivery
systems, where the official (Western) health services
reach only a fraction of the population.

It has become increasingly clear that indigenous
healing strategies do not represent a rural phenomenon,
which is bound to decline with increasing Westernization or modernization. Many patients prefer to be
treated by a traditional doctor or in addition to, a
Western trained doctor. This is especially interesting
given that several of the more popular traditional
doctors are also some of the most expensive, charging
in many instances, much more than a Western styled
physician would (Lieban 1976).

By 1977, at least 2.3 billion people or 56 per
cent of the World's population continued to rely upon
local indigenous health care services for treatment of
a wide variety of physical and mental illnesses (Good
1977). The continued reliance upon traditional medicine is deeply rooted in the beliefs, values, social
organization and customary behaviour patterns of each
community (Fabrega 1974). Providers and users are
interconnected through a shared "psychological reality"
which constitutes their culture (Hallowell 1955). Indeed, as Suchman (1973: 206) pointed out, since illness
is a frequently recurring phenomenon which generates

190

fundamental concerns and anxieties, significant group
norms and mores have been evolved which strongly influence individual attitudes and behaviour in the health
area. Illness has meaning for the patient and those
around him, and it is ordered by that meaning (Parsons
1951). It is above all, an undesirable human condition
which is responded to with compassion and not modern
medicines as such (Friedson 1970:20). All societies
have always done what they could to alleviate pain and
suffering, and over time have evolved systems or strategies of healing.

African healing strategies, however, have not been
properly understood because of continuing pent-up
suspicion and prejudice which has built up over the
years, and which has been supported by modernization
theories of development that as a whole, have tended to
be hostile towards what they have poorly defined as
traditional societies and tradition in general. These
theories have tended to suggest that African traditional ways and thought are particularly lacking in objectivity, and in the systematic pursuit of knowledge.
Unlike European ways and thought, African ways are said
to be replete with mystification, ceremony and ritual
and, more so than any other, tend to promote the non-
rational as the predominent mode of explanation of
natural phenomenon. Thus, the separation of facts from
fiction, dreams from reality, and the subjective from
the objective is not a distinguishing feature of the
African way of life.

This type of thinking has tended to stand in the
way of clear thinking about African ways and the
methodology resulting therefrom has led to spurious
findings about indigenous African systems, including
findings on African healing systems. But, just as the
spread and support of Western medicine by governments
all over the world was not based on prior proof of
overall superiority over competing medical systems,
contemporary interest in traditional African or Chinese
medicine does not necessarily reflect or represent an
acknowledgement of their overall compatibility, let
alone superiority, over Western medicine. In addition,
the fact that Western medicine is indeed the most
technically sophisticated product of a collaborative
group of highly trained scientists and engineers, it
has not as a result achieved astonishing results in the
overall improvement of the health of populations. It
has nevertheless been promoted simultaneously with the
discrediting of competing systems.

"There is demonstrable evidence that the academic
observers in Africa and other continents look at
African traditional medicine with rather poorly
disguised suspicion. Our western-based criteria

of judgement acquired during the many years of
Anglo-American university education, and social-
isation into western value systems, determine what
we see, what we want and what we eventually
choose. We approach traditional African medicine
the way interogators face their suspects, who have
to prove their innocence. In our best moods the
traditional health practitioner is like a job
seeker who has to show proof of his ability to do
the job well, in addition to demonstrating his
honesty and reliability. The standards we set
cannot be matched by the traditional medical
practitioners. In many ways they are right to
treat us suspiciously. We thinly hide our biases
under the guises of cloudy rhetoric and
obscurantist pseudo scientific standards. Thus we
hide our own inadequacies and misunderstandings"
(Mburu 1983: 2).

Before we proceed any further, it is important to
especially emphasize that there are many modes of life
which pass under the label African, when in fact their
basis is as foreign as the system of administration
currently in vogue across Africa. In addition, what is
really African, and what is not, often proves, upon
close examination, to be a universal phenomenon.
Furthermore, it should be pointed out right from the
beginning that mystification, ceremony and ritual are
not characteristically traditional as opposed to
modern; nor are they peculiarly African as opposed to
European. In Europe and the West in general, just as
anywhere else, the realms of religion, morals and politics remain strongholds of irrationality. Even Western
scientists convinced of the universal reign of law in
natural phenomena, may pray to a suernatural being for
rain and a good harvest (Wiredu 1980:42).

When a modern, western educated African or European presides in a High Court, he wears a wig and other
uncommon garments. Truly speaking, these do not add
anything to his knowledge or ability to make a rational
judgement. They belong to the realm of legal mystification, not so much because they are traditional to the
Courts of law, but because they have no rational connection to the abilities of men to achieve harmony in
human relations by the method of objective investigation. Similarly, modern University ceremonies are not
despised because they involve elaborate ritual which
has no objective relationship to the achievements,
knowledge or abilities of their participants. The
truth is that mystification is not the preserve of
traditional societies or a peculiarity of the African -
just as rational knowledge is not the preserve of the
modern West. The conquest of the religious, moral and

political spheres by the spirit of rational inquiry
remains a thing of the future, even in the West. Even
if certain ceremonies are peculiarly African, ceremonial pomp and mystification is not in any intrinsic,
inseparable sense, African. But a comparison of
African traditional thought and Western traditional
thought is still not possible until anthropologists
first learn in the same detail about the folk thought
of their own peoples as they have those of Africans.
Such comparisons may well turn out to hold less exotic
excitement for the anthropologist than present practice
would suggest. Without fair comparison, Westerners and
Africans alike, will continue to go about with an exag-
gerated notion of the differences in nature between
Africans and the people of the West.
     In other parts of the world, if you want to know
the "philosophy" of a given people, you do not go to
aged, illiterate peasants, but to the individual
thinkers in person or in print.

> "A reference to British philosophy is unlikely to
> be interpreted as alluding to the communal
> weltanschauung of say, British rural communities.
> Indeed, even when one speaks of traditional
> British philosophy, this will be taken not in an
> anthropological sense, but to refer to the line of
> British empiricists stemming from Bacon. On the
> other hand, African philosophy is usually taken in
> the sense of the traditional folk thought of
> Africa" (Wiredu 1980: 37).

     Since most knowledge about Africans has been of
this kind, even the African of today, motivated by a
genuine desire to preserve the indigenous culture of
his people, must contend with the fact that the traditional, non-literate character of his culture has been
for a long time contrasted with the culture of the
literary Bacons and Newtons, and not with its European
non-literate traditional counterpart. The result has
been an image of African traditions which does not meet
the criteria of modern science based thought.
     African medicine conjures images of witchcraft,
sorcery and superstition. The fact that there are
numbers of white men in London today who proudly proclaim themselves to be witches, does not suggest to the
African that witchcraft is a widespread European phe-
nomemon. Wiredu (1980: 42) notes that if they read,
for example, Trevor Roper's historical essay on
"Witches and Witchcraft", they might come to doubt
whether witchcraft in Africa has ever attained the
heights to which it reached in Europe in the sixteenth
and seventeenth centuries. Similarly, an African
visiting America might participate in, or observe, the

large scale celebration of Halloween and even import it
to his homeland without seriusly connecting Halloween
with witchcraft. Even if he did, he would customarily
not, by the same token, take note that similar celebrations associated with witches, even on a small scale,
are not known in his home country. He will continue to
believe that more so than anywhere, the African child
is reared in a world where ghosts are more real than
men, a world in the control of spirits of the dead, and
where magical conceptions and magical causations are
the only facts of his knowledge.
     But the belief that sickness is supposed to be
caused by the action of ancestral spirits or fabulous
monsters, and that the pleasure or anger of the spirits
are the causes of all diseases, famine, death, etc., is
not a monopoly of Africa. Europeans, however, have
made it appear that their own people never believed and
practiced these things; yet it is not rare to find a
woman living in the country plains of modern England,
who for her after birth pains, takes horse dung in wine
without a prescription from a doctor (Kalulu 1977: 5).
A play reflection of what people believed in is well
illustrated by the Witches of Macbeth, who knew full
well the potency of a nauseous mixture:

> "Fillet of penny, snake in the cauldron, boil and
> bake. Eye of newt, the toes of a frog, wool of a
> bat and tongue of a dog, adder's fork and blind
> worm's sting, lizard's leg and howlet's wing. For
> a charm of powerful trouble, like a hell-brogh
> boil and bubble. Scale of dragon, teeth of wolf,
> witch's mummy, maw and gulf of the ravined salt-
> sea shark, root of hemlock dugg'd in the dark,
> liver of blaspheming Jew, gall of goat and slips
> of yew, silvered in the moon's eclipse. Nose of
> Turk and Tartar's lips, finger of birth-strangled
> babe, ditch delivered by a drab, make gruel thick
> and slab, add thereto a tiger's chaudron from the
> ingredients of our cauldron, cool it with a
> baboon's blood, then the charm is firm and good"
> (Kalulu 1977: 6).

Despite the apparent similarities in folk beliefs,
African custom were attacked by Europeanan missionaries
who were concerned, according to Moffat (1869:235), to
sweep away refuges of lies, prostate idols and altars
in the dust, abolish rites and ceremonies, and trans-
form babarous and antiquated judicial systems, and,
after apostolic example, "turn the world upside down".

The Main Challenge To Tswana Medicine

In order to comprehend the dilemman of Tswana
traditional medicine it is important to put it in a
wider, global context, rather than do a microscopic
analysis of a system which in reality exists as part of
and has been influenced by a much wider worldwide
context. Developments in nineteenth century European
society are especially relevant to an understanding of
Tswana healing strategies. For one thing, British
medicine was technically not far removed from Tswana
medicine, yet this did not encourage a belief by Europeans that there were more similarities than differences between the two. The supposed inherent inferiority of "natives" and their medical system was not being
subjected to empirical tests, but rather, more than
being taken for granted, it was ideologically popularized as part of a larger strategy to change African
society and to replace African ways with European ways.

Tswana healing strategies were, in the nineteenth
century, shaped by an historical environment which
proved hostile to African customs and (though somewhat
reluctantly and hypocritically), to communal traditional institutions in general. To be sure, missionaries preached a message of brotherhood and love for
mankind. Nevertheless, they systematically crushed
Tswana customs and the authority of the Tswana doctors
and took over their highest positions as advisors to
the political leadership, mainly because Tswana doctors
were a major, ideological, moral, and political force,
capable of inducing collective rejection and influence
against missionaries and their overall goal of cultural
imperialism and domination.

Long before colonialism, the Christian missionaries were the pioneers of western cultural penetration
in Botswana, and they set a foundation as well as a
support system for later European involvement in Botswana. Missionaries soon labled all traditional doctors
as witches and wizards, and the more acceptable among
them were called "witchdoctors". They were generally
regarded as part of the dark evil and mainly nocturnal
world, and their elimination was regarded consistent
with the spreading of the "light", and the saving of
the lost heathens in the "dark interior". One of the
major aims of Christianity was to stamp out all traditional Tswana customs. Christianity was presented as
the only true religion and any other doctrines were
considered misguided, if not inspired by the devil
himself.

The spread of Christianity was ethnocentrically
conceived to be a British prerogative and the London
Missionary Society had the monopoly over the spheres of
influence. Insignificant missionary competition was

present, but this was limited to the Barolong, who were
missionized by the Wesleyan Missionary Society. The
prominence of the London Missionary Society, L.M.S.,
was to a large extent due to the fact that it was the
first British Missionary Society to work among Batswana. The L.M.S. missionaries, who did not represent a
particular church, acted, first and foremost, as British agents, rather than proponents of a formally established church doctrine. Since the L.M.S. was founded
as an interdenominational religious organization, its
resource base and support system at home was more
national than religious and denominational. According
to Gelfand (1957), one of its popular missionaries to
the Batswana, David Livingstone, for example, believed
that the British people were the most suitable to be
entrusted with the conversion of the African heathen.

Just as Berman (1975) suggests, many of the early
explorers embellished their accounts to increase book
sales. The missionaries, on the other hand, distorted
the image of Africa in order to win the support of home
parishioners for overseas work. The darker the picture
of Africa, the more necessary the work of the missionaries. Furthermore, the ethnocentric belief in the
innate inferiority of Africans, coupled with the belief
that Satan was at work among the natives, convinced the
L.M.S. missionaries that they would have little difficulty persuading Africans of the superiority of the
Christian gospel and European ways of life.

Europeans supported the missionaries yet, they
themselves, lived in a period when religion was
questioned and when the tenents of the doctrine that
"science equals progress" were being formulated. It
was not the teachings of Luther or Calvin, encapsulated
in the Protestant ethnic which mattered in Europe, but
rather the belief, not just in reason and the natural,
but in science and its wonders, that would lead to
civilization, modernization, and progress. With the
institutionalization of this doctrine, it appeared that
there was little that science could produce that would
not be of benefit to the larger society.

Progress in all fields, including health care
delivery, was soon to be firmly associated with progress in scientific knowledge and the improvement of
health was taken to be the result of the application of
science and technology. Little was made of the fact
that by the time medical science had really come of its
own and medical technology had applied the scientific
discoveries, most of the improvement in the health of
peoples in European countries had already taken place.
The decline in the death rate in England that began in
the mid-eighteenth century, was little affected by
medical measures. Turshen (1975) argues that the nineteenth century decline was probably most influenced by

rising standards of living, especially improved diet.
All the same, it is significant to note that major
improvements in health have occurred without capital
intensive sophisticated medical technology in Europe.
Similarly, improvement in the health status of Africans
was never contingent upon the development of sophisticated medical services and did not, and does not,
depend on the westernization of Africans by European
agents.

Livingstone was impressed by the comparatively few
diseases present among the Tswana. He treated only one
case of tuberculosis and observed that venereal disease, although it had already reached the Batswana,
seemed to him incapable of permanence in any form in
persons of pure African blood anywhere in the center of
the country (Seeley 1973:81). The diseases most prevalent were those promoted by sudden changes of temper-
ature, which became rare as people adopted European
dress - not medicines. Other ailments were more severe
just before the rains, again confirming the significance of weather on morbidity.

Despite these observations, the missionary, like
the contemporary health education worker in Botswana,
as elsewhere, attempted, with great success, to alter
African traditional ways by demonstrating the advantages of European ways. The decision that the African
system was "wrong" had already been made. By definition, what the missionary had to offer was deemed
better than that which already existed. Development
and progress was seen as the process of change toward
those types of social, economic and political systems
that had developed in Western Europe. The development
of medical services was evaluated by their proximity to
institutions and values of Western societies. Traditional medicine was despised in part because the
admission that it was similar to British medicine would
have run counter to the imperial ideology that Victo-
rian civilization was the acme of human development.
Besides, Africans were simply regarded as primitive,
unenlightened, barbarian pagan heathens. Their medicine could only be labelled "witchcraft", or African
"Black Magic". As we shall see, the missionaries
rejected traditional medicine because it was also in
direct competition with the faith they wished to propa-
gate.

European Medicine In The 19th Century

From 1775, when the L.M.S. was established,
medical effort was not perceived as constituting a
significant aspect in christian teaching (Mushingeh
1982: 94). In Britain, the knowledge of "tropical diseases" hardly existed and any idea of the role played

by such insects as mosquitoes, tampans and tsetse flies
on the transmission of disease, was not yet conceived.
At the time when Moffat commenced his missionary work
at Griqua Town (Kuruman), Southern Africa had only one
L.M.S. medical doctor, Van der Kempt, who practiced at
Bethelsdorp in South Africa. From 1820 to 1840, Kuruman had no trained medical or nursing missionary.
Realizing that they would be working in isolation and
far from medical skill, Moffat and his colleagues were
compelled to learn whatever medical remedies they
thought might be of assistance to them. As a result,
they only learnt the more simple medical treatments,
mainly for personal use at the mission station. Medical treatment and care for the sick was not yet an
important part of missionary work. The L.M.S. Headquarters in London did not yet realize the importance
of medicine for the missionaries' struggle to spread
their religion. European medicine, which the missionaries originally intended to keep for themselves, was
only extended to Africans as an inducement to accept
Christianity, after years of personal efforts to
evangelize had failed.

     Despite their opposition to Christianity, Batswana
readily accepted missionary medicine in part because of
the similarities between their own healing strategies
and those of the missionaries. Secondly, they believed
that the missionaries possessed similar powers as their
own doctors. In addition, the Tswana belief that a
foreign doctor or one from distant lands might possess
special healing powers, led them to experiment with and
allow strangers as doctors in their midst. Furthermore, having been used to their own medicines, they
wanted to try something new with the hope that it was
more potent. Seeley (1973: 75) points out that every
one of the L.M.S. missionaries gave medical assistance
in some form or another to the tribe with whom they
came into contact. But the medicine they practised was
far removed from medicine as it is known in the Western
world today, and did not even meet the standards of
nineteenth century British medicine - primarily because
the practitioners, i.e. missionaries, traders, and so
called travellers, were simply not doctors.

     The missionaries, with the exception of the
qualified Livingstone, were men of humble background
and little education. The medical profession itself
did not exist, since the current organisation of the
medical profession in England emerged only after the
Industrial Revolution. Turshen (175) notes that at the
beginning of the nineteenth century, there was little
differentiation within British medicine beyond gross
class distinctions, with upper class born physicians on
top and barber surgeons and apothecaries, who were less
qualified, serving the middle and lower classes.

Overall, British medicine in the nineteenth century was a little more than a fairly sophisticated folk system (Dennis 1978: 57). Technically, there was little difference between missionary medicine and Tswana medicine. Both were based on the ministration of herbal remedies, accompanied by a limited knowledge of surgical technique. In addition, the missionaries' claimed that their healing powers came from their God, just as Tswana doctors claimed that their healing powers came from Modimo (God). Formalized medical training was available at Oxford and Cambridge as well as in the Scottish Universities and some hospitals to which Medical Schools were attached. Nevertheless, training involved little more than a period of apprenticeship to become an established doctor (Seeley 1973). This system of training was substantially not different from the apprentice system which the Tswana doctors were already accustomed to.

During the course of the Industrial Revolution, however, scientific knowledge grew and was applied to medical practice. Specialization began to appear and there was a tug-of-war for patients between physicians and general practitioners. Physicians and surgeons took over the voluntary hospitals and general practitioners, unionized in the British Medical Association, remained in the community to serve an increasingly middle class clientele (Turshen 1975).

Before the Medical Act of 1958, which provided a national register of regular practitioners and a central Council to examine all those applying for licence, most British doctors did not have formal qualifications (Seeley 173). This fact, however, did not present any serious barrier to those who chose to practice as doctors, and it was estimated that only one third of practitioners in Britain possessed formal qualifications of any kind.

It is worth emphasizing that, when Livingstone qualified in 1840, and went to settle for some thirteen years among the Tswana, British medicine was far from medicine as we know it today. Gelfand (175) points out that the study of biochemistry had hardly begun. Although the microscopic study of living tissues had commenced with the introduction of the archromatic lenses in 1920, selective strains were not employed until the latter part of the nineteenth century. At this point, knowledge of the causes of disease was still highly speculative.

Like the unqualified Moffat, Smith and some of the travellers, hunters and traders before him, Livingstone, with a licence of the College of Physicians and Surgeons from Glasgow, used the method of bleeding the affected parts of the patients in many of his treatments. Livingstone's reason for the use of this method

was to relieve what he believed to be congestion and
irregular distribution of the blood (Mushingeh 1972:
110). In Tswana medicine, there was a belief that illness was caused by "bad blood", "dirty blood", "thin
blood", thick blood", or foreign objects in the blood.
Cupping was often used to remove quantities of blood
and the supposed causative agents in the blood. Persons with "good blood" were often not only said to be
healthy, but were also regarded as favourably well
disposed to fortune.

Despite their well documented arrogance towards
Tswana medicine, missionaries sometimes sought medical
help from African doctors, owing to the insignificant
nature of their medical facilities. Mushingeh
(1982:101) notes that when Smith arrived at Kuruman in
1835, he found Moffat waiting for an African woman
doctor, reputed in the art of cupping, to come and
treat his wife who was suffering from both post-natal
sickness and migraine. Thus, when illness hit among
the missionaries, the question of their superior ways
was often forgotten. They displayed the same desparate
health seeking behaviour as the Africans. Their concern then, was with basic survival than with ethnocentric arrogance. Africans were no different in this
regard. Many of them came to Smith for treatment of
Kwatsi (anthrax), and smallpox. His treatment included
bleeding the patients.

"After bleeding one or two... almost the whole
kraal made application to have the same operation
performed. One man had a pain in his loins and he
was very anxious to have the blood taken from his
foot. ...Mr. Moffat informs me that he has been
permitted time after time to bleed them, and with
him they showed the same desire to lose great
quantities" (Mushingeh 1982:98).

European medicine was sought in addition to,
rather than instead of, Tswana medicine. Similarly,
Tswana medicine was sought by Europeans. Livingstone's
friendship with many African doctors helped him to
learn about the insights of African strategies in
dealing with illness. In typical European fashion,
however, Livingstone's motivation was not so much as to
use African medicine as it was to check its credibility. Although he knew that African medicines worked,
the assumption that they were inferior led him to seek
ways of improving them. But the fact that he was even
willing to build on African medicine indicates that he
was aware of the insufficiency or inadequacy of his own
medicines. Thus, rather than waging an outright war
against African doctors, he was willing to work with,
and learn from them. He knew that the African doctor,

like doctors everywhere, had an assymetrical relationship with respect to other members of society. Because
they possessed knowledge of relieving suffering, they
were held in high esteem and possessed powers to control the ordinary citizen, as well as the leadership.

Because of the technical similarity between Tswana
medicine and European medicine, practitioners from both
sides often worked together. When in 1859 Thomas
Baines, for instance, visited the brother of Chief
Khama III, Kgamane, to treat his eight-year old son who
had sore eyes, Baines was assisted by a local Tswana
nurse (Mushingeh 1982). There was more interdepen-
dency than the often assumed African dependency on
European medicine. With regard to snake bites, for
example, Europeans for a long time depended on African
remedies. At least for fifty years, missionaries and
other Europeans proved unhelpful to African victims of
snakebites. The situation only changed in the 1950's
when Charles Croft of Grahamstown in the Cape, successfully developed "Crofts Tincture of Life", as an
effective cure of snakebites (Mushingeh 1982:118).

Many fundamental ingredients of western medicine,
as we know it today, were still not known in Britain,
and those that were known, were still not yet marketable on a large scale. Surgery was, in the first half
of the nineteenth century, characterized by the performance of many daring operations, executed with
astonishing speed necessitated by the lack of anesthe-
tics. Ether was introduced two years after Livingstone
qualified and chloroform appeared five years later
(Gelfand 1957: 2-3). Gelfand notes that the discovery
and application of anticeptics (carbolic acid spray)
was not to take place for twenty-five years after
Livingstone graduated. Even the part played by insects
in the transmission of disease was not yet conceived.
One of the few firmly established facts, was the knowledge, since William Harvey's (1578-1657) discovery,
that blood circulated in the body (Burrows 1957: 18).
This may have accounted for the Europeans belief in
bleeding their patients.

The introduction of ether in 1842, and of chloroform in 1847, opened the way for advances and developments in surgical techniques, and in 1848, the first
appendectomy was performed (Seeley 1973: 76). Seeley
points out that, although the introduction of general
anesthethics alleviated much suffering on the part of
the patient, it indirectly increased mortality because
of the resultant post-operative infections, for it was
not until 1864 that Lister discovered and developed
antiseptics. Pathology was at a speculative stage and
though, as an increasing number of diseases were specified and differentiated, it became possible to seek for
causative factors, the aetiology of disease was a sub-

ject of much controversy. The study of cellular pathology was not published until 1858 by Virchow, and the
foundations of bacteriology were laid by Pasteur and
Koch in the 1870's. The relationship between insects
and transmission of disease was not conceived until
1898 for malaria, and 1902 for yellow fever. The
causes of disease was still a subject of serious debate
and speculation.

"Some favoured the belief that disease resulted
from the inhilation of noxious miasmas, some
supported the contagion theory, and others
elaborated a monistic pathology in terms of simple
or uncomplicated gastroenteritis. The widespread
support of the last theory accounts for the
popularity of tHe application leeches for the
bleeding of the head or abdominal wall in an
attempt to cure or prevent gastroenteritis"
(Seeley, 1973: 76).

Livingstone believed that the heavy menstrual discharge
of African women accounted for their lower mortality
from malaria, whose source he, and John Mackenzie,
attributed to "marshy miasmata", as it provided a means
by which the poison could be carried out of the system
(Seeley 1973: 80). Thus, the early missionaries, many
of whom had little formal education let alone medical
training, and being men with no skill other than that
which they had developed by common sense and experience, suffered very much, not only from a variety of
diseases, ranging from fever, eye diseases and
dysentery, but also from great ignorance of medicine.
Their success was more a product of cultural arrogance
than pure scientific, and, by implication, superior
knowledge. In addition, they were hampered by
competing theories of diseases as much as by lack of
medical instruments. Those medical instruments which
were being developed in the nineteenth century, were
still not firmly established as part of the usual
medical bag.

Livingstone's Surgical Instruments	
Thermometer	scapels
tourniquet	artery forceps
trephines	spatual
probes	surgical needles
forceps	knives
lion forceps	bone saws
dental forceps	ligature silk
tooth extractor	tissue forceps

```
     umbilical scissors              curetts
     surgical scissors               catheter
                                     catheter introducers
Source:   Seeley 1973:80
```

The stethescope was introduced in 1817, but was not
universally accepted and employed for some time.
Gelfand (1957:24) noted that Livingstone, who is reputed to be one of the first doctors to use the clinical
thermometer, nearly failed his qualifying examinations
as a doctor at Glasgow because of his support of the
stethescope whose usefulness his examiners doubted.
Seeley (1973) notes that the President of the Royal
College of Physicians was aware of the great gap in the
then knowledge of therapy.   While it was reasonably
well known what doctors were dealing with most of the
time, they did not know so well how to deal with it.
Symptoms, not causes, were treated and few specifics
were available.   The ingredients of medicines were
mainly herbal.   In the light of this, Seeley (1973),
concludes that it was with some justification that the
TIMES, on April 3rd, 1856, remarked that: "The President of the College of Physicians is nearly on a level
with the nearest herbalist".
     The above increases the strength of our argument
that there was little difference between Tswana medicine and British medicine in the nineteenth century.
British medicine was not based on purely scientific
principles and consequently was not in conflict with
tradition.   It was at an experimental and speculative
stage, and its basic tenets were surrounded by
conflicting and contradictory theories and opinions.
Tswana medicine was experimental to a certain extent in
that it was able to admit of and allow foreign methods
of treatment from non-Tswana practitioners, yet at the
same time, was supported by a coherent and circumscribed traditional philosophy relating to the causation and
treatment of illness.   The Christian rationale which
accompanied the medical practice of the missionaries,
corresponded closely to the integrated nature of Tswana
religion and medicine.   This contributed to the
Tswana's recognition of missionary medicine and their
ascribing to the missionary the title and role of Ngaka
(doctor).
     One area of technical similarity between Tswana
medicine and British medicine was in the art of innoculation against smallpox.   Livingstone seems to have
been the first missionary to acknowledge and report on
the Tswana practice of innoculation, having seen it for
the first time among the Bakwena in 1845.   The process
involved the transfer of smallpox virus from infected
to uninfected persons.   The virus was mixed with other
medical compounds to make it more effective.   He noted

that for a long time before he came to Botswana,
innoculation was popular among Barolong, Bahurutshe,
Bangwaketse, Bakwena and Bangwato; among whom it was
done either in the leg, arm or shoulder. Mushingeh
(1982:72) notes that Bangwato doctors innoculated their
patients on the forehead, knee or leg.

   Herbert (1975), however, attributed the presence
of innoculation in Southern Africa to Portuguese
activities at Delagoa Bay. She argues that innoculation might have spread in the interior of Southern
Africa as a result of the trading contacts between the
Portugueses and the Tswana. Mushingeh (1982), on the
other hand, aruges that the basic problem with
Herbert's argument is that it exaggerates the nature of
the trading contacts between the Tswana and the Portugueses. He notes that in the first half of the nineteenth century, Shaka's monoploy of trade with the east
coast reduced any chances of trading contacts between
the Twsana and the Portuguese. The Twsana communities
in the hinterland were unaffected by the traffic of
whites who travelled between Europe and the Orient.
What is more, Portuguese innoculation was done in the
arms, while that of the Tswana ranged from leg to forehead, and in gerneral, there were no similarities in
the preparation of the medicines. Finally, Chapman
(1968) notes that Livingstone saw innoculation as one
of the most important local innovations and he defended
it throughut his career. The decline in use and popularity with innoculations among Batswana, increased
with age, as the older members of the community progressively considered themselves immune from earlier
attacks. Smallpox Sekgwaripane, was said to attack
young people. Adults believed that they were immune,
and therefore, if it reoccurred, it would kill if
"intended" to kill. To cure Sekgwaripane involved
introducing the disease in a patient and local innoculation had helped to reduce epidemics. But with age,
both local and European forms of innoculation were
resisted by adults. During the 1862 outbreak of smallpox at Shoshong, Mackenzie found that local innoculation, as well as his methods, were to some degree
resisted by the people (Mackenzie 1971).

Comparative Medical Training and Knowledge

   If Tswana doctors were, accordig to modern western
criteria of judgement, not trained and therefore not
qualified, so were more than 90 per cent of the Europeans who came to assume, with impunity, the Tswana title
of Ngaka. Rather than being alarmed or annoyed by the
title, missionaries enjoyed an profited from the obviously false title. unlike the missionaries, however,
Tswana doctors were, like British doctors, products of

some apprenticeship under an established doctor. What
is more, Tswana apprenticeship was often a much longer
period than that of their British counterparts. The
Tswana doctor was more often than not born into a
family of doctors and learnt his trade throughout his
youth and most of his adult life. He therefore had a
much more internalized knowledge of his profession.

The training of doctors in other European countries was in the nineteenth century, not anywhere
similar to what we know today. In Holland, only the
physicians graduated from a University. The surgeon
was a product of the guilds. The Physician or doctors
received no practical training during their three year
course; this had to be obtained in postgraduate work
(Burrows 1957: 19). The surgeons on the other hand,
were reared in the hard, practical school of experience, by apprenticeships to established doctors, among
whom the Dutch East India Company chose its medical
men.

The seventeenth century had seen the relocating of
the educational center of medicine from the Mediterranean to Leyden. The information had rendered the French
and Italian schools less popular and non-Catholics were
being excluded from Italian universities by Papal
decree. Since Leyden's doors were open to all students
and the lectures held in Latin, it drew an international class to its portals. But the ancient beliefs died
slowly and, as Burrows (1957) points out, the leading
surgeon in England believed in the Royal Touch for cure
of scrofula ("surgical" tuberculosis).

In the United States, any man or woman with an
elementary education could become a doctor by taking a
course for a winter or two, and passing an examination.
Even as late as 1900, there were many medical students
who could not have gained entrance to a good liberal
arts college (Mechanic 1978:317). Mechanic notes that
it was not until Osler and Welch formed their group at
Johns Hopkins in the 1890's that there was any development in the United States of which foreigners took
note. Medicine was largely a private practice, similar
to that found among nineteenth century Tswana doctors.
Medicine was not institutionalized, and even at the
time when the first hospital was established in
Philadelphia in 1751, it was set up under voluntary
auspices and was privately run.

Like in Tswana society, beliefs about illness was
largely governed by religion and morality. Rosenberg
(1962:40) notes that during the cholera years 1832,
1849 and 1866, many ordinary Americans believed that
cholera was a consequence of sin; man had infringed
upon the laws of God, and cholera was an inevitable and
inescapable judgement. Medical opinion was unanimous
that cholera was a scourage, not of mankind, but of the

sinner; the intemperate, the imprudent and the filthy,
were particularly vulnerable. Knowledgeable Americans
were convinced that only those of irregular habits had
anything to fear from the desease:

> "It was clear, proclaimed the Governor of New
> York, that an infinitely wise and just God (had)
> seen fit to employ pestilence as one means of
> scourging the human race from their sins, and it
> (seemed) to be an appropriate one for the sins of
> uncleanliness and intemperance" (Rosenberg, 1962:
> 41).

It was believed that a few days of moderation
could scarcely undo the physical ravages of a life time
given over to drink and gluttony. Sexual excess as
well, left its devotees weakened and, "artificially
stimulated"; their systems defenceless against cholera.
Whenever any person of substance died of cholera, it
was an immediate cause of consternation, a consternation invariably allayed by reports that this ordinarily
praiseworthy man either had some secret vice, or else
had indulged in some unwanted excess. Cholera, the
flood and the plague of locusts, were temporal means by
which the Lord achieved the world's moral purification.
Overall, the major contribution of American traditionalism to health, was the sanitary and hygienic regula-
tions that it had helped to institute. Such laws were
worth more to Americans than it is customary to acknowledge. Similar sanitary and preventative public health
measures were prevalent in African traditionalism.
Because African doctors had general control over their
social systems, their influence over basic social
conditions was profound. General social conditions are
especially important in the study of medicine, because
they have greater impact on disease and mortality than
do therapeutic practices. Feierman (1983) notes that
in the years before colonial conquest, African healers
from across the continent and the political leaders
with whom they were allied, had a much wider range of
control over the social conditions of health than they
have had ever since. In a study of pre-conquest Asante, Maier (1979) has shown the importance of street
cleaning, careful maintenance of latrines and variola-
tion for smallpox, along with the organisation of healers under the stool of the Asantehene's doctor. In
Malawi, traditional doctors at times, compelled people
to plant particular crops, and restricted fishing and
grazing so as to protect fragile resources (Schoffeleers, 1978). Thus, traditional practice helped to
balance the eco system. Ford (1971, 1979) noted that
Chief Mzila understood the ecological relationship
between tsetse fly, trypanosomiasis or sleeping sick-

ness, and vegetation cover. He compelled his followers
to draw near the King in concentrated settlements in
order to establish a tsetse free zone, and ordered the
establishment of a game reserve outside which all wild
animals (as trypanosomiasis hots) were hunted. Feierman (1982) also noted how healers of the Shambaa
Kingdom in the Usambara Mountains, in cooperation with
Chiefs and local elders, controlled a wide range of
basic health conditions. They coordinated the cleaning
of irrigation ditches and the distribution of water,
with thousands of hectares under irrigation. Local
people, with the advice of traditional doctors, chose
village sites in high locations to keep them free of
insect pests and diseases. This is how Moshoeshoe and
the people of Lesotho lived.
        In Botswana, despite the flatness of the country,
villages were placed on higher altitudes. A vivid
example of this settlement pattern is to be seen in
Kanye, where, like in other villages, the tribal headquarters are at the strategic ko ntsweng (at the hill
top). Kanye is a significant example because, even at
the turn of the century, Europeans believed it to be
the healthiest spot in the Bechuanaland Protectorate,
where weakly officers could be taken for recovery.
        Africans understood that mosquitoes caused malaria
and tried to avoid long stays in the mosquito-infested
lowlands. People who, according to African tradition,
were regarded as impure or afflicted by an uncommon
disease, were isolated from the rest of the community,
either by sending them out of a village, or by
restricting them to one home or hut. Among the Shambaa
(Feierman 1983), the Kungwi - a traditional instructor
who had been initiated and had survived smallpox - was
regarded as safe and immune, and could carry food and
drink to the afflicted. Feierman (1983 notes that in
fact, anyone who had already suffered smallpox was
called a kungwi, and therefore could carry food to the
sick.

Tswana Medicine in the Missionary Context
        At first, European medicine did not threaten
Tswana medical practice. Tswana doctors, Dingaka tsa
Setswana, were well accustomed to the presence of rival
dingaka from other African groups. To increase their
medical repertoire, dingaka also apprenticed themselves
to their professional equivalents from non-Setswana
tribes, thus acquiring new and foreign skills. Europeans, and the missionaries in particular, only augmented
their numbers, presenting no immediate threat to the
local practice of the indigenous healers. Seeley
(1973) argues that the basic electicism of Tswana
medical beliefs and the pragmatic attitude which was
taken towards the seeking of treatment, allowed the

AFRICAN HEALING STRATEGIES

missionaries to be assimilated into the ranks of the
dingaka at the local level, without invalidating the
indigeous healers in the eyes of the people, or depriv-
ing them of their power and influence. By assuming the
role of ngaka, missionaries operated within the traditional Tswana medical system. Their new or different
methods provided additional alternative treatments, and
not something to replace Tswana medicine.

Among the Tswana, the average ngaka doctor was not
distinguised from other citizens. His ability to treat
disease did not isolate him from the rest of society.
Mushingeh (1983) notes that the art of healing was not
a symbol of specialization. When not engaged in healing activities, the ngaka led exactly the same life as
the other members of his community. He cultivated,
built up his hut and looked after his cattle with members of his family in customary fashion. The amount of
time the ngaka spent on his healing activities largely
depended upon the nature and extent of disease referred
to him by the affected families. On the average, however, the ngaka had a fair amount of spare time on his
side to perform other social functions.

The degree of respect accorded to a ngaka by his
community depended largely on his professional skill
and success in the treatment of disease. Through his
skill, the ngaka exercised authority and influence over
others, but only in the sphere of treating disease, an
area which many people had some general knowledge. The
main difference between most adults and the ngaka was
that, unlike other members of the community, the ngaka
was known to be specially trained.

"The instruction is called 'teaching to dig',
because most medicines and charms are obtained
from plants which are dug up in the fields... So
the Bechuana lecturer takes his pupil or pupils
with him to the open country one day, and to the
mountains the next, and shows him where the
healing plants are to be found. In the course of
time, he communicates to his pupil all his
knowledge" (Mackenzie 1971:381).

The training of a ngaka involved long and close
observation. Because of the length of training,
apprentices were usually members of the family who, in
addition to learning medicine, were taught other family
responsibilities. By attending consultancies in which
his mentor was told many confessions and confidential
information by clients, the apprentice, from an early
age, learnt all the "secrets" of his community. He
grew up not only knowing ailments of families in the
community, but the various social, economic and other
hardships of most of his fellow villagers. The young

ngaka learnt to guard the secrets of his clients and by being a walking bank of the community's sensitive information, he also learnt to be diplomatic and professional. At the same time, the knowledge possessed of his people, raised his status and prestige. Because of the sensitive and privileged nature of this profession, permission of the village leaders, including the Chief and household heads, had to be granted before training as a ngaka could begin. The real difference between a ngaka and his fellow citizens was in the degree of exposure and experience with medicine. Another feature of the ngaka was his ability to throw bones, go thela bola, commonly referred to as to divine or diagnose. But it was possible for one to be a "diviner" without necessarily being a ngaka and vice versa. Those doctors who did not "divine", diagnosed patients by taking their medical history from members of the family or directly from the patient, or by "guessing" the disease on the basis of the patient's appearance.

Divination by the use of ditaola (bones) was especially employed when unusual diseases or deaths were confronted. Campbell (1968:9) notes that ditaola were employed by a large proportion of the population at all moments of crisis or decision, particularly to seek the cause of inexplicable occurances, or sickness, or to determine the right steps to be taken to bring a doubtful issue to a successful conclusion. They were used for the purpose of making a difficult judgement or prediction where no hard evidence or testimony existed or was difficult to obtain. Their use was not a secretive matter to be understood only by those with special gifts, such as that of interpreting the supernatural. Most old men, though not "diviners", knew the names of the bones, what they represented and could interpret many of the throws. As amateurs, however, they were unable to give a comprehensive picture, having only a rudimentary knowledge.

The use of ditaola is likely to increase rather than decrease during times of rapid social and economic change, which are often times of great uncertainty. At all events which happened to disrupt the community, such as war-time, drought, relocating in a new village, etc. ditaola, and those dingaka that had built a good reputation using ditaola, were sought.

However, the use of ditaola, while commonly associated with traditional Tswana doctors, is not an essential or necessary feature in the traditional context of treating patients. Ditaola belong more to the religious side of Tswana custom than to indigenous medical practice. Their use follows from the religious attribution of illness, death or misfortune, to the supernatural. This is not a peculiary Tswana or Afri-

can phenomenon. Campbell (1968) argues that at times
of stress and uncertainty, people turn to some form of
support, particularly religion, which offers spiritual
security. Religion also helps to present a world view
which is consistent with peoples' beliefs. An illumi-
nating comparison would be to see in what different
ways the belief in the supernatural is employed by
various peoples in an attempt to achieve a coherent
view of the world, especially in times of stress. In
such specific differences will consist the real
peculiarities of African traditional thought in contra-
distinction to, say, European traditional thought.

The religious interpretation of illness, death and
misfortune, via ditaola, did not mean that these
phenomena were never accepted as natural events and
only attributed to the supernatural intervention of
some external agent by Batswana. The employment of
herbs and the administering of natural remedies for
illnesses, are a clear indication of the rational or
naturalist conception of illness. Indeed, no society
could survive for any length of time without basing a
large part of its daily activities on beliefs derived
from empirical evidence. The association of Tswana
medicine with ditaola and divination is, in part, a
result, more of stereotyping than of careful study.
Part of the problem may be attributed to intellectual
laziness and a general disrespect for the so called
traditional culture. Part of the problem is due to the
self protective mystification associated with all
marketable professions. And, no doubt, Tswana medicine
is indeed marketable.

Strickly speaking, there is no mystery in ditaola.
Go laola, to control, to command or give orders,
essentially refers to a diffuse prophetic lawlike
prediction or judgement, which renders its subject
consciously or unconsciously committed to obeying the
principle of the command to expect the outcome of the
taolo. It is essentially a religious rather than a
medical prediction or judgement.

In Tswana tradition, go laola is an ability which
comes from Modimo (God), or badimo (ancestors). Dennis
(1978:55) notes that the legitmate bone-thrower acknow-
ledges that his powers of "divination" come from modimo
(God), and that it was the badimo (ancestors) of the
ngaka (doctor) who spoke through the bones. Similarily, Brown (1926:122) notes that both the bone-thrower
and herbalist alike believe that their ability to heal
emanated from modimo, who gives them blessing to work
so that their "doctoring" is helpful to mankind.

Although the bones are commonly associated with
diagnosis, in reality, they are called upon more for
non-diagnostic, religious and ceremonial purposes. A
bone-thrower might be consulted to ascertain prospects

of a journey or a marriage, the whereabouts of missing
cattle, or before building a new hut or tribal court.
The correctness of the bone-throwers judgement was, to
a large extent, based on his extensive knowledge of his
community and the many secrets of each family and
individuals in the community. At the national level,
the Chief would invariably seek the advice of royal
bone-throwers, dingaka tsa morafhe, before holding a
tribal ceremony; before entering into battle; or before
selecting the site of a new capital (Dennis 1978). Few
decisions were taken by the Chief without consulting
his dingaka. Surely these dingaka were not in any
sense performing medical duties. They were, so to
speak, doctors of political, religious and cultural
affairs. They were the leading intellectuals who acted
as consultants for personal, as well as national,
affairs. If they made a poor policy, they could be
punished by the Chief. Dingaka carried a heavy responsibility, especially those among them who acted as
prophets for their society by foretelling the outcomes
of a seemingly complex future.

The Chief was head of the dingaka and as such was
the ngaka supreme of the tribe. Certainly this did not
mean that he could cure any diseases as such, yet he
possessed tshitlho, or "medicine" believed to secure
protection for the tribe and combat hostile influences.
The Chief's tshitlho was contained in two horns: (1)
Lenaka la bogosi (the horn of Chiefship); and (2)
Lenaka la ntwa (the horn of warfare). Only the Chief
could possess these horns. Like all symbolic regalia,
the horns "took a life of their own", and gave the
Chief a sort of supernatural or divine right to rule.
If the Chief could assume the title of ngaka when
it was well understood that he possessed no healing
powers or knowledge beyond that which was equitably
distributed among elderly members of his society, it
should not be too far fetched to imagine that any other
persons of authority could, in Tswana tradition, be
given this somewhat honorary title. Furthermore, a
person could be known as a ngaka without necessarily
being a medicine man.

In his role as ngaka paramount, the Chief performed many major national ceremonies, such as rain making,
doctoring of agricultural fields, and fortifying of his
village. In doing so, he acted es a religious leader,
rather than a medical man. To suggest that the Chief
was a rain maker in an objective sense, is, however, a
bit misleading. In Tswana belief, rain is made by God.
Rain making is no more than a prayer for rain. When a
modern African leader, together with his Cabinet, leaders of the community, including foreign diplomats,
gather at the National Stadium, as it were, to perform
a rain making ceremony, it is unlikely for a modern

observer to attribute any real rain making powers to
such a ceremony or people. In fact, such gatherings
are hardly known to be ceremonies, let alone rituals.
Such occasions, strictly speaking, symbolize a
national concern and deep desire for rain, especially
in a country such as Botswana where drought is common-
place. Similarily, when missionaries prayed for rain,
they did not believe themselves to have any power of
their own to cause rain. In all cases, only God
(Modimo) could cause rain. The mystification associated with rain making, therefore, should be understood
correctly as a desperate attempt by communities to deal
with uncertainty and to insure survival.
In all mational ceremonies, Chiefs were, like all
modern leaders the key figures who "blessed" the occasion. The Chief was supported and assisted by dinagka
tsa morafhe and dingaka tsa kgosing (dingaka of the
nation and of the royal court, respectively). In Praying for rain, the Chief was assisted by baroka, usually
referred to as rain makers - but who essentially were
praise-singers, poets, and reciters of oral tradition.
The ceremonial and religious aspects of Tswana
medicine were to be main causes of suspicion as well as
rallying points against Tswana doctors by missionaries
and the colonial government. These were the more
clearly cultural aspects of the Tswana which came under
fire and which were to be scorned by Europeans who
themselves, acknowledged that their healing powers also
came from their God, just as dingaka acknowledged that
their healing powers came from Modimo (God). Although
their emphasis on the efficacy of faith and prayer was
compatible with Tswana integration of religion with all
aspects of life, they set out to stamp out Tswana
religious beliefs. In their place, they introduced
their own - Christianity.
Christianity taught that Jesus Christ died and
that through his death mankind would be saved. The
converted were baptised and could "eat the body of
Christ", as well as "drink His blood". In addition,
the new African Christians were taught that Christ was
the Healer, and by praying to Him, not only would they
be, in a difuse sense, saved from all sin, but would,
in addition, receive good health. Traditional prac-
tises, including indigenous medicine, were alleged to
be pagan, uncivilized and would surely lead people to
eternal damnation and punishment through an everlasting
fire.
The Tswana were taught that their dead ancestors
could not save them. Only the death of Jesus Christ
could, and Jesus was no ancestor. In this and many
other ways, the Tswana were subjected to all sorts of
cultural imperialism, thereby forcing them to despise
and reject their own traditions, which were the results

of many years of experience and practice. Kalulu (1977) argues that this made the African wear a countenance of an inferiority complex that led him to believe that he was a member of a low and sub-human race that could do nothing good in the world.

The missionaries, with their limited knowledge of medicine, could not support their methods of treatment in terms of a rational scientific explanation of either the causation of illness or of the pharmacology of their medicines (Seeley 1973). They condemned the traditional agents of illness and substituted the Christian concepts of divine retribution and the "Will of God". But the attempts of the missionaries to provide a Christian philosophy were seen by the Tswana as being merely a shift of emphasis to a compatible system. There was a close correspondence between the rationale surrounding the act of healing as presented by the missionaries, and that existing within the Tswana belief system. When Livingstone informed the Kwena that, "It was God alone who could make rain", they answered:

"Of course, we know that, and never entertained any other ideas, but it is God who cures diseases too... We pray to God by means of the medicines which he has given to us. We don't make the rain, he does" (Schapera 1960:300).

It is clear that both the Tswana and the missionaries believed in God. What is more, both believed that, although ultimately it was God who healed or provided rain, the credit, reputation and honour of curing diseases and causing rain to fall, was enjoyed by both the missionary and ngaka. If the missionary prayed for rain, he was the rain maker, and if he cured a patient, he was the ngaka. It was to him that supernatural powers were attributed, and it was him who enjoyed the credit. The same was true for a Tswana doctor. If the Tswana doctor sang and danced to praise God for his success, so did the missionary. The missionary then sought, in challenging Tswana tradition, to replace ritual with ritual, mystification with mystification, religion with religion, worship with workship, and therefore one set of traditional customs with another.

But contrary to what one might be tempted to think, the embracing of Christianity by large sections of the Tswana population has not modernized or simplified ceremony or ritual; on the contrary, it has brought new complications. For, in addition to all the traditional celebrations, there are now-a-days Christian services and ceremonies which have been added and have extended the length of many traditional Tswana ceremo-

nies - and have added a particularly expensive phase to
funerals, weddings, naming of children, etc.   Conversion to Christianity in Africa has not generally meant
the exchange of the indigenous religion for the new
one, but rather an amalgamation of the two, made the
more possible by their common belief in spirits.   It
should always be noted in discussing African religion,
that Christianity too teaches of a whole hierarchy of
spirits, starting from the Supreme Threefold Spirit,
down to angels and the lesser spirits of the dead
(Weridu 190:44).   Where African and Christian ceremonies converge, unless one happens to be rich, he is in
for hard financial times (after all the elaborate and
extended refreshments to the often large community of
Christian brothers and sisters, customary family
friends, and members of the extended family go their
merry way).

Missionary Strategy to Undermine Tswana Custom and Medicine

a)   **Political Strategy**:   The policy of the London
Missionary Society depended on the ability of an
individual missionary to colonize the mind and heart of
a Chief.   Judged comprehensively, it was political and
not religious control which proved to be the key source
of the missionary power over the people.   This provision of medicines and the conversion of the African
masses, were, in that order, preceded by political,
diplomatic and militarily strategic promise that the
missionary had for a given Chief.   This was especially
significant in the light of the turbulent environment
in which the missionary found Southern Africa, and in
the light of the impact of such political turbulence on
the stability of Tswana society, territorial integrity
and sovereignty.
Indeed the prospects of facing a Matebele _impi_
single handed on the battle field troubled each Tswana
Chief.   The _impis_ had been established by Shaka during
a period known as the _Difagane_ or _Mfecane_ (meaning the
shattering or forced migration).   They were known
throughout Southern Africa as the fighting regiments
(Mephato in Tswana) that went about conquering every
African group on sight.   The Tswana Chiefs knew of the
impis and had themselves suffered for many decades,
periodic invasions by one of Shaka's rebellious _impi_
leaders, Moselekatse.   Faced with shuch conditions,
Tswana Chiefs soon found in the missionary, a reliable
source of intelligence information, an astute negoti-
ator and, above all, an ally as well as a source of
arms and ammunition.
Although Robert Moffat had wished to separate the
spheres of religion and politics, he was the first to

set the precedent for political intervention by the
missionary. In 1823, when the mission station at Kuru
Although Robert Moffat had wished to separate the
spheres of religion and politics, he was the first to
set the precedent for political intervention by the
missionary. In 1823, when the mission station at Kuruman and the Tlhaping people were being threatened by
Chieftaines Mantantisi, Moffat enlisted the help of
Chief Waterboer, who provided him with mounted Griqua
riflemen (Seeley 1973:71). The following year, he
promised Chief Tawana of the Rolong similar help
against Mantantisi and the Ngwaketse. It became known
by other Tswana Chiefs that missionaries were good
mediators who could solicit help to protect their people against whoever the enemy might be. The missionaries were also a source of arms and ammunition needed
for self defence. So great was the identification of
missionaries with the provision of arms   and ammunition, that Moffat, on meeting the Ngwaketse
Chief Sebego, was compelled to inform him that:

> "We as missionaries came for the purpose of
> instructing them about God and their immortal
> souls, and not to give, or be the means of giving
> or procuring for them either guns or ammuniton"
> (Seeley 1973:73).

Despite such clarifications by missionaries, Kuruman
acted as a distributing point for fire arms and Moffat
supplied Livingstone with the guns which he exchanged
with the Kwena for food and other commodities.   It
should be noted also that as long as David Livingstone
resided at the Kwena capital of Kolobeng, the Boers
refrained from attacking the tribe.
    As conflict between the Boers and the British
escalated, the missionaries took sides with their
countrymen and acted to prevent control of Tswana
Territory and the "missionary road" to the north. The
protective capacity of the missionary became increasingly more obvious to Tswana Chiefs. Local Tswana
advisors were not able to make fruitful negotiations
with the British and every Chief did all he could to
secure the presence of a missionary in his headquarters. Seeley (1973) argues that missionary paternalism
was not governed by motives of imperialism. She notes
that by the 1850's when the Boer's Great Trek north-
wards had gathered momentum, it became evident to the
missionaries that the Tswana tribes would benefit from
British rule and the L.M.S. missionaries became united
in their support of the annexation of Bechuanaland on
moral and humanitarian grounds. History however, does
not support this argument. For the most part, missionary interests were not only imperialistic, but were

paternalistically in search of a wider cultural victory
over the Tswana.

The success of the missionaries was, as Mackenzie
acknowledged, the work of conquerors (Dachs 1972:468),
and the result of the practical strategies which have
been noted by Dachs (1972) as "Missionary Imperialism
in Bechuanaland". They consisted of the exchange of
secular benefits between missionaries and the Chiefs.
The relationship between the two parties became a
relationship of trading partners in which firearms were
critical for influencing a Chief's attitude towards a
given missionary. Evangelism took a subordinate position in the line of priorities.

The very first missionaries to the Tswana, Edwards
and Kok who settled among the Batlhaping in 1801, were
concerned more with trade in ivory and cattle than with
evangelism. Edwards later, using his acquired wealth,
retired on a farm in the Cape and Kok was murdered by
his Tlhaping servants for withholding their wages
(Moffat, 1969). In 1816, James Read gave generously to
Chief Mothibi Molehabangwe of Batlhaping in order to
secure permission to outspan. Mothibi had asked Rev-
erend John Campbell in 1813 to send missionaries to
his capital Dithakong, but when Evans and Hamilton
arrived at Dithakong in 1815, they met with opposition
from Mothibi himself. Mothibi made it clear that he
would only approve of the men to live among his people
as traders and would on no account allow them to preach
or teach his people. While missionaries came at the
request of the Chief (Schapera 1970:38), their eager
acceptance was governed by motives of political expediency, and modified by rumours of the changes in custom
which resulted from missionary presence in other tribes
(Campbell 1815:206).

The rejection of religious teaching created tacti-
cal problems in the missionary strategy. Their evange-
listic aims, and aims at general social and cultural
changes, were being frustrated by the intransigence of
Tswana society. The Tswana knew that the Scottish
Mission to the Xhosa and Tembu in South Africa had
openly challenged the authority of the Chiefs and
decreased their control over their people who could
take political assylum in a mission station (Wilson and
Thompson 1969). The Tswana knew that missionaries had
introduced the questioning of traditional African
authority elsewhere and, at the same time, it was known
that they were influential in shaping diplomatic relations with stronger outside forces. Thus, while on one
hand missionaries provoked a reaction from established
authority, the Chiefs saw some benefits in associating
with missionaries. Overall, the Chiefs remain ambivalent, yet pragmatic, in their relations with missionaries.

The average Motswana, at first strongly resisted the disturbance of his cutomary way of life by the missionary. Change meant more uncertainty and uncertainty called for an increased dependence upon the command-like prophetic interpretation of life through the use of ditaola. Go thela bola, throwing the bones, became prominent, especially at the national and ceremonial level, for only ditaola could give meaning to the new unknown ways of the missionaries whose longterm as well as short-term consequences were as uncertain and intriguing as the changes themselves. Those who were quick to see some benefits in the new ways, nevertheless remained ambivalent and often reverted back to the traditional Tswana ways of doing things. The Tswana strategy was to dip one foot in the missionary ways while careful not to alienate themselves from the well beaten and stable path of tradition and custom.

The chief of the Bakwena, Sechele, was one such man, who although for some time he remained the only Chief to profess such a favour for Christianity as to request baptism, reverted to polygamy within six months of his baptism. In adopting the missionary ways, he had put aside four of his five wives. But by converting to Christianity, he began to see the immediate weakening of his secular authority, and the more he moved away from tradition, the weaker his authority became. By attributing the drought which befell his territory to his conversion, his people convinced him to yield to tradition and defend his secular authority. Neighbouring opponents of the Gospel enjoyed plentiful rain, while Bakwena were suffering from the ravages of the drought. After he reverted to his old ways, Sechele

> "assured his people that he had only
> requested baptism in order to see and
> know all that the white men do, and to
> become as wise as they are; and he comforted
> his headmen by resuming relations with them"
> (Dachs 1973: 1-2).

The kind of back sliding and lack of commitment exemplified by Sechele's actions led missionaries to take more resolute measures to produce change; win converts and break down the intrasigence of Tswana society. To achieve their mission, they looked to the secular power of the British military force (Dachs 1972).

From the middle of the nineteenth century, they called upon the British government to preserve their mission field and their hosts, the Tswana, from Boer expansion. So important were political developments in Southern Africa, that David Livingstone actively di-

rected his efforts to the north to occupy the interior
before the Transvaal settlers could enter their claims,
to the exclusion of the missionaries. For him, preoccupation of the interior was the only remedy to the
encroachment of the Boers. Missionaries believed that,
in terms of secular politics, the road along the
Bechuanaland mission stations was the key to the
balance of power between the British colonies and Boer
Republics. When Livingstone demanded the exercise of
British military force to protect British missionaries
(Dachs 1972:469), he was aware that missionary settlement, imperial security and commercial interest rein-
forced each other. Thus, he could make an appeal to
the British public and government as a citizen of the
Imperial Government. Ignoring the rights of British
residents and the interests of British commerce would
have been the most un-British policy. For this reason,
the missionaries at Kuruman welcomed the British
military.
      The mission station at Kuruman (established 1824
by Robert Moffat), became the headquarters for the
British military. In addition, the mission press
printed notices calling on the Tswana to surrender to
British rule (Dachs 1972). The same mission station
had been established as a centre for training African
Evangelists-teachers, and had served as a refuelling
station for missionary journeys into the "unknown" interior (Thema 1969). Thema argues that it was in this
same mission station that the conception of missionaries as the sole agents of civilization, whose efforts
were to be extended to almost every field in which the
life of the African revealed defects, was consolidated.
      Since 1816, the year Robert Moffat was sent to
Africa by the London Missionary Society, he commission-
ed himself to learn the Tswana language. By 1829, he
had finished translating Luke's Gospel, and in 1830 it
became the first complete book of the Bible in the
language of the Tswana. The complete New Testament
appeared in print with 497 pages in 1840, and was the
first full New Testament in the language of any African
people south of Ethiopia (Sandilands 1971:1), and when
Livingstone first sailed for the Cape in 1841, he took
with him five hundred copies of the Testament. The
small hand-operated press in Kuruman continued to
produce selected books in the Bible until 1870 when the
first single-volume, complete Bible in Tswana was
published. But when the missionaries realized that the
instruction and teachings of the Bible were not sufficient to produce the desired changes, natives were made
to surrender personally to missionaries like John Mackenzie, who, encouraging private leasehold and individual tenure, resettled the Tswana on farms where he
gave them orders, including when to plough. Resettle-

LAMIN SANNEH holds a Ph.D from the University of London and is at present Assistant Professor at Harvard University. He has previously taught at Ibadan, Nigeria, at Fourah Bay College, Freetown, Sierra Leone, and at the Universities of Ghana, Legon, and Aberdeen, Scotland. He is the author of two recent books and over twenty articles in scholarly journals.

CAROLYN SARGENT is Assistant Professor of Anthropology at Southern Methodist University. She received her M.A. (Econ.) at the University of Manchester, England, and her Ph.D. from Michigan State. She is the author of *The Cultural Context of Therapeutic Choice: Obstetrical Care Decisions Among the Bariba of Benin.*

NATALIE S. SMALL, M.S., Ed.S. is a licensed Mental Health Counselor in the Department of Social Work Services at Shands Hospital of the University of Florida where she counsels pediatric families adjusting to life-threatening illness. Her interest in cost-effective methods of counseling have led to the development of multi-media helath education presentations, a study tour of health and family life in China, consulting in Nigeria and work as a doctoral student in counseling at the University of Florida.

PARKER A. SMALL, JR., M.D. is Professor of Immunology and Medical Microbiology and Professor of Pediatrics at the College of Medicine, University of Florida. His research efforts are currently divided between the development and testing of new methods of teaching immunology. He has published over 100 articles, most in the area of immunology. His Patient Oriented Problem-Solving (POPS) system of teaching immunology is in use at over half the U.S. medical schools. The University of Lagos College of Medicine brought the Smalls to Nigeria in 1982 to advise them on immunology education and research and cost-effective counseling methods. In 1983 Dr. Small returned to Lagos, Kenya, and Saudi Arabia. The Smalls have three children.

ANITA SPRING is Associate Professor of Anthropology and Associate Dean, College of Liberal Arts and Sciences, and is affiliated with the Center for African Studies at the University of Florida. She received her Ph.D. from Cornell University, her M.A. from San Francisco State University and her B.A. from University of California, Berkeley. She has done work on health care, religion, and gender roles in Zambia, and in agricultural development and farming systems in Malawi and Cameroon. She co-edited *Women in Ritual and Symbolic Roles* (Plenum Press, 1978, with J. Hoch-Smith), and has written articles on population, symbolic systems, refugees, and women in farming. Most recently she directed a USAID project on women in agricultural development Malawi.

ROBERT STOCK is a medical geographer employed as a Postdoctoral Fellow in the Department of Geography, Queen's University. He has studied at the University of Western Ontario (B.A.), Michigan State University (M.A.) and the University of Liverpool (Ph.D.). He has undertaken considerable research on health care systems in Nigeria and the health care behaviour of the Hausa of Nigeria.

ment was conditional on political surrender and, as
Mackenzie reported to Colonel Warren, head of the
military at Kuruman mission station, "Every native who
gave himself up was asked if he was (willing to give
himself up), (and the answer was) invariably in the
affirmative (Dachs 1972:652).

To make Bechuanaland Christian, Mackenzie and
other missionaries had decided that they first had to
make it British. They campaigned for imperial rule,
arguing that their only hope to civilize the Tswana
depended on their ability to save Bechuanaland from the
Transvaal, both for the sake of the missionary interests to preach the Gospel, and for the sake of protecting the natives against foreign intrusion by the Boers.
The ultimate purpose, however, was to safeguard the
strategic interests of Great Britian, militarily,
commercially and politically. The missionaries efforts
culmunated into a powerful combination of imperialists
and merchants, who claimed imperial protection for the
Tswana and for British trade in Southern Africa. In
1883, Macknezie and his supporters founded the South
African Committee (Dachs 1972:654) whose first Chairman, W. McArthur, M.P., was a former Lord Mayor and
Cape merchant, as well as committee member of the
Wesleyan-Methodist Missionary Society.

In 1884, Mackenzie had a formal relationship with
Colonel Warren at Kuruman, and in 1885, he formulated
an offer by Khama to open his Ngwato country to English
settlement and accept Britisn protection. Dachs (1972)
notes that Mackenzie deliberately concealed his own
handwriting of the offer, but openly rejoiced at his
action, "in furtherance of one great work which God
would establish in his own time - the peaceful opening
of South Africa under Her Majesty's Government". Ten
years later,in 1895, another missionary, Willoughby,
negotiated with the British South Africa Company and
the British Colonial Office for the transfer of parts
of the Bechuanaland Protectorate to Company rule. As
the London Mission Society claimed, in its centenary
report of 1885:

> "The only way to get a just estimate of
> the missionary history of the past century
> is to read with it the story of material
> progress and territorial expansion... The
> extension of trade, the facility of colonization,
> the enlargement of territory, the scientific
> knowledge of the world and its peoples, the
> suppression of international wrongs, the
> possibility of free and useful intercourse
> between the different races, have been largely
> helped by the earnest labours of the band of
> unassuming missionaries" (Dachs 1972:657).

Botswana was not economically attractive throughout
much of the nineteenth century, and continued to be of
no interest to the British Government, except perhaps
as part of the road connecting the north and the south,
even until independence in 1966. It should be clear,
therefore, that colonialism in Botswana was not so much
instituted by what the Imperial Government thought or
intended. It was the missionaries who brought colonialism to Botswana explicitly, at first through
informal imperialism with its religious objectives and
later, more resolutely, through formal imperialism.
From the very first days of missionary settlement, they
threatened local authority and social structures as a
practical strategy of overall imperialism. Furthermore, Mackenzie's doctrine of formal imperialism was
the outcome of more than half a century of missionary
frustration and practical experience of the resilience
of Tswana resistance.
    Indeed, the missionaries found great difficulties
in converting the Tswana. For example, Robert Moffat,
who settled at the head-station of Kuruman in 1821,
only made his first Tswana convert in 1819 (Dachs
1973:2), the year he finished translating Luke's Gospel
into Setswana (Sandilands 1971:1). In another case, it
is charged that, in his entire missionary career,
Livingstone converted only one man (Chief Sechele), who
apostasized by reverting to polygamy within six months
of his baptism (Dachs 1973:1). Livingstone justified
his failure as an evangelist by proclaiming that it was
not fruitful to spend an age on one tribe of people.
According to Livingstone,

> "Those who have never heard the Gospel are
> greater objects of compassion than those who
> have heard it for seven years and rejected it"
> (Dachs 1973:4).

Livingstone was much more of an explorer than an evangelist, and his work was important for the scientific
detail with which he reported on: geography, agricultural potential, and other subjects, which were of
primary significance to merchants and scientists.
    The failures of missionaries as evangelists is
little known and hence little is said about it.
Perhaps it could be argued that since missionaries
controlled the press, and since it was not in their
interest to acknowledge or publish their failures in
what presumably was their major mission (evangelism),
much of this data was suppressed or distorted. It
should also be argued that, if missionaries had found
no difficulties in converting Botswana, they would have
not found it necessary to formally invite the intervention of the Imperial Government. On the other hand, it

might have been easier to interest British commerce to
a people who had no objection to foreign cultural
domination. It is difficult to support the latter two
speculations. What is clear, is that the establishment
of a formal British Protectorate was the work of over
10 years of practical missionary strategies among the
Tswana.

b. **Medical Strategy**: Despite formal cultural domination by the Europeans, Tswana traditional life persisted and traditional doctors continued to survive. The
presence of and conversion to Christianity, did not
eliminate, but restricted traditional customs. As one
traditional doctor argued with Livingstone:

> "I use my medicines, and you employ yours;
> we are both doctors, and doctors are not
> deceivers. You give a patient medicine.
> Sometimes God is pleased to heal him by means
> of your medicines; sometimes not, and he dies.
> When he is cured, you take the credit of what
> God does. I do the same. Sometimes God grants
> us rain, sometimes not, when he does we take the
> credit of the charm. When a patient dies, you
> don't give up trust in your medicine; neither
> do I when rain fails. If you wish me to leave
> off my medicines why continue your own?"
> (Dachs 1973:3).

But, because they strove to abolish the initiation
ceremonies, bogadi or bride price, polygamy, fortifica-
tion of villages and rain making ceremonies, in which
the traditional doctor was the key figure, missionaries
were motivated to break the influence of the ngaka who
was the custodian of a social order which they regarded
as sinful, pagan, and above all, the great barrier to
civilization. European medicine was largely meant to
disuade Africans from depending in any way on their
dingaka for anything. Missionaries fully recognized
that as long as the ngaka retained his pre-eminence in
his society, his influence would continue to overshadow
theirs, and thereby hinder their progress in cultural
penetration. Mushingeh (1982) argues that, whereas the
ordinary Tswana eventually accepted western medicine,
the conflict remained between the ngaka and the
missionary, both occupying important offices, and both
fighting to outdo each other in supremacy in the same
constituency. Rain makers were considered the most
inveterate enemies, who had to be confounded before any
real progress was made in their duty of evangelism
(Moffat 1869).
      Moffat and Livingstone took advantage of their
roles as rain makers. After a series of prayer meet-

ings for rain, which were followed by copious rainfall,
Moffat was asked by many Batswana to make rain for
them. Livingstone also took advantage of his reputation as rain maker and hoped to use his irrigation
scheme at the Kwena capital to persuade the tribe of
the rain making powers of the Christian God.

> "The natives were quite delighted with the idea
> that I could make rain (the doctor and the rain
> maker are one and the same), and by this
> means, I hope they will see the folly of
> trusting any more to their rain doctor"
> (Schapera 1959:53).

Despite the fact that the missionaries possessed the
requisite qualifications to be regarded as rain makers
and doctors alike, they launched attacks on Tswana rain
making. The Tswana were, however, able to defend themselves by referring to the basic shared premises.
Livingstone questioned the power of the ritual employed
by the rain maker to make rain for the tribe, but soon
it was the missionary who performed the role of tribal
rain maker, utilizing his own form of ritual - Christian prayer. With the conversion of the Chief to
Christianity, Tswana ritual was replaced by Christian
ritual.
    Once the political maneouvres of the missionaries
had led the Chief to rely on them for matters in general, the medico-religious strategies became much
easier to implement. Sechele, against the wishes of
the tribe, took up his missionary's suggestion that the
tribal capital be moved to Kolobeng (Seeley 1973:15).
The Chief also adopted Livingstone's ideas and ordered
the tribe to assist the missionary in the construction
of the necessary canals and dams.
    Unlike Sechele, who adhered more to tradition than
to Christianity, Khama and his brother, Sekgoma, were
adamant Christians who rejected the traditional customs
of their people. But, when trouble came, tradition was
employed.

> "In 1862, the Ngwato found themselves once
> more under threat of attack by the Matebele.
> Sekgoma performed the ceremony of the doctoring
> of the army, arrayed himself with calabashes
> containing protective medicines, and threw the
> bones to ascertain the outcome of the battle.
> Mackenzie, supported by two Christian Chiefs,
> organized a prayer meeting for the assembled
> army... a protective ritual performed within a
> Christian context" (Seeley 1973:111).

The early days of Khama's Chiefship were characterized
by a battle of ritual wits between the traditionalists,
led by the tribal ngakas, the royal advisors and the
traditional councillors against the Christians, led by
the Chief and his missionary, James Hepburn. Seeley
19973) notes that the royals and councillors were anti-
Christian because the reliance of the Chief upon his
missionary had deprived them of their traditional positions of influence. Even the educational role, which
the initiation schools had performed within the traditional context, was being appropriated by the mission
schools. In 1875, the traditionalists arranged an
impressive bogwera initiation ceremony against Khama's
advice. On the day when the initiation began, some
rain fell in the territory, but this was the last rain
that the Ngwato were to see in a long time, and the
year that followed the initiation ceremony was marked
by one of the worst droughts in Ngwato history. This
led Khama to refuse any further bogwera. As the
drought became worse, Khama was asked by the traditionalists to organize a rain making ceremony.

"Following the advice of his missionary, Hepburn,
Khama agreed to the rain making ceremony, but at
the same time, he and Hepburn organized an
equivalent Christian ceremony - a week of
prayer for rain. The rain making ceremony was
held, a week passed, but no rain fell. The
traditionalists and the Christians both placed
the blame on the ritual of the other. On the
seventh day of prayer, rain fell and continued
to fall for 27 days. The productive ritual of
the missionary had proved effective; the fortui-
tous cloudburst was interpreted as demonstrable
proof of the power of the Christian God.

The traditionalists were defeated and Khama proceeded to Christianize other traditional ceremonies, just as he had transformed the traditional
rain making ceremony. At his installation,
instead of being ritually doctored by the dingaka
tsa morefe, he had Hepburn officiate at a Christian service held in the Chief's Kgotla. Khama
abdicated his role as high priest of the tribe,
renounced all claims to supernatural powers and
refused to acknowledge the healing or ensorcelling
powers of dingaka, as he had refused to consult
them in their traditional advisory and ritual
capacity. The Chief continued to officiate at
tribal ceremonies advised by his Christian priestdoctors, the missionaries, but the traditional
content of these ceremonies had been replaced by
Christian ritual... the function and purpose of

the ritual remained constant, the tribe continued
to ask for rain, for protection against the ememy
for good crops and to give thanks for the harvest.
To the people, the missionaries were now the
dingaka tsa morafe, performing the productive and
protective rituals formerly carried out by their
traditional predecessors. Further, they were the
dingaka tsa kgosing, for the Chief depended upon
them, not only as ritual assistants, but as
advisors on personal and political matters".
(Dennis 1978:58).

It is interesting to note that, whereas both traditionalists and the missionaries performed parallel rain
making rituals, success was attributed to the missionary, and not to the cummulative impact of the efforts
of both groups. Secondly, missionaries, who were known
locally, and who themselves accepted the title of ngaka
(doctor), had performed rituals which had no medical
significance, yet this did not discredit their reputation. To the contrary, it enhanced their endeavour to
supplant all forms of traditional authority and ritual.
Thirdly, the Chief and missionary were allies, almost
indispensible for each others existence. On one hand
the Chief benefitted from the missionaries who enhanced
his position by supplying guns and ammunition and for
British help and protection against opposition and
possible extinction. The missionaries on the other
hand, relied on the Chief's power over his people and
specifically on his ability to command and institute
enforceable changes which the missionaries, by their
own power, could not institute. The abandoning of
traditional customs and the removal of dingaka tsa
Setswana from positions of influence was the major role
that a Christianized Chief could perform.
     According to Dennis, tribal rites were finally
abolished, and by 1920 were no longer performed by any
of the tribes living in the Protectorate. Dingaka tsa
Setswana no longer had any official function at the
tribal or national level. As early as 1889, Khama
announced that there was to be no more divination or
use of protective and pructive medicines. Other Chiefs
made laws to limit traditional doctor's practice.

"The laws passed by the Chiefs were made with a
view of limiting the number of dingaka and to
bringing their practice under closer jurisdiction.
Chief Kgamanyane of the Kgatla (1848-1875) had the
sole right of selection of those to be trained.
His grandson, Isang (1921-1929), insisted on being
notificed of all new dingaka working within his
tribe... In 1913, Chief Seepapitso of the
Ngwaketse decreed that any man seeking the

services of ngaka, must first consult the Chief;
and in 1916, he announced that in the future, he
alone would select those dingaka permitted to work
among his people. In 1929 his son, Bathoen II,
declared that he wanted no foreign dingaka in his
tribe and that same year drafted his 'melao ya
dingaka - laws for doctors'... These required
headmen to give the Chief the names of trusted
dingaka, to whom the Chief then gave a permit to
practice, and they regulated the etiquette and
content of that practice" (Dennis 1978:59).

The restrictions excluding foreign doctors by Bathoen
did not refer to the missionaries, despite the fact
that they also were regarded as dingaka of foreign
origin. The missionaries had already done their job on
the Chiefs. Their success was, as we have seen, the
work of conquerors.

Bongaka, traditional Tswana medicine, was officially no longer practiced at the national level. It had
been replaced by Christian ritual and its practitioners
ousted by the priestdoctors of Christianity. As a
defence mechanism, traditional doctors mystified themselves, practiced in secrecy, and engaged in increasingly more religious and non-national practices in an
effort to explain both their defeat and to preserve
their clientelle. In addition, the medical practices
and religious beliefs of the missionaries were absorbed
into traditional Tswana medicine. As we noted earlier,
it was customary for Tswana doctors to learn from foreign doctors. Seeley (1973) points out that the
repeated failure of one method, in no way invalidated
its support on a future occasion, and thus the traditional belief system remained in tact and unquestioned.
To the Tswana, presenting oneself to one doctor and not
another, did not invalidate the expertise or therapeutic value of another doctor's medicines. Batswana were
not opposed to everything the missionaries introduced,
and history shows that, despite their defeat by
missionaries, Tswana doctors continued to learn from
European medicine, and the occasional conflicts between
the missionary and the Tswana did not deter them from
availing themselves of Western medicine. Throughout
history, Batswana adopted pragmatic attitudes in their
relations with hostile neighbours and strangers. One
of the major cut-backs to the advancement of their
medical profession was in their reification of mystification which resulted as they battled to keep their
healing strategies in tact. They moved gradually away
from naive openness to rugged protectionism; a development which has tended to lead to spurious findings
about traditional African medicine in general.

Christian missionaries produced an abrupt break
between the ngaka and the milieu of the patient's daily
life. With time, the ngaka came to lose his knowledge
of the families, who in turn have come not to know the
healer and have become less willing to cooperate.
Slowly but surely, society no longer invested in the
ngaka the role of "restorer of social balance". Uncertainty about the position healers occupied and the
degree of credibility that could be accorded them, has
increased with time. Many of them have reacted to this
uncertainty by adopting the accoutrements of western
medicine, while others have emphasized the mystical or
magico-religious aspect of their practices, intending
thereby to affirm their specificity. But given that
the organization of medicine and society in general has
been moving in an increasingly "rational" bureaucratic
direction, Tswana medicine, in so far as it operates
mainly within the principles of "traditional authority"
it will prove inconsistent with modern bureaucratic
institutions and therefore inconsistent with the
official structure of the Ministry of Health.

Conclusion

By employing historical materials, we have tried
to suggest a way to look at African healing strategies
which does not isolate them from developments within a
comparative global context. Historical data seems to
support our earlier conclusions (Fako 1977, 1978) which
suggested that indigenous healing strategies do not
represent a rural African phenomenon which is bound to
decline with increasing westernization, urbanization
and modernization. Furthermore, there seems to be
sufficient historical evidence to strongly suggest that
African healing strategies were not far removed from
European strategies in the nineteenth century.
The case of Botswana shows that, although the
authority of African medicine was crushed by missionaries, there was very little difference between
missionary medicine, nineteenth century European medicine, and that which was found among the Tswana.
Missionaries crushed Tswana medicine, not because it
was fundamentally at odds with their presumably more
enlightened systems of health care, but mainly because,
as a system, it competed as a major ideological, moral
and political force, capable of inducing collective
rejection of the missionary and his ways.
Acceptance of European medicine by the Tswana, was
not based on scientifically demonstrable overall
superiority, but on a subjective fondness for medicines
from distant lands. Likewise, the spread of European
medicine by missionaries was more the result of politi-

cal and military maneouvering than that of fair market-
ing tactics or demonstrated overall superiority of
European medicine. Their strategy was to supplant
traditional doctors by taking their highest positions
of political and medical authority, as well as their
positions as advisors to the political leadership.
This facilitated the introduction of an overall
system, together with a curative medical system which
systematically individualized and depoliticized all
problems, including health problems.

Traditional Tswana doctors were forced by the new
circumstances to adopt rugged protectionism, as uncertainty about their credibility and positis as healers
increased with time. As a defence mechanism, they
became secretive and mystified their practice so that
it could not be easily penetrated by both local and
foreign hostile elements. Latter day doctors continued
the mystification of their practice as a given, and
thus gradually, the reification of mystification process evolved so that by the time anthropologists came
to study African Societies in the early twentieth
century, Tswana traditional medicine was no longer in
any intrinsic inseparable sense, peculiary African, let
alone Tswana.

Although the ngaka lost his position of "restorer
of social balance", Tswana medicine did not adopt the
individualized curative perspective from the missionary. The Tswana have always wished for and sought out
effective cures for specific ailments, as well as
individualized protection against the group. The
collectivity orientation existed side by side with the
self or individualistic orientation. European medicine
did not present truly fundamental changes or expectations.

The major point of departure is that, once weakened by missionaries, Tswana medicine was forced to
become increasingly non-rational. But, given that the
organization of the official Western health care system
and that of society in general has been moving in an
increasingly rational bureaucratic direction, Tswana
medicine has failed to effectively adapt to the newly
imposed conditions which have come to predominate.

REFERENCES

Berman, Edward, H. African Reactions to Missionary
    Education. New York: Teachers College Press,
    Columbia University. 1975.
Brown, J. T. Among the Bantu Nomads. London. 1926.
Burrows, Edward, H. A History or Medicine in South
    Africa: Up to the end of the Nineteenth Century.
    Medical Association of South Africa. 1957.

Campbell, A. C. Some Notes on Ngwaketse Divination.
    Botswana Notes and Records. Vol. 1. 1968.
Campbell, J. Travels in South Africa Undertaken at the
    Request of the London Missionary Society London.
    1868.
Chapman, James Travels in the Interior of South Africa
    London. 1868.
Dachs, A. J. "Missionary Imperialism - The Case of
    Bechuanaland". Journal of African History, Vol.
    13, No. 4, 647-658.
Dachs, A. J. Livingstone: Missionary Explorer.
    Salisbury: Central African Association. 1973.
Dennis, C. "The Role of Dingaka tsa Setswana from the
    19th Century to the Present". Botswana Notes and
    Records, Vol. 10, 53-66. 1978.
Fabrega, H. Disease and Social Behaviour: An
    Interdisciplinary Perspective. Cambridge, Mass.:
    M.I.T. Press. 1974
Fako, T. T. "Traditional Medicine and Organizational
    Issues in Botswana". National Institute for
    Research in Development and African Studies.
    Documentation Unit Working. Paper No. 20.
    Botswana July, 1978.
Feierman, Steven "Village Healers, Specialized
    Healers, and Health in Tanzania: A Study of Tonga
    Region". International African Institute,
    Conference on the Professionalization of African
    Medicine. Gaborone, Botswana September 1983.
Ford, John The Role of Trypanosomiases in African
    Ecology. Oxford 1971.
Ford, John "Ideas Which Have Influenced Attempts to
    Solve the Problems of African Trypanosomiases".
    Social Science and Medicine, Vol. 13b, No. 4,
    269-275, 1979.
Freidson, Eliot The Profession of Medicine: A Study
    in the Sociology of Applied Knowledge. New York:
    Dodd, Mead and Company. 1970.
Gelfand, Michael Livingstone the Doctor: His Life and
    Travels. A Study in Medical History. Oxford:
    Basil Blackwell, 1957.
Good, Charles, M. "Traditional Medicine: An Agenda
    for Medical Georgraphy". Social Science and
    Medicine. Vol. 11:15-16 705-713. (November)
    1977.
Hallowell, A. I. Culture and Experience. Philadel-
    phia: University of Pennsylvania Press, 1955.
Herbet, W. E. "Smallpox Innoculation in Africa".
    Journal of African History, Vol. 16 No. 4,
    539-559, 1975.
Kalulu, S. Traditional Medicine and its Role in the
    Development of Primary Health Care in Zambia.
    (Opening Speech of the Workshop), Zambia, 5-8, May
    1977.

Lieban, Richard W. "Traditional Medical Beliefs and the Choice of Practitioners in a Philippine City". Social Science and Medicine, Vol. 10, No. 6, 289-296, June 1976.

Mackenzie, John Ten Years North of the Orange River from 1859-1869, 2nd Edition, London, 1971.

Maier, D. "Nineteenth Century Asante Medical Practices". Comparative Studies in Society and History, 21:63-81, 1979.

Mburu, F. M. "Professionalization and Differentiation of Traditional Medicine in Kenya". International African Institute, Conference of the Profession-alization of African Medicine, Gaborone, Botswana, September, 1983.

Mechanic, David Medical Sociology. New York: The Free Press. 1978.

Moffat, Robert Missionary Labours and Scenes in Southern Africa. London, 1869.

Mushingeh, A. C. S. Aspects of the History of Disease and Medicine in Botswana. (Unpublished Disserta-tion for the Diploma in Historical Studies. St. John's College, 1982).

Parsons, Talcott The Social System. Glencoe: The Free Press. 1951.

Rosenberg, Charles E. The Cholera Years: United States in 1832, 1849 and 1866. Chicago: University of Chicago Press, 1962.

Schapera, Isaac (ed.) Livingstone's Private Journals, 1851-1853. London, 1960.

Schapera, Isaac Rainmaking Rites of Tswana Tribes, Leiden, 1971.

Schoffeleers, J. M. (ed.) Guardians of the Land: Essays on Central African Territorial Cults. Gwelo: Mambo Press, 1978.

Seeley, C. F. The Reaction of the Tswana to the Practice of Western Medicine. (Unpublished M. Phil Thesis, University of London, 1973).

Suchman, E. A. "Social Patterns of Illness and Medical Care" Journal of Health and Human Behaviour, Vol. 6, Spring, 2-16, 1965.

Thema, B. C. "The Church and Education in Botswana During the 19th Century". Botswana Notes and Records, Vol. 1, 1-14. 1968.

Turshen, M. The Political Economy of Health: With a Case Study of Tanzania. (Ph.D. dissertation, University of Sussex, 1975).

Wilson, M. and Thompson, L. (eds.). The Oxford History of South Africa. Oxford: 1969.

Wiredu, Kwasi Philosophy and an African Culture. Cambridge, 1980.

CHAPTER 13

PRACTICAL ORGANIZATION OF HEALTH SERVICES FOR DISEASE SURVEILLANCE IN AFRICA

Arlan L. Rosenbloom

Introduction

The title of this paper is taken from the Third Annual Disease Surveillance Conference of the Program to Strengthen Health Delivery Systems in West and Central Africa (SHDS) which took place during February 1984 in Freetown, Sierra Leone. SHDS is an AID sponsored program, working with the World Health Organization, that is involved with twenty countries of West and Central Africa in the development of infrastructures for health, including health management, curricula for primary health care teachers, epidemiology training, the development of health information systems, and the development of primary health care research efforts including training programs in research methods. This is essentially a horizontal program primarily concerned with training local health workers in health management, primary health care program development, and epidemiologic methods. Sharing the coordination of the conference with SHDS was the program Control of Childhood Communicable Diseases (CCCD). This project encompasses most of Africa, is also AID sponsored, and is based at the Centers for Disease Control in Atlanta. In contrast to the SHDS program, CCCD is considered a vertical program, committed to control of preventable diseases largely responsive to immunization, tetanus, tuberculosis, measles, diphtheria, pertussis, and poliomyelitis. In addition to these conditions responsive to immunization, the program is also concerned with the control of diarrheal diseases through oral rehydration therapy and the control of malaria mortality through treatment of childhood fevers with single-dose chloroquin. CCCD also deals with other locally prevalent diseases, such as yaws and yellow fever. The SHDS and CCCD programs overlap and compliment each other in more ways than would be suggested by simply describing these as horizontal and vertical programs. Both are interested in the training of health workers, development of operational research, health information systems, health management, and surveillance activities.

230

The goals of the conference reflected this common
interest:
1) Emphasize importance of disease surveillance
   in planning at local and national levels.
2) Emphasize practical and appropriate methods
   to achieve surveillance.
3) Share experience with surveillance
   activities in a workshop setting.
4) Provide "hands on" microcomputer experience
   using surveillance program teaching tools.
5) Identify means of achieving epidemiologic
   surveillance goals with limited resources,
   including the carrying out of comparative
   studies.
There was a wealth of experience and wisdom among
the attendees at this conference representing Somalia,
Kenya, Sierra Leone, Nigeria, Liberia, Ghana, The
Gambia, and the United States. The conference was both
an exhilarating and a sad experience. Exhilarating
because of the talent represented by the public health
physicians and others who participated, the creativity
they demonstrated in trying to achieve public health
goals for their countries, and their honesty and openness in dealing with the problems and failures of their
efforts. The sadness comes from the tremendous obstacles they must confront and the frustration of their
tasks.

Importance of Disease Surveillance

Disease surveillance can be defined as the systematic collection of data to monitor the disease burden
of a country or region for planning, evaluating, and
managing health services or to carry out comparative
health studies. The concept extends beyond simply
disease surveillance to include the monitoring of
program indicators and the carrying out of special
studies. This fundamental concept, that surveillance
must be intergral to any effort to improve health, is a
major residual of the highly successful smallpox eradication program in West and Central Africa in the late
sixties and early seventies. In 1967, for example, we
discovered that vaccination coverage in the endemic
areas of Northern Cameroon was determined by numbers of
vaccinations given, not by any systematic survey for
take rates, easily determined by vaccination scars.
The SHDS project was developed because the twenty
countries collaborating in the West African Smallpox
Eradication Program approached AID with a proposal for
ongoing collaborative efforts incorporating epidemiologic methods.
Surveillance is, of course, especially important
in Africa because of limited resources. This has a

dual aspect. Disease surveillance must be used to
apropriately allocate resources and emphasize the
enormous cost benefits of preventative approaches.
Secondly, the disease surveillance activity itself must
be low cost. A typical budget in West Africa for
health, both curative and preventive, is under US $ 2
per capita. For a country of 3 million persons this is
less than the annual budget of my university department
of pediatrics.

The steps for planning a surveillance program have
been outlined by Parker (1984) and provide an idea of
what is necessary to do an efficient and appropriate
job with surveillance:

1) Define surveillance objectives. These may
   vary from management of a health system to
   outbreak recognition.
2) Identify management-evaluation questions.
3) Identify decision options. For example, one
   must consider at what level one defines an
   epidemic of a specific disorder.
4) Intervention. Define criteria. One seldom
   has the luxury of laboratory confirmation of
   a diagnosis but for many, if not most
   purposes, this is seldom necessary. For
   example, the local population may be able to
   define a case of cerebrospinal meningitis
   with high reliability.
5) Select indicators.
6) Develop standards.
7) Define data needs.
8) Identify data sources, flow, and analysis.

Problems Affecting Disease Surveillance

The various country presentations underscored a
commonality of problems affecting disease surveillance:

1) Unrealistic comprehensiveness. This is a
   traditional problem involving long lists of
   diagnoses which cannot possibly be verified
   or even known to the local individuals responsible for reporting. Those individuals
   who are capable of making most of the
   diagnoses are unlikely to have the time to
   complete comprehensive reports.
2) Verification and supervision. There is a
   lack of supervision of primary data collectors which makes for highly suspect data
   and a lack of opportunity to train the
   collectors.
3) Parallel systems. This results in waste.

4) Lack of analysis-intervention. Data may
    accumulate without being used, even though
    it could be quite good data, as in Ivory
    Coast.
5) Multiplicity of forms. A recent consulting
    team noted 56 different forms being used for
    data collection in Bombali district in
    Sierra Leone.
6) Lack of feedback. Feedback is important to
    assure the quality of data. People need to
    know why they are collecting data and must
    see it used to reach decisions which will
    help them in the field.
7) Lack of qualified personnel. Such person-
    nel, when present, may not have the time to
    keep the necessary records.
8) Communication breakdown. This is a result
    of fuel shortages, drought (hydroelectric
    power failure), and lack of spare parts.
    The inability to supervise noted earlier is
    perhaps more a function of these transport
    and communication difficulties than a
    shortage of supervisory personnel.
9) Outside support can be a mixed blessing.
    Programs can get under way with enormous
    outside support but cannot be sustained nor
    exported.
10) Attrition of village health workers. This
    is generally because of a lack of community
    support or an elevated self-concept and
    desire for improved monetary return. The
    impediments to volunteerism and the
    encouragements to cynical self-interest are
    mounting in Africa as elsewhere.

These problems, reflecting the general decline in
the economic situation in West Africa, have led to the
resurgence of previously controlled public health
problems, such as yaws and yellow fever in Ghana.
How are countries dealing with these enormous
problems and what more can they do? Several recommen-
dations emerged from the presentations and discussions.

1) Selective reporting. The usual approach is
    to pick the ten most important problems for
    primary health care intervention and concen-
    trate the data collection on these. These
    would be the conditions for which primary
    health care workers would be trained (skill
    specific training). This is the approach
    being used in the Bo district in Sierra
    Leone. There the list includes neonatal
    tetanus, measles, tuberculosis, malaria,

234   AFRICAN HEALING STRATEGIES

> whooping cough, polio, pneumonia, anemia of
> pregnancy, tuberculosis, diarrhea, and
> undernutrition. The list may vary from one
> country to another, for example, to include
> yellow fever or yaws.
>
> 2) The use of sentinel sites instead of global
> reporting, permitting supervision and
> verification.
>
> 3) The use of microcomputers. Microcomputer
> use for data management and analysis is an
> exciting tool. However, there are numerous
> concerns. The selection of a computer must
> begin with a careful definition of what one
> wants the system to do. Compatability
> country-wide is extremely important. The
> availability of service personnel is an
> important consideration in the U.S. and
> absolutely crucial in Africa. The greatest
> value of the introduction of computers may
> be that it forces people to look at the kind
> of data that they want and how they want to
> analyze it, resulting in simplification of
> data collection. In fact, it is important
> to design a system that is not dependent
> upon the computer but that can use the
> computer for efficiency, as a tool.

A delightful example of simplified data collection was
provided by The Gambia. Pictorial forms are used for
disease reporting by illiterate primary health care
workers.

Relatively simple measures carried out at the
village level can have profound impact on health, but
their sustenence requires surveillance, initally to
demonstrate need, then to monitor the effect and
dictate needed changes in approach, and finally,
ongoing surveillance to avoid resurgence of problems.
For example, one can readily document that up to 2/3 of
the mortality in the first five years of life in many
areas is due to diarrheal diseases and measles. As
shown in Figure 1, a measles vaccination and oral
rehydration therapy program resulted in a further 23%
reduction of child mortality over a period of a year
and ongoing surveillance demonstrated but there was no
change during the subsequent year. Between 1979 and
1980, more intensive ORT efforts based on home visits
by health workers resulted in a further 40-50% drop in
program areas where this was carried out (Mobarak
1982).

The refugee health program in Somalia demonstrates
the value of well thought out surveillance efforts in
controlling a complex and potentially disastrous situation. The Refugee Medical Unit (RMU) was developed to

deal with the 700,000 refugees coming into a country
with a population of 3,000,000. A one page surveillance form identified the principal problems which
require action. Identifying the principal problems in
the population which accounted for disease and death
permitted direction and control of the outside
assistance. Their disease control objectives were
diarrhea, respiratory disease including tuberculosis
and EPI (Extended Program of Immunization) diseases -
diphtheria, pertussia, tetanus, polio, and measles.
Surveillance also permitted the development of a list
of essential drugs. The outcome of this effort was an
improved health status for the refugees compared to the
rest of the Somalian population. The achievements of
the RMU were possible as a result of considerable
outside aid, resulting in a substantial increase in
public health expenditure compared to the rest of the
Somalian population. The RMU also had the advantage of
a concentrated population with inherently better
discipline and cooperation with authority.
      A further example of a remarkable use of limited
resources was provided by a visit to the Bombali
district of Sierra Leone. The ministry of health and
non-governmental organizations (NGOs) attained some
impressive primary health care goals despite many of
the constraints and problems previously noted. They
have improved the community health effort with maternal
and child health microclinics under mango trees,
comprising supervision by traditional birth attendants,
immunization of babies, and some medical care. In
addition, health centers have been developed which are
run by nurses and these units relate to the hospitals
in the area. School teachers are trained as village
health workers to become agents for primary health care
and to teach their students to be such agents, as part
of their curriculum. Villages have built pit latrines,
compost fences, protected wells, animal pens, and
clothes lines and poles. The simple device of drying
clothes in the air rather than on the ground can
markedly reduce the incidence of neonatal tetanus.
This system is supervised through overlapping commit-
tees at four levels; subsection, section, chieftancy
and district. Coordination of primary health care and
other clinical services is assured by the district
medical officer being chairman of the PHC committee.

Conclusion

      I have attempted to outline the importance of
surveillance in attempting to achieve primary health
care goals in West Africa, despite stultifying limita-
tion of resources. The development of information
systems which are simple, responsive to the planning

and program development needs in primary health care,
and independent of complex and costly technology is a
realistic goal, because of the talented and dedicated
workers in these countries. Our commitment must be to
provide assistance and training to help establish disease surveillance and preventative programs. The
lessons learned can, in turn, be applied to more wisely
allocating health resources in the more developed
countries.

NOTE

Dr. Rosenbloom is partially supported by a contract with the Department of Health and Rehabilitative
Services of the State of Florida for a Diabetes
Research, Education, and Treatment center. The Program
to Strengthen Health Delivery Systems in West and Central Africa is a USAID contract with Boston University,
Health Policy Institute, directed by Dr. David French,
MD, MPH. Jean Shaikh, MPH (Associate Director SHDS),
Dr. Ronald Waldman (CCCD) and the author shared the
coordination of the conference on which this paper is
based.

REFERENCES CITED

Mobarak, A. B. et al. Diarrheal disease control study –
    1980. Strengthening Rural Health Delivery
    Project, Ministry of Health, Cairo, Egypt, 1982.
Parker, R. L. Surveillance in diarrheal disease control
    programs. Proceedings of Third Annual Disease
    Surveillance Conference; Freetown, Sierra Leone;
    February 27 – March 2, 1984 (in press).

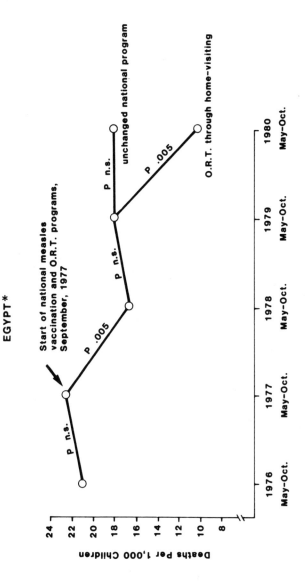

CHILD MORTALITY BETWEEN ONE MONTH AND FIVE YEARS OF AGE
BY MODE OF O.R.T. PROGRAM DELIVERY
(MAY THROUGH OCTOBER 1976 THROUGH 1980)
EGYPT*

MOBARAK, ET AL. (1982)*

FIGURE 1

CHAPTER 14

IMMUNIZATION IN THE THIRD WORLD: A DILEMMA IN THE TRANSFER OF TECHNOLOGY

Parker A. Small, Jr.
Natalie S. Small

Introduction

A World Health Organization poster states that
"The health of a nation can be better judged from the
number of water taps per person than from the number of
hospital beds per person." The health of the majority
of people in Africa is more dependent on the quality of
their water supply and the way they dispose of their
excrement than on access to modern medicine. Their
health is much more dependent on adequate nutrition
than on access to modern drugs; Africans need engineer-
ing and agricultural help more than they need medical
help. However, once one moves from consideration of
sanitation and nutrition into the realm of medicine, it
is absolutely clear that preventative medicine is the
subdiscipline that has the most to offer. Diseases
like measles, polio, and tetanus that are rarely seen
in the U.S. are major causes of death in Africa.
Immunization has enabled us to totally eliminate smallpox, one of the most vicious killers and maimers ever
known to mankind, and has made measles, polio and
tetanus rare diseases in the developed world. Yet
these diseases continue to be major killers in the
developing world.
    The purpose of this paper is to discuss the prob-
lems associated with the use of immunization techniques
in the Third World. These problems fall into three
categories: As illustrated with tetanus, the first
problem is the logistics of getting vaccine administered to the people. The second problem, as illustrated
by polio, is choosing the vaccine that is most likely
to be effective in the Third World environment. The
third problem, as illustrated by measles, is the development of new approaches to immunization because those
in use in the developed world are not optimal for the
Third World.

The widespread introduction of immunization would
be one of the most cost effective ways of improving
health in the Third World, but what would be the
effects of this improved health? First, there is the
obvious problem of population growth. We believe that
this effect is an unavoidable short term problem, but
necessary in the long run, since infant mortality must
be controlled before a population will control its
birth rate. Second, if we can eliminate measles and/or
polio from the world we will be able to stop immunizing
all the children of the world against these diseases,
as we have already done for smallpox, and thereby save
a great deal of money and suffering.

TETANUS

      Figure 1 is a picture of an 11 year old Nigerian
girl taken at the General Hospital in Lagos, the capital city of the most affluent black nation in Africa.
She has tetanus or lockjaw. About three weeks before
the picture was taken she cut her foot (see insert for
healed wound). The wound became infected with a
bacterium, Clostridia tetani, which is found in soil
throughout the world. The bacteria grew in the wound,
produced a toxin which spread through her body and
affected her nervous system causing her muscles to go
into spasm. Since the muscle for closing the mouth is
much stronger than that for opening the mouth, one of
the first symptoms was her inability to open her mouth.
Hence, the name lockjaw. As the disease progressed and
muscle spasm became more general, the stronger back
muscles "out pulled" the weaker abdominal muscles and
she developed the arched back and head observed in the
picture. She will probably die due to spasm of her
respiratory muscles and the resulting asphyxia. The
tragedy is that this unnecessary scenario is repeated
hundreds of thousands of times a year in the Third
World. In the total U.S. we have at most a few hundred
cases a year. The hospitals in Lagos treat more tetanus patients in a year than all the hospitals in the
U.S.A. combined! The difference is attributed to just
one thing: almost everybody in the developed world is
immunized and few in the developing world are. The DPT
(diptheria, pertussis or whooping cough, and tetanus
baby shots and booster shots give protection against
tetanus so it is possible to prevent this terrible
disease. Why then does it persist?
      The problem is a logistic one and perhaps a
political/social one. How do you get simple health
care to the people of the developing world? How can
the goal of the World Health Organization, "Health care
for all by the year 2000" be met? The primary need is
not for highly trained doctors to provide sophisticated

care for a few, but for health care workers trained to
provide simple care for the most common problems of all
the people.   In Lagos we learned of one such program
which was able to reduce infant mortality by 70%!   It
consisted of teaching a lay person (even an illiterate
one) from each village simple things which they could
use to teach and treat others.   The four simple procedures were: 1) to sponge children with fevers with
tepid water to prevent convulsions; 2) to give anti-
malarial pills for any fever, as most fevers are caused
by malaria and the drugs do little or no harm if it
isn't malaria; 3) to diagnose malnutrition by measuring
the circumference of the arm at the biceps and comparing the measurement with a simple chart; 4) to treat
infant diarrhea with a simple solution made by filling
a beer bottle, the universal measure of volume, with
water (boiled if possible) and adding two cubes of
sugar and a half teaspoon of salt.   Giving the children
all the liquid they will drink saves the lives of most
of them.   This program could have been introduced
throughout Nigeria for much less than a million dollars. However, instead of instituting this outstanding
program, the government was spending or planning to
spend tens or hundreds of millions of dollars on the
construction of elaborate hospitals.   They have bought
the latest X-ray equipment for the hospitals and it
sits out in the rain while waiting to be installed.
But it would not matter, because if they had installed
it properly, they still would not have had anybody who
could have read their X-rays, assuming there would have
been any X-ray film.   Why were they building these
relatively useless, massive buildings instead of doing
what the nation needed?   The answer was that when they
bought material, such as the X-ray equipment, there
were at least four or five middle-men and each middle-
man made a 15% commission.   Thus it appeared to us that
it was the combination of graft, corruption, and mis-
management that took place in Lagos, and Nigeria in
general, that made it nearly impossible to introduce
the kinds of programs that would meet the needs of the
people.   However, before we appear to be too critical
of their system and its limitations on meeting the
needs of the Nigerian people, we must remember our own
defense budget, especially the money we spend on building more nuclear arms.   The developed world spends more
money on the arms race in 5 hours than was required to
eliminate smallpox from the earth.
    Returning to tetanus, it is also possible to train
health workers to immunize children, but the task is
more complex than the 4 steps outlined above for the
reduction of infant mortality.   The health workers
would have to be given syringes, needles, and vaccine
and taught the rudiments of sterile technique.   The

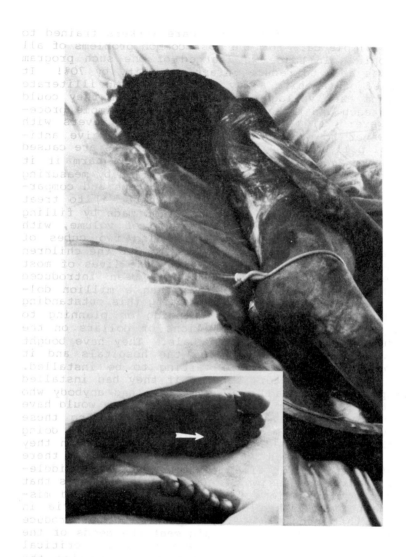

Figure 1: 11 year old Nigerian girl with tetanus. Note the arched back due to spasm of her back muscles. The inset shows the healed wound on the sole of her foot which is the portal of entry of the bacteria which will probably kill her.

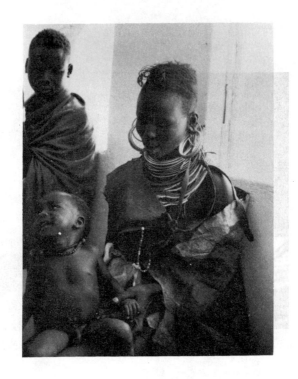

Figure 2: Infant of the Pokot Tribe with poliomyelitis. He has a flacid paralysis of both legs. The
picture was taken in the Rift Valley in Kiwawa, Kenya.

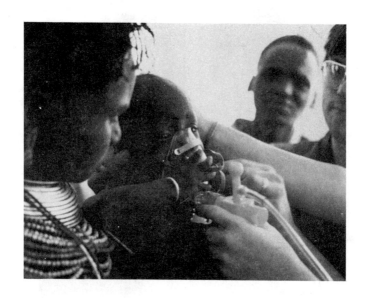

Figure 3: Pokot infant receiving an aerosol. The source of air pressure is a Coleman 12 volt "Inflate-all 150" air pump powered by a car battery.

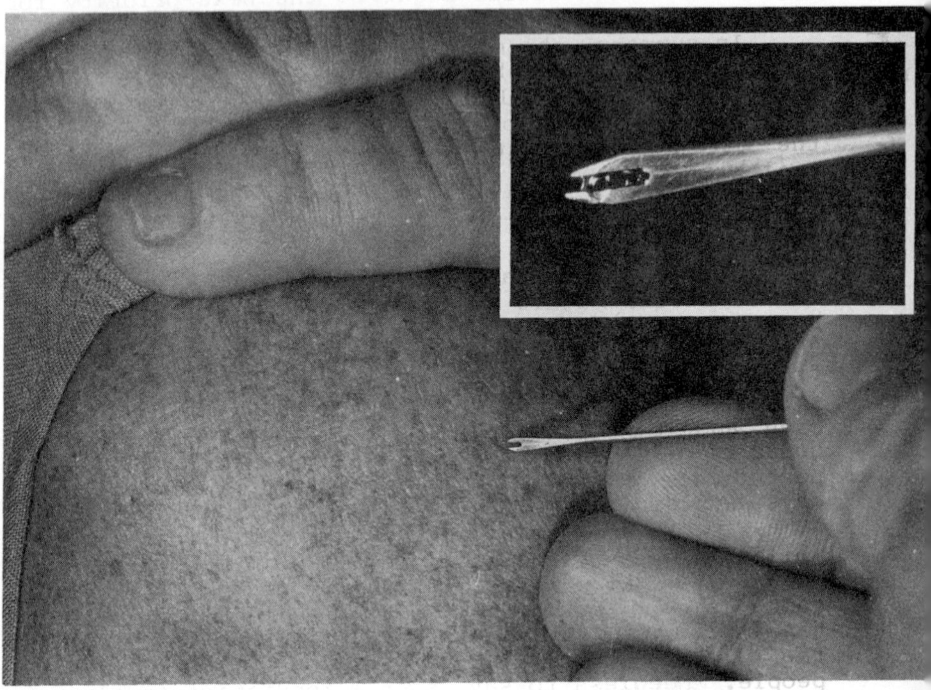

Figure 4: The bifurcated needle being used to vaccinate a patient. The insert shows that when the needle is dipped into a solution of vaccine, the correct amount is taken up between the prongs.

vaccine would have to be properly transported and stored. This should be a high priority, certainly higher than the construction of many hospitals, but providing each village with a health worker knowledge-able about the 4 procedures is obviously the highest priority. Once the latter system is established, add-ing immunization skills might be the next priority for the villages.

In summary, the major challenge is creating a sys-tem that will bring health care to the people of the Third World, especially those in the villages. When such systems are in place, immunization will be one of the more cost effective methods for preserving the health of the people.

POLIOMYELITIS

Figure 2 shows a young Pokot boy who was brought to the Kiwawa clinic in Kenya because of paralysis of both his legs. The clinic is in the Rift Valley about 20 miles from the Uganda border and more than 100 miles from the nearest electric or telephone line. It is staffed by two dedicated missionary couples, one physi-cian and his wife. We do not know the boy's age because there are no calendars or birthdays in this part of the world. The boy's mother told us that some days ago her son developed fever, became very irrit-able, vomited and over the last few days lost the ability to move his legs. He cries a lot and appears to be in pain. She brought him to clinic, because there is word among the Pokot that a paralytic disease has been spreading among them and that the doctor at the clinic had treated and cured some paralysed tribe people. Needless to say, such a reputation is a strong incentive to seek help and mothers walk for several days carrying their sick children to seek the aid of Dr. Larry Banta. He is the first to admit that he has no cure for polio. His reputation is based on the natural history of the disease. The paralysis is transitory in some children so they arrive unable to walk and over a few weeks regain that ability. Dr. Banta is able, however, to teach the mothers to give physical therapy to minimize the damage and try to prevent contractures. He does what he can, but ideally he would like to prevent polio.

Poliovirus replicates in the gut and is spread either directly by oral secretions or indirectly by fecally contaminated water or food which is ingested by the next victum. Unlike the ubiquitous <u>Clostridia tetani</u>, polio can only be found where there are infect-ed people. The virus can replicate and cause disease in other primates, but they are not important in main-taining the presence of the virus. Once over the acute

phase of the illness neither animals nor man continue
to shed virus. Thus, it is theoretically possible to
eliminate polio from the earth. The requirement would
be to immunize the people who might be exposed to the
virus and thus break the chain of person to person
spread. Because the virus can survive in water or food
supplies for months, potentially infectable people must
either be immunized or restricted from entering potentially infected areas.

So the potential gain with polio immunization is
even greater than with tetanus because there is the
Evidence that such an approach could work is provided
by the fact that, unlike in earlier years, poliovirus
cannot now be isolated from the sewerage sage of many
large developed world cities. However, the problem is
somewhat more complex because there are two polio vaccines: the killed Salk vaccine which is injected and
the live Sabin attenuated virus vaccine which is given
orally. In order to understand why one is far superior
to the other for the Third World. One must know a
little more about the viruses. The killed vaccine has
a large dose of inactivated virus which, when injected,
stimulates the body to make antibodies and thereby pro-
tects the person from infection with the wild poliovirus. The live oral vaccine contains much less virus.
In order to successfully immunize the person, the virus
must replicate in the person's gut and thereby produce
enough virus to stimulate antibody formation. Superfi-
cially, it would seem better to use the oral vaccine
because of its ease of administration. However, this
advantage pales in light of the need to keep oral vaccine frozen prior to use. Getting frozen vaccine into
places like Kiwawa and then keeping it frozen, without
electricity, is very difficult. If the vaccine is not
kept frozen it dies and then it will not replicate in
the person's gut nor produce immunity. There is, however, an even more difficult problem with the oral
vaccine. Most Third World people have chronic gut
infections caused by a variety of virus, bacteria, and
parasites. These infections stimulate the formation of
interferon which will prevent the poliovirus from growing and thereby immunizing.

Therefore, with polio appropriate and inappropriate technology is available. Unfortunately, the
wisdom to pick the right vaccine is not universally
available. In Kenya the mdical missionaries were being
supplied with Sabin vaccine but should have been provided with there stable Salk killed polio virus, which
would be effective irrespective of the state of the
recipient's gut at the time of administration. Even
hen vaccine is properly supplied, the main problem is
establishing a network of health workers in the field

who are capable of administering the vaccine to the
people of the Third World.

MEASLES

Another major killing disease is measles. In
parts of Africa, over 50% of the children will get
measles before they are a year old and as many as 20%
will die. In these areas 10% of all live births die of
measles by one year of age. That figure does not
include severe side effects that come with the disease.
The optimum age for immunization against measles in the
U.S. is 15 months. Because so much measles occurs
before that time in the Third World, measles epidemics
will not be eliminated unless new approaches are developed. The reward for eliminating measles from the
Third World is great. Measles like polio only affects
man and primates. Man is the only reservoir. Unlike
polio, measles virus cannot survive in water or food
and must be spread directly from an infected person to
a susceptible person by nasal secretions, usually in
droplet form. As with most infections, once well, the
person no longer sheds the virus. Thus, if the chain
of person to person spread could be broken throughout
the world for one month, we would eliminate measles, as
we have eliminated smallpox.

It is important to realize why our standard
measles immunization is given at 15 months of age.
Like the live polio, the measles vaccine is a live
virus but it is injected. Mothers today have either
had measles in childhood or have been immunized themselves. That means they have protective antibody to
measles which they transmit through the placenta to
their child. Injecting the live virus into infants
while they have their mother's antibody present is
ineffective because the antibody neutralizes the virus
and thereby prevents replication. Thus there is not
enough virus to stimulate the infant's antibody production. In places like Nigeria and Kenya studies have
been done to determine the earliest time that the
average child can be immunized (around 8-9 months), but
even this approach is flawed because there is a wide
variation in this time from child to child. Thus, some
children will still get measles before this time and
others will be injected but not protected since their
residual maternal antibody will have neutralized the
virus. There are, however two new approaches to this
problem which offer hope.

One possibility for success in the Third World
would be to spray the virus directly into the respiratory tract rather than injecting the virus. The antibody that the mother passes through the placenta does
not get into secretions. If the virus is put into the

respiratory tract in the form of an aerosol, the virus
reaches the cells lining the respiratory tract, infects
them and gains a "beachhead" before the antibody can
neutralize it.   Dr. Sabin and his colleagues (1983)
have shown that chilren as young as 5 months of age can
be immunized by aerosol and thereby stimulated to make
their own antibody which should protect them. This is
an exciting breakthrough, but several questions remain.
Is it feasible to aerosolize children under very prima-
tive conditions?   Will the mothers accept the procedure? Technically, how does one get compressed air in
places like the Rift Valley?   Figure 3 shows the
answers to some of these problems. Mothers who trust
the staff of the Kiwawa clinic will readily accept the
aerosol procedure.   It consists of having the baby
breath a vapor from the apparatus shown.   The problem
of obtaining compressed air was quickly solved by Mike
Courtney, one of the missionaries. He plugged the 12
volt air compressor he uses for filling flat tires into
the car battery and showed that the aerosol device
delivered a volume of fluid very similar to that
delivered under controlled laboratory conditions.
Thus, it seems aerosol immunization is quite possible
even in the bush. However, the problem of maintaining
the vaccine in a frozen state and the relatively "high
tech" delivery system presents serious concerns when
one considers the possibility of a worldwide campaign
to eliminate measles.
      There is another approach which eliminates all the
refrigeration and "high tech" problems.   With the
advent of molecular biology and its recombinant DNA
technology it is now possible to create new vaccines
that were previously unheard of and even unimaginable.
For example, Dr. Bernard Moss and his colleagues at
NIH, have put a gene from the influenza virus into the
smallpox vaccine virus (vaccinia), vaccinated hamsters
and shown that they were protected from influenza viral
pneumonia (Smith, Murphy, and Moss, 1983). It is theoretically possible to put 10 to 20 new genes into
vaccinia.   Much additional research is necessary to
work out the details, but before the year 2000 it may
be possible to vaccinate children in the first year of
life, i.e., before they have lost their maternally
derived protection, with a recombinant form of vaccinia
and protect them from measles, mumps, rubella, and
perhaps polio, hepatitis, herpes, tetanus, diphtheria,
pertussis, and maybe even malaria. Long before the
year 2000 it should be possible to know whether a
recombinant vaccinia virus containing a measles gene
can prevent measles. If so, this new vaccine could
lead to the total elimination of measles from the earth
just as has been accomplished for smallpox. The recom-

binant vaccinia approach has several advantages over
the aerosol immunization approach:

1) The vaccinia virus when lyophilized (freeze
dried) can be kept for months without refrigeration
even at temperatures of 40° C and not lose its effectiveness. Health workers can take the vaccine into
remote areas without the need for the equipment that
would be required to keep the measles vaccine frozen.
2) Large quantities of recombinant vaccinia virus
can be produced in cows whereas measles vaccine must be
produced in tissue culture and the cost of the recombinant vaccinia virus should be much less than the cost
of the measles virus.
3) The vaccinia virus has been administered using
the inexpensive and simple bifurcated needle, rather
than the expensive and complex aerosol apparatus (see
Fig. 4). This means that the necessary personnel
require less training, equipment failure in the field
will be rare and cost of administration will be much
less than with the aerosol approach.
4) Finally, there is a precedent for such a worldwide campaign to eliminate measles. Smallpox has been
eliminated using the same techniques. The World Health
Organization has the technical and political knowledge
necessary co successfully undertake such a campaign.
The next critical step in this campaign is the development and testing of the recombinant vaccine containing
the appropriate measles gene.

Summary

The introduction of immunization procedures into
the Third World requires that the scientific community
develop some new approaches for diseases like measles.
For other diseases, like polio, it requires choosing
the technology that is most appropriate for the local
conditions. But the major problem for all immunization
programs is the creation of an effective delivery system which must be founded upon a detailed understanding
of the political and social structure of each country.
In spite of the great difficulties inherent in
providing appropriate immunization for the peoples of
the world, it is very important that the developed
world actively pursue this goal. The reasons are both
humanitarian and selfish. A vigorous and effective
worldwide program for measles and polio immunization
could eliminate these diseases from the earth. The
cost of the immunization program would be recovered
many times over, as it has been for smallpox, due to
the savings from not having to ever again treat or
immunize any child for measles or polio.

References

Sabin, A.B., A.F. Arechiga, J.R. de Castro, J.L. Sever,
D.L. Madden, I. Shekarchi, and P. Albrecht.
Successful immunization of children with and without maternal antibody by aerosolized measles
vaccine. 1. Different results with undiluted
human diploid cell and chick embryo fibroblast
vaccines. Journal of the American Medical
Association, Vol. 249:2651-2662, 1983.
Smith, G.L., B.R. Murphy, and B. Moss. Construction
and characterization of an infectious vaccinia
virus recombinant that expresses the influenza
hemagglutinin gene and induces resistance to
influenza virus infection in hamsters. Proceedings of the National Academy of Science (USA)
Vol. 80:7155-7159, 1983.

CHAPTER 15

HEALTH PLANNING FOR AFRICAN COUNTRIES: THE QUESTION OF PRIORITIES AND APPROPRIATE METHODOLOGIES

Peter D. Reuman
Alice C. Reuman

Introduction

Discrepancies between the health status of less developed countries (LDCs) and that of developed countries (DCs), including associated discrepancies in the amount of funding available for health care, are well known. Differences in the underlying causes of mortality and morbidity in LDCs and DCs are less well known. What is clear is that international efforts to address the health care needs of LDCs through health related aid programs reflect an apparent widespread belief that health care policies, priorities, and tools in LDCs should be modeled on those of Western DCs. Experience has shown, however, that many such efforts attain consistently poor results. It is the thesis of this paper that the major failures of health planning for African and other LDCs are attributable to an inadequate decision-making framework resulting in inappropriate health related programs and policies. We propose to develop a decision-making framework based on the social and economic developmental level of a society within which appropriate health inputs for developing countries can be determined. Methods will be presented by which current conditions in developing countries can be correlated with analogous historical conditions of present day developed countries. The basis for this approach is the proposition that sound health care practices evolve through time in tandem with the social and economic evolution of a society or societies. Health policies and programs that are out of step with the social and economic developmental level of the society will either be ineffective or counterproductive in the long run. The aim of this paper is to propose a decisional framework and methodology for developing countries which will lead to health related efforts that are appropriate, functional, cost-effective, and development inducing.

The methodological framework presented here is
developed in a step-by-step fashion. First, background
information is presented outlining differences in the
health problems and common causes of mortality and
morbidity in LDCs and DCs. These differences are evaluated in the context of divergent levels of funding
available for health care in the developed and less
developed nations. Present directions in health planning are then reviewed. At this point our proposed
developmental approach to health planning in developing
countries is outlined as the theoretical basis of this
article. The history of health development is briefly
traced, followed by a discussion of the various measures of development that can be used to compare
present conditions in LCDs with historical periods of
western social development. Western (European) history
serves as the reference point here both because of
available documentation over serveral centuries of time
and because current role models for the LDCs in setting
health care policy appear to be those of the developed
western health care systems. Finally, the framework
developed is used to discuss present conditions in
African LDCs and to propose appropriate health related
inputs for ongoing health planning efforts in developing African nations.

Background: Health Problems of Developing African
Countries
     The diseases of highest prevalence, morbidity, and
mortality in African and other LDCs are very differnt
from the common diseases of European, North American,
and other DCs. Diseases of LDCs are primarily infectious diseases, whereas diseases of DCs are primarily
degenerative. Diarrheal diseases, respiratory diseases, malaria, measles, whooping cough, tetanus, and
diptheria account for 60 to 70% of the overall mortality in LDCs (Walsh and Warren 1979). In contrast,
arteriosclerotic heart disease and neoplastic diseases
account for 60 to 70% of deaths in Europe and North
America (Centers for Disease Control 1981). In LDCs
the infectious diseases of highest morbidity and mortality affect young children much more than adults
(Dyson 1977). One of the reasons for this large
contribution of the young population to the overall
morbidity and mortality of LDCs is the population
structure (Figure 1).

Figure 1. Percentage of total population in each of
four functional age groups in eight major world areas
(Baker 1977).

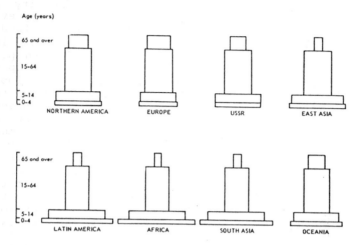

In African and in other LDCs a much higher percentage (commonly up to 20%) of the population is under
five years of age. One-third to one-half of these
children die before reaching five years of age (greater
than 97% of deaths that occur worldwide in the under
five age group occur in LDCs (Morley 1973). Another
characteristic of disease in Africa and other LDCs is
its predominant occurrence in rural reas. This is
true, as Morley points out, because the majority of
children live in rural areas, whereas the children of
DCs live primarily in urban areas (Figure 2). In
summary, diseases of underdevelopment are primarily
infectious diseases of children living in rural areas.

(Figure 2). Proportion of under-fives living in rural
areas. (Morley 1973).

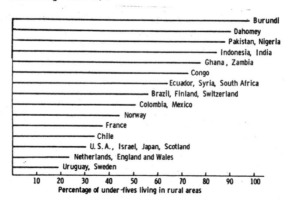

There are a number of factors associated with the
poor health of the rural pediatric population of African and other LDCs (see Morley 1973 and King (ed.)
1966). These factors are intimately connected with
overall social development. Although these factors are
commonly listed as separate entities, they are intimately intertwined (Figure 3). For example, malnutrition can thwart brain development and lead to poor
intelligence (Jelliffe 1968); diarrhea, measles, and
respiratory diseases can worsen malnutrition (Scrimshaw, et. al. 1968); malaria and schizophrenia can
affect work output (Teadem, et al. 1978); lack of
adequate housing can lead to crowding and increased
transmission of airborne infectious disease (Health
Hazards 1972); prevention and treatment of disease can
lead to increased body size and increased population
size with consequent increased demands on nutrition
(Scrimshaw et al. 1968); ignorance can lead to continued use of contaminated water supplies and improper
waste disposal which in turn can lead to more disease
(Wagner and Lanoix 1958 and 1969). Although only
health related entities are listed in Figure 3, it has
become clear that these health factors are intimately
connected to non-health related factors important for
the development of a country.

Figure 3. Interconnections among health-related factors important in development.

                        Nutrition

        Water Supply   Waste Disposal

Housing, Clothing   Population Size
Shoes, Crowding   and Body Size

    Ignorance and   Production and
    Mental Development   Work Output
                        Infectious
                        Disease

It is a common opinion among westerners that the
high morbidity and mortality in African and other LDCs
is simply due to the lack of modern medical weapons and
good doctors (See Morley 1973); King (ed.) 1966; and
Bryant 1969). It is true that the great killers of the
rural children in Africa are largely beyond the reach

of modern medical weapons and that most mothers of these children are unable to reach a doctor. However, even if these mothers were able to reach a doctor, the methods used by the doctor often can do little without extensive expenditures of time and money. The effect of malnutrition and the other factors listed in Figure 3 on infectious diseases frequently makes supportive treatment difficult or futile (Morley 1973: Scrimshaw, et al. 1968; and Wittmann and Hanson 1965). Such extensive expenditures are far beyond the per capita health allowance of many African countries. Providing modern medical equipment and training modern doctors is not appropriate for the majority of LDC settings.

Background: Health Expenditures in African Countries

In order to determine the shape of any health services for African countries, it is also necessary to consider the money available for provision of health services in these countries. The most widely used indicator of development is the gross national product (GNP). By calculating the GNP on a per capita basis, useful international comparisons of the money available for health expenditures may be made (Bryant 1969). Present annual per capita expenditures on health are small for LDCs, averaging from $1.70 for most African countries (the least developed countries) to $6.50 for other developing countries (Figure 4). In contrast, the per capita expenditures on health in the U.S. are $700 per person annually (Health in the U.S. 1981). Some African countries could spend their entire budget on health care and still not equal the per capita health expenditures of some DCs. The health expenditures of LDCs have been projected to increase at a much slower rate than projected per capita health expenditures for DCs. This widening gap between developed and underdeveloped countries will make it harder to provide for health services in African countries in the future (Kahn and Weiner 1967).

Present Directions in Health Planning for Africa

At present the choice of aid efforts used for the overall development of African nations as well as other LDCs has been left to what has been termed the "intuitive approach" (Bryant 1969). Such a strategy attempts by unknown methods to relate health to development in the "broadest possible way." For example, it is felt to be better to fund supplies to rural clinics than to build an addition to the central hospital since the former would result in an improvement in the health of the average citizen, whereas the latter would serve only a small segment of the population. In fact the "intuitive approach" is fairly random in that it takes its direction primarily from the opinions of national

leaders and the particular leanings of the form of
national government. In addition, the opinions of the
DCs offering aid have had an impressive effect on the
developmental directions taken.

Figure 4. Health and related socioeconomic indicators
(Global Strategy for Health 1981).

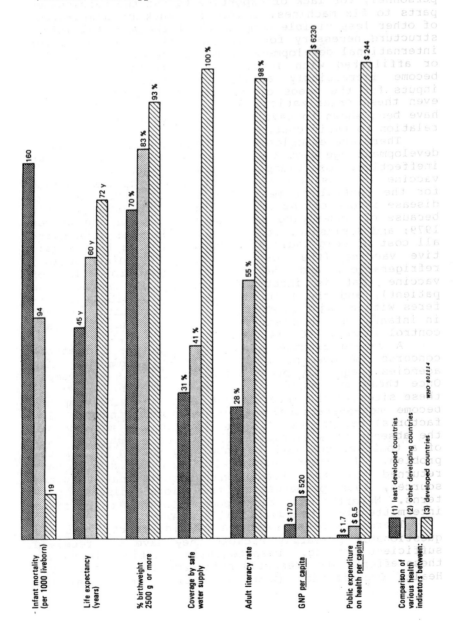

In spite of a thirty year history of aid aimed at stimulating development in LDCs, much of this aid, in the form of materials and training, has not fulfilled its purpose. The national governments of LDCs are often at fault. Large central hospital complexes with expensive, up-to-date equipment are commonly constructed only to be left to dust and rust for lack of trained personnel, for lack of expertise to run the machines or parts to fix machines, and/or for lack of a multitude of other less visible components of the societal infrastructure necessary for this operation. Agencies for international development, based in developed countries or affiliated with international organizations, have become increasingly attuned to picking appropriate inputs for the needs of developing nations. However, even these organizations persist in some efforts that have been shown to have marginal benefit overall or in relation to their cost.

There are examples of continuing efforts funded by development agencies that have consistently been shown ineffective. One example is measles vaccine. Measles vaccine in consistently touted as the optimal method for the control of measles disease in LDCs (measles disease is one of the top ten killers in LDCs, probably because of underlying malnutrition, (Walsh and Warren 1979; and Scrimshaw, et al. 1968). However, the overall cost of cold chain maintenance of this heat sensitive vaccine (the cost of transport, distribution, refrigeration, and the cost of that proportion of vaccine that is inactivated before it reaches the patient), and the fact that maternal antibody interferes with a major proportion of its protective effect in infants, has demonstrated that this form of disease control in many LDCs is questionable.

A second example of an inappropriate aid effort concerns improvement made in water supplies. Aid agencies frequently provide money for wells and pumps. Once these are supplied, it is common to return to these sites months later only to find that the pump has become non-operational or is not being used. The factor(s) responsible for the lack of use may include the absence of a simple part, such as a nut, the lack of a tool, or the lack of knowledge needed to fix the problem. In other cases, villagers may simply have returned to the traditional, contaminated water sources, thus perpetuating traditional disease patterns. Nevertheless, these pumps continue to be fixed intermittently with additional aid money.

There are other examples of aid efforts that are questionable primarily because they have not received sufficient testing. Despite their questionable value, these efforts are presently being advanced by the World Health Organization (WHO) as optimal techniques for

dealing with certain disease entities on a worldwide
scale. WHO, as well as many other aid agencies, is
stressing that the most appropriate method for dealing
with the problem of diarrhea in an underdeveloped setting is the use of home-made fluid and electrolyte
solutions (Pierce and Hirschhorn 1977). Although it is
clear that fluid and electrolytes made properly and
given orally can save a child from death by dehydration, it is not at all clear that this method is
appropriate for home use in African and other LDCs.
The problems involved with oral rehydration are multiple but are not clearly identified by present developed
country agencies and experts. These problems include
the lack of clean water, the inability of the lay
person to clearly differentiate between the diarrhea of
malnutrition and infectious diarrhea (Brown and MacLean
1984), the need to continue breast feeding during diarrhea (interruption of breast feeding leads to further
malnutrition and dehydration), and the lack of refined
foods (sugar and salt) in many households in LDCs. The
poorest households, in which diarrhea is most commonly
found, would be the least likely to have refined foods
such as sugar and salt, and fuel is too precious a com-
modity to use for boiling the frequently contaminated
water supplies. Oral rehydration may work in a clinic
setting, but whether it provides a useful home remedy
and whether its drawbacks outweigh its benefits are
issues requiring more study.

A second example of a questionable health input
stressed by international edict concerns another very
common problem in African and other LDCs: lower respiratory disease. It has recently been recommended by
WHO that penicillin injection be used for all lower
respiratory tract disease (LRT) indentified in rural
clinic settings (Denny - personal communication). Such
therapy has not been tested and is open to question.
It is already known that lower respiratory disease
found in LDCs is closely associated with respiratory
viruses which are unaffected by penicillin therapy
(Bulla and Hitze 1978; and Sobeslovsky, et al. 1977).
Measles is another virus closely related to these
respiratory viruses and commonly producing lower respiratory tract disease in LDCs. Penicillin therapy has
been studied and found ineffective and possibly detri-
mental for treating measles pneumonia (O'Donovan and
Barma 1973; and DeBuse, et al. 1970). Although this
example and the others above represent only a few cases
of inappropriate application of health care policies,
the fact that these few examples are presently being
advanced for use on a worldwide scale suggests that
other health inputs are being in appropriately directed
as well.

Cost is another factor that is not adequately considered in formulating health care policies. Although
many inexpensive methods are available today for
prevention and therapy of individual diseases, the
additive effect of each disease-specific measure
becomes uneconomical in the present circumstances of
most African countries. For health inputs to have
sufficient developmental impact without losing cost-
effectiveness, they must ideally have broad effects.
The more specialized and disease-specific the health
input, the lower its overall cost-effectiveness. The
present developmental level of most African countries
does not permit the luxury of separate methods of disease control for separate diseases.

The need to develop a general, rather than
disease-specific, approach to health care is LDCs tends
to be thwarted by government aid agencies. Government
agencies whose purpose is development aid have aimed
their efforts at health priorities established by
experts from developed countries. These aid agencies
have been organized into programs and specializations
that are generally accepted divisions of labor within
developed county, et al. 1977). Measles is another
virus closely related to these respiratory viruses and
commonly producing lower res of diseases (e.g., diarrheal diseases, viral diseases or helminthiases), or
categories of public health efforts (e.g., environmental health, maternal and child health, nutrition,
vector biology and control, water supply and waste disposal, and others). In developed countries such an
organizational framework functions because it has
evolved through decades of increasing specialization
and public awareness of health issues. But in LDCs the
system is unwieldy and inappropriate. The result is
excessive governmental bureaucracy lacking the underlying social and organizational framework and the
necessary checks and balances to ensure sound policy
debate and development. the present burden of excessive government bureaucracy in African and other LDCs
thus originated from DCs and from the specialized funding orientation of the international aid organizations.
Excessive specialization of health-related efforts
creates bureaucracies with competing and inappropriate
orientations and with an inability to adequately see
the broader perspective of cost-effective developmental
efforts.

Complex interrelationships between health and
other socioeconomic factors often make it inappropriate
to isolate health from the rest of the developmental
process. Fragmented approaches to planning at the
national levels can lead to expenditures which solve
few problems at the local level. In general, those
methods that cost the least and produce the best re-

sults in overall living conditions for the common man
are the most appropriate methods for development. However, a common problem in developing countries is the
lack of any clear and simple methodology for choosing
these methods.

A Developmental Approach to Health Planning for African
Countries
     From our personal experience with African coun-
tries and from our dealings with international aid
organizations that operate within these countries, we
have found that no simple and clearly explained methodology is available for development planning or for
related health planning efforts. Present methodology
is usually stated in general terms, such as "improving
the health of the average citizen" or providing "appropriately directed health care and technology" (Bryant
1969; and Schumacher 1973). Although international aid
has become more appropriate in its development orientation in recent years, there is still lacking a simple
framework within which the appropriateness of health
inputs can be evaluated. Are all developmental or
health related inputs of equal cost equivalent? How
does an agency for international development choose
between different health related inputs? Which health
input is more important: improvements in agriculture
or the funding of vaccines and antibiotics for use in
local health centers? Organizations for development
aid have avoided answering these questions largely
because of the limits posed by their specialized
bureaucracies. Ideally the health impact of any non-
health directed efforts should always be evaluated as
part of any development methodology. We propose to
derive such a development methodology from an examination of the history of social development.
     The proposition on which the central organization
of this paper rests is that, in a broad sense, social
ontogeny recapitulates social phylogeny. That is,
although every human culture includes multiple unique
aspects as it evolves over time, the larger social
evolutionary processes follow a common pattern. This
pattern is represented by the stages of development
summarized in the following section outlining the history of health development. Each level of development
outlined in that section carries with it a level of
cultural understanding and practice of health related
phenomena that builds on prior stages. Development aid
that is out of synchrony with the developmental stage
of a particular society will either fail or backfire.
The objective, then, is to develop measures by which
the level of development of a particular nation or

region can be determined in order to match aid policies
and programs to this level. This paper argues that no
model exists to carry out this task and that many
development aid efforts are misguided as a result. We
propose a basis for a model and show how to begin to
develop parameters for its operation. We do this by
summarizing with broad strokes the major advances in
western health development over the past 4 or 5 centuries and keying these to objective measures of health
status available for those times (e.g., mortality
statistic, GNP, and so on). These objective measures
are then applied to present-day LDCs to determine their
levels of health development and the developmental
needs historically associated with those levels. These
developmental needs are then translated into appropriate aid program orientations. Although we use western
civilization as our model (primarily for reasons of
convenience, familiarity, and relative availability of
historical data), we believe any culture that developed
prior to the era of massive aid intervention would
demonstrate a similar developmental pattern.
     To illustrate the importance of using the history
of social development in the development planning
process, let us turn to an example. USAID and other
international agencies have in the past provided hand
pumps and wells for villages that normally use surface
water from a river or pond. Shortly after installation, as previously pointed out, these pumps are commonly not used. Their lack of use is usually secondary
to something simple such as the lack of a nut or tool
or the inability to make simple repairs. In addition,
villagers may not have been given the framework to
recognize and understand the improvements offered by
well water. Without materials and knowledge and without the framework to support and motivate continued use
of a new practice or idea, such development aid efforts
and monies come to no avail.
     Historically, improvements in the usage of water
occurred in incremental steps. As each step was taken,
it led both to an improved water supply and to improved
health. The first source of water used by man was the
surface water of rivers and ponds. As populations
spread from these sources, the distance to water became
increasingly difficult to traverse. Men may have noted
that water could be reached in dry river beds or ponds
by digging for it. Presumably holes were dug in the
ground deeper and farther from the pond or river to
provide easier access to water. From such a man-made
water hole each family would draw its own water using a
separate container owned by the family. Perhaps with
tribal or community cooperation one container was left
at the water hole. Water retrieved by each family with
this common container would be poured into personal

receptacles for transport to each household. Alternatively, each family may have dug its own water hole.
Either of these changes in water usage, although small,
would have resulted in a decline in the contamination
of well water. Such a slight change in methology would
have resulted in an overall improvement in the health
of the tribe or community.

Further improvements in water usage might have
included methods designed both to keep sand and soil
out of the receptacle that was used and to retain the
structure of the water hole. Although these improvements were motivated primarily by practical problems,
they led to improvements in health by decreasing both
contaminating particulate matter and the runoff of
contaminated water from the surrounding ground into the
well. Although these changes were not perceived as
health related at the time of their initiation, they
brought with them the benefits of improved community
health.

It has only been within the last 200 years that
the hand pump was introduced into western society. The
introduction of the hand pump came only after many
prior steps that were incremental and integrated into
the social framework of the society. In fact, the hand
pump was introduced only after western society had
become industrialized. Without this supporting industrial framework at the time of the pump's introduction,
it would not have been developed or used. It would
instead have been discarded as were other inventions
that were developed before their time. For example,
the first steam engine was invented in ancient Greece
(McKeown 1979), although it did not come into general
usage at that time in that pre-industrial society. Two
thousand years later, in a society with a developing
industrial framework, the steam engine was reinvented
and used. Knowledge concerning the details of the
surrounding social framework within which improvements
occur is not only necessary, but mandatory, in order to
avoid development efforts that become useless or detri-
mental expenditures.

The Historical Development of Health

Although limitations of time and space preclude
review of overall social development from primeval
times to the coming of the industrial state, we will
attempt in this section to outline briefly the historical development of health in western civilization. The
pattern which emerges from this review will then be
used as a model for comparison with present-day LDCs.
Throughout the following discussion, it should be
recognized that this outline primarily covers large
national events and only lightly touches on developments that were occurring at the local level and in the

the mind of the average man. Although we do not spend
time on such local changes, it is these changes and
their historical and social contexts that are of utmost
importance to a clear understanding of the development
of health. Incremental changes at the local level
which become incorporated into the fabric of everyday
life and culture are the essence of an evolving social
order. However, we are aware of no historical discussions integrating the developmental steps that occurred
at the local level with the broad historical context
within which these social changes occurred (McKeown
1979; and Basch 1978).

If we exclude the brief interludes of the Greek
and Roman cultures, the majority of the human populace
prior to 1500 A.D. lived in settings that were similar
to the settings now found in many African countries and
other LDCs (McKeown 1979). The overall health status
of the general populace prior to 1500 A.D. was more or
less static. Food supplies were gererally precarious,
there was a general lack of education, and communication and travel were difficult. Almost all changes in
health that took place occurred only at the upper
levels of society. Health was never recognized as a
national objective. Any change in overall health that
did occur was sporadic and associated more with religious edicts than with governmental institutions. Very
little is understood concerning the history of the
development of health during this period in western
history. This is unfortunate since it is this period
to which the present conditions in most African countries are analogous. It is this period in the history
of developed countries that is most fertile for insights into appropriate developmental efforts in LDCs.

To categorize health development prior to 1500
A.D., the most instructive division is based on way of
life: nomadic versus agricultural. Hominidae have
been on this earth for approximately 10 million years.
During most of this time, man's ancestors have lived as
nomads, dependent for food on hunting, fishing, and
gathering fruit. Under nomadic conditions, the earth
could support no more than a few people per square
mile. During these times the total population of the
earth was probably well below 10 million. Life was
short and there was a high mortality rate because of
food shortages, disease, and predation.

It has only been for the last 10,000 years, or
about one-1000th of our existence on earth, that
cultivation and domestication of plants and animals
have been known. With this transition to an
agricultural way of life came a ten-fold increase in
the world's population. This increase was small and
slow considering that it occurred over a 10,000 year
period prior to 1500 A.D. The reason for this slow

increase in population despite a settled way of life
has been attributed to the balance between infectious
disease and nutritional status (Scrimshaw, et al.
1968: and McKeown 1979). The relationship between man
and microorganisms was finely balanced and this balance
continued over 10,000 years. An increase in the prop-
agation and transmission of microorganisms as a result
of the expansion and aggregation of agricultural populations was balanced by improvements in nutritional
status. An improvement in nutrition would tip the
balance in the favor of the parasite. Further improvements in food supplies were a necessary condition for
any substantial reduction of mortality from infectious
disease d for coincident improvements in health.
     After 15 A.D. and for the next 150 years, the
world's population again increased in size, but more
rapidly. This expansion in population occurred with
little evidence for any improvement in life expectancy
(Sobeslovsky, et al. 1977; Bulla and Hitze 1978; and
Hobson (ed.) 1979); thus it occurred primarily because
of decreased infant mortality. The factors leading to
this decreased infant mortality and increase in population size are not entirely clear but may be deduced
from an assessment of the major changes occurring during this period. Factors that can contribute to an
altered host-parasite balance in favor of the host
include: a) immunization and therapy, b) decreased
disease transmission, and c) improved nutrition.
Neither immunization nor effective therapy was available during this period and thus neither played a role.
Methods for decreasing transmission of disease using
hygienic practices (e.g., handwashing, isolation, and
so on) were also not known or practiced. There have
been no studies of the extent to which coincident
changes in social practices and in the environment
might have led to decreased transmission. Thus the
possible contribution that such changes in hygiene
might have made is not known. This leaves the last of
these three factors, nutrition, as probably the most
important contributor to health and the decline of
infant mortality from 1500 to 1650. Although nutrition
appears to be the most important factor for the ontogeny or development of health during this time period,
there is only indirect evidence for this. This evidence consists of the general knowledge that food
supplies kept pace with the population expansion and
that there were advances in agriculture and the transport of food during this historical period.
     A transition period occurred from 1650 to 1800,
during which time western society evolved into a pre-
industrial society. With this period came the dawning
of the era of problem solving. A few great minds began

writing about Utopian schemes and the general populace
began to perceive that social improvements were possible (Hobson 1979). It was during this period that
rulers first conceived of the idea that people themselves were the natural wealth of a country (McKeown
1979; Basch 1978; and Hobson 1979). Rulers began to
take steps to preserve the life and health of the
populace so as to increase their own estate. With
these glimmerings came further improvements in health
and associated population growth. The population of
England and Wales increased from 5.5 million in 1700 to
8.9 million in 1800. Since exports and imports of food
during this period were relatively small, food production must have doubled to sustain this increase.   In
spite of these changes and improvements, the average
life span of the common man remained essentially
unchanged: approximately thirty years (no different
from that of a Grecian city dweller from 400 B.C.).

   After 1800, infant mortality declined still
further and the population continued to grow. But now
life expectancy began to show a rise. This occurred
coincidentally with industrialization and urbanization.
The hospital was introduced and medical therapy began
to take shape. Along with the increased emphasis on
hospital-based medical care, doctors began to connect
ill health more specifically with pollution of the
environment. Local citizens began to see the need for
public measures of disease control; state and local
governments focused their attention increasingly on the
need for sanitation. But although local and national
governments became involved in public health issues,
there was little scientific basis for their action.

   At the beginning of the twentieth century evidence
supporting the germ theory of disease was increasing.
Public health laws and methods followed one another in
bewildering succession (Hobson, et al. 1979). As local
governments grew in importance, health officers and
sanitariums were utilized in increasing numbers. With
the bacteriologic concept of disease, the growth of the
modern hospital, and the evolution of professional
nursing came the teachings and simple laws of antisepsis that were preached as household hygiene (McKeown
1979; Basch 1978; and Cohen 1984). This emphasis on
health practices in the home has been promulgated only
for the last 100 years.

   These changes in household and community hygiene
were exceptionally powerful tools for preventing a
variety of infectious diseases and improving their
associated morbidity and mortality. Figure 5 presents
graphs of mortality from 1800 to 1950 attributable to
different diseases in England. Despite the lack of
antibiotics, the lack of vaccines, and the lack of
knowledge of disease mechanisms and supporting thera-

Figure 5.   Disease-specific mortality for the last 100
years (McKeown 1979).

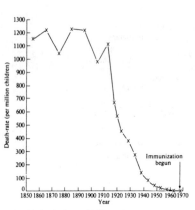

Measles: death rates of children under 15: England and Wales.

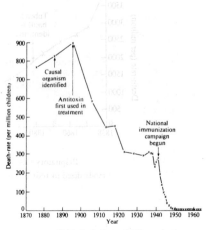

Diphtheria: death rates of children under 15:
England and Wales.

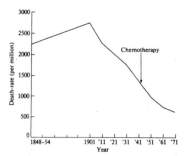

Bronchitis, pneumonia, and influenza: death-rates
(standardized to 1901 population): England and Wales.

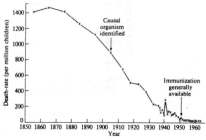

Whooping cough: death rates of children under 15:
England and Wales.

Figure 5.   (cont'd)

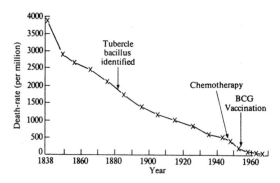

Respiratory tuberculosis: mean annual death-rates
(standardized to 1901 population) · England and Wales.

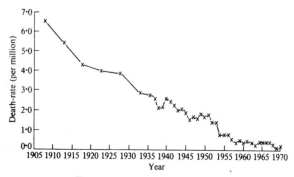

Tetanus: mean annual death rates: England and Wales.

pies, mortality from these diseases declined continually after 1900. This disease-specific decline cannot
be attributed to the doctor until after 1940. Prior to
1940, the doctor's powers were primarily those of
providing solace and relieving pain. Between 1900 and
1940, then, the majority of the disease-specific
improvements in health were probably attributable to a
variety of public health factors including: a) better
hygiene (soap and water), b) better housing (ventila-
tion and light), c) better nutrition (improved jobs,
better food distribution, higher agricultural output),
d) improved waste disposal (sewage, garbage, etc.), e)
improved food handling methods, f) insect control, and
others. These factors as practiced in the home appear
to have been promulgated through education and proven
to be effective, cheap, and long-lasting in effect.
    Beyond simple hygiene measures, the more sophisti-
cated methods of health care have come about only
during the twentieth century and have been used effectively against agents of disease only over the last
forty years (Bulla and Hitze 1978; Sobeslovsky, et al.
1979; and Hobson (ed.) 1979). It is unlikely that
personalized medical care had a significant effect on
mortality before 1940. Although medical care alleviated morbidity and mortality due to some diseases, it is
clear that medical contributions accounted for only a
small portion of the decrease in deaths before 1940.
After antibiotics (sulfonamides, penicillins, and
others) came into widespread use. It has only been
over the last twenty years that viral immunizations
directed at some of the biggest contributors to
mortality in LDCs have become available. It is also
within this same time period that developed countries
have begun to see the importance of the health of the
world as a whole.
    In summary, the historical development of health
appears to have gone through four states. The first
stage, from prior to 1500 to 1800, primarily involved
nutritional improvements which included both changes in
agricultural methods and improvements in the transport
of food. The second stage, from 1800 to 1940, involved
primarily those health inputs concerned with public
health and hygiene. The third stage, from 1940 to
1960, involved curative approaches to health, the most
important of which was antibiotics. Finally, the
fourth stage began in 1960 with the development and use
of new vaccines and their widespread distribution to
prevent infectious disease. Each of these stages in
health development and the supporting societal framework were intimately dependent on the preceding developmental stage. For development to occur that is self
supporting, development stimulating, and stable, both

health and social improvements must evolve through
these four stages.
   Historically, the social framework of western
societies has been able to support the development and
use of the curative and preventive methods of health
care only over the last 100 years. Does it make sense
to use these advanced methods of medical science today
outside of the social framework required for their
development, distribution, and economic support? Are
not the methods that led to improved health prior to
the initiation of antibiotics and vaccines more
important, more appropriate, and more cost-effective
than these more advanced modern techniques?

Measures for Estimation of a Nation's Level of
Development
   The history of social development provides the
necessary framework within which the development plans
of present LDCs can be modeled. If the present level
of development of an African country can be closely
matched to an analogous level of historical western
social and health development, many insights into
present problems of development can be gained. Such
correlations are necessary both to determine the most
appropriate type of health aid input as well as to
determine the extent of development that can be expected for a given amount of resources contributed.
   Less developed countries vary in their stages of
development. To be able to utilize the knowledge
derived from the study of the history of social development, it is necessary to have simple measures to
compare the current stage of development of each LDC
with that of historical levels of development. Few
measures are available. Historical improvements in
health were primarily measured by population characteristics. Other overall measures of health improvement
may exist but few are available. Some measures are
best used at one end of the social development scale
and other measures at the other end of this scale.
Ideally more study of social development is needed in
order to provide for optimal correlations and to
suggest applications in present LDC settings.
   Kahn and Weiner (1967) categorized countries of
the world according to per capita GNP. Their five per
capita GNP divisions included 1) pre-industrial, 2)
partially industrialized or transitional, 3) industrial, 4) mass consumption or advanced industrial and
5) post-industrial societies. Such per capita GNP
divisions provide a measure spanning the development
spectrum to more closely correlate the level of each
LDC with an analogous level in the history of western
social development. However, there are several difficulties with this approach. The major difficulty

concerns the accuracy of correlations between present
and historical per capita GNP values. In addition,
economic statistics are less available and less accurate in earlier historical periods.
     Another index of the level of development of
African or other LDCs may be mortality statistics. As
has already been pointed out (Figure 5), the mortality
for a variety of diseases has declined since 1900.
Historical levels of disease-specific mortality could
easily be matched with the present level of disease-
specific mortality of an African country. Such a
matching method would help determine the analogous
historical period of health development and identify
appropriate health related developmental inputs. However, such a methodology can only be used for those
LDCs that show levels of disease mortality below levels
occurring prior to 1900 in western societies, since
disease specific mortality was relatively stable at
high levels before that time (Figure 5). Thus, African
countries that have disease-specific mortality at or
above the 1900 level require use of other measures for
valid developmental comparisons.
     Correlations to western development levels preva-
lent between 1800 and 1900 could be obtained using
overall mortality statistics, depending on their availability. Overall mortality statistics, as opposed to
disease-specific statistics, are available as far back
as 1800, but are spotty. For earlier comparisons,
population growth rates and life expectancy estimates
might be used, but again depend on the availability of
statistics. In historical pre-industrial societies
with no population statistics, other measures need to
be sought. It appears that the level of development of
many African countries in fact corresponds to an historical period with few recorded population statistics.
This characteristic indicates the need to develop
additional measures that are both simple and easily
quantified.
     In summary, correlations between present LDCs and
historical time periods in western social development
must use different measures for different time periods.
Each measure is best used within its specified time
period or correlating LDC development level. After
1900 correlations can be drawn using disease-specific
mortality statistics, infant mortality statistics, or
GNP, depending on the availability of these statistics
for the LDC in question. From 1800 to 1900, overall
disease mortality is probably the most available and
most reliable statistic. From 1650 to 1800, population
growth, life expectancy, and other factors such as food
exports, might be useful measures. Unfortunately, the
present development level of many African countries
falls outside of the periods for which the obvious

statistical measures of development are available.
Until such time as studies can determine appropriate
measures for performing earlier historical correlations, development assessments in countries with the
lowest levels of development will remain somewhat
subjective.

Appropriate Directions for Health Aid in Africa

Appropriate directions for health aid in African
and other LDCs, as stated in the preceding sections of
this paper, may be derived from historical studies of
the development of today's more advanced societies.
For proper correlations to be drawn between the present
status of LDCs and other countries at various steps in
their historical development, the primary limiting
factor is the availability of proper statistics for
comparison. Once analogous historical periods are
identified, generalizations can be drawn concerning
health related issues of an individual country. Figure
6 shows the present average life expectancies in various LDCs. Thes statistics can be compared to the life
expectancies recorded for various historical periods
(Table 1). As can be seen, many African countries have
life expectancies or overall levels of health that correlate with historical time periods from prior to 1850
to about 1940 in western societies. During these
historical periods (as is the case today in these African countries), there was a high infant mortality rate
and high incidence of infectious disease and malnutrition in children under five years of age.

The development models obtained by drawing correlations between present-day African countries and
historical time periods can be used to obtain insights
into appropriate inputs for health improvements without
lags in development. Table 2 illustrates the use of
these historical correlations for health planning. At
the top of Table 2, four possible disease control
efforts are listed along with the historical time
periods with which they were associated. On the left-
hand side of Table 3 are listed three disease categories: gastrointestinal, respiratory, and skin
diseases. For each category listed in Table 2, one
might ask which form of disease control is optimal for
a particular African country. Presently most inputs
suggested by aid organizations for use in African
countries are those listed in the right hand side of
this table. This orientation should be questioned.

By using present estimates of life expectancy for
African countries (Figure 6), past life expectancies of
a western society (Table 1), and the timing of disease
control options (Table 2), several implications can be

Figure 6.   Estimates of life expectancy, 1980-1985
(Source: World Health Statistics 1983).

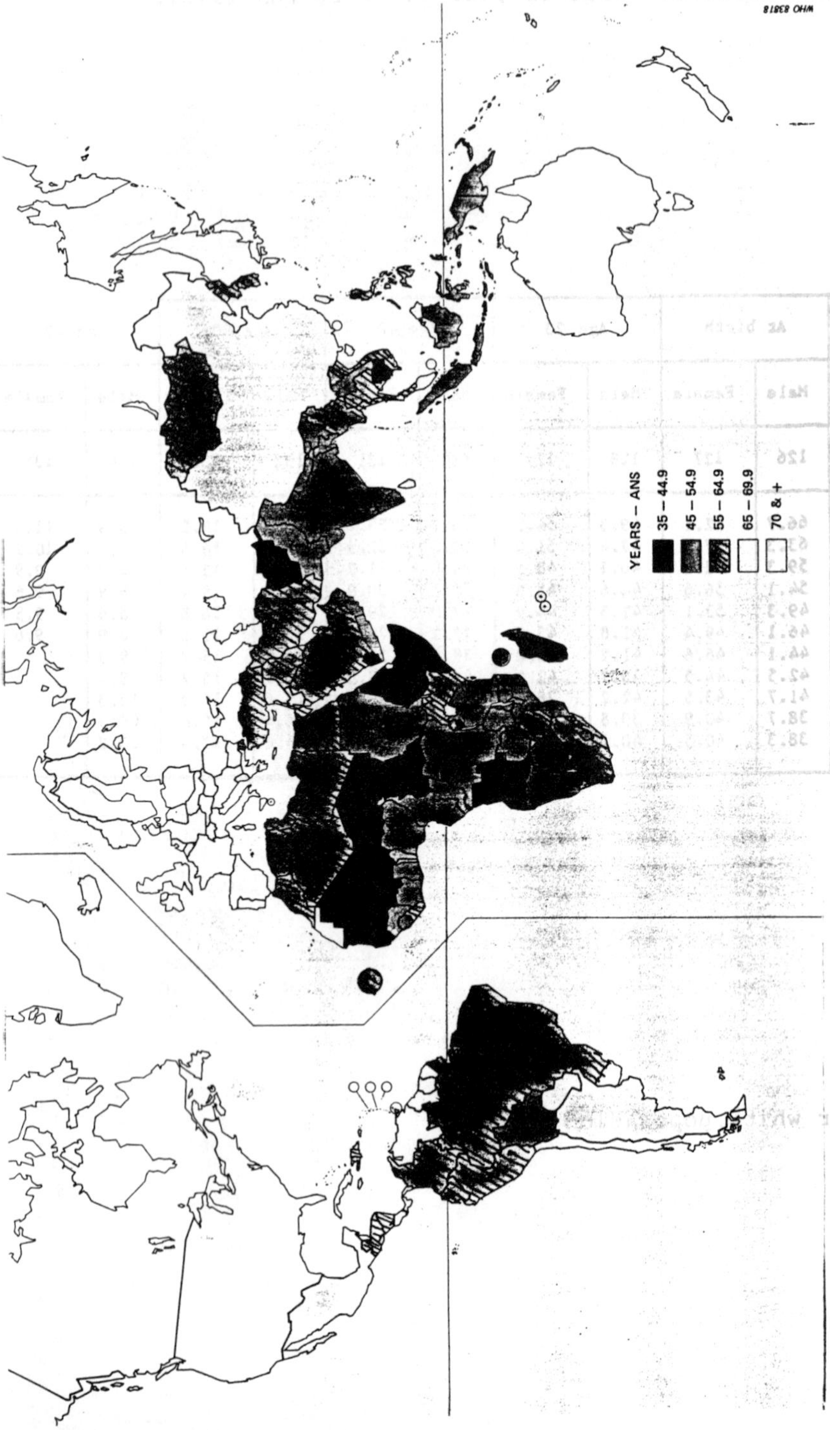

HEALTH PLANNING

Table 1. Expectation of life at birth, by sex, for
Massachusetts: 1850 to 1949-51 (Preston 1976).

Year or Period	At birth		Age 20		Age 40		Age 60		Age 70	
	Male	Female	Male	Female	Male	Female	Male	Female	Male	Female
	126	127	128	129	130	131	132	133	134	135
1949-51	66.7	72.1	49.3	54.2	30.7	35.2	15.4	18.3	9.9	11.6
1939-41[1]	63.3	67.6	47.4	51.0	29.3	32.6	14.5	16.4	9.1	10.2
1929-31[1]	59.3	62.6	46.1	48.5	29.0	31.2	14.3	15.8	8.9	9.9
1919-20[1]	54.1	56.6	44.6	45.5	28.8	30.0	14.4	15.4	8.9	9.6
1909-11	49.3	53.1	42.5	44.9	27.0	29.0	13.4	14.8	8.6	9.5
1900-02	46.1	49.4	41.8	43.7	27.2	28.8	13.9	15.1	8.9	9.6
1893-97	44.1	46.6	41.2	42.8	27.4	29.0	14.4	15.7	9.3	
1890	42.5	44.5	40.7	42.0	27.4	28.8	14.7	15.7	9.4	
1878-82	41.7	43.5	42.2	28.9	28.9	30.3	15.6	16.9	10.3	
1855	38.7	40.9	39.8	39.9	27.0	28.8	14.4	15.6	(NA)	
1850	38.3	40.5	40.1	40.2	27.9	29.8	15.6	17.0	10.2	

[1]For white population only

Table 2.   Disease control options.

Disease Category	Possible Disease Control Efforts and Approximate Historial Periods of Importance			
	Agricultural Nutrition Prior to 1800	Preventive Hygiene 1800-1940	Curative Medicines 1940-1960	Preventive Vaccines 1960-Present
Gastrointestinal Diarrhea, polio	Calories and protein	Soap and water, sewage disposal, etc.	Fluid and electro- lytes	OPV, (Rotavirus)
Respiratory Viral pneumonia, measles, pertussis diphtheria, TB	Calories and protein	Soap and water (32,33), housing and ventilation, covering the mouth, isolation, etc.	Antibiotics, fluid and electrolytes	DPT, MMR, (Influenza) (RSV) (Parainfluenza
Skin Ulcers, tetanus, hookworm, malaria schistosomiasis	Calories and protein	Soap and water, shoes, clothing, sewage disposal, screens, etc.	Antibiotics, antiparasitics anti-fungals	Tetanus (malaria) (schisto- somiasis)

drawn for health planning in present day African countries. Those African countries that are least well off
and have a life expectancy below 45 years of age
(Figure 6) correspond to a historical period prior to
1850 (Tables 1 and 2) and, in most cases, prior to
1800. In such African countries health related aid
efforts should be directed almost entirely to improvements in agricultural output. On the other hand, those
countries that have climbed to a life expectancy range
of 45 to 55 years (Figure 6) are ready for industrialization and should be assisted in developing hygienic
improvements and non-vaccine preventive efforts. Both
of these groups of African countries would not benefit
economically by budgeting money for curative medicines
or preventive vaccines. On the other hand, the group
of African countries with an average life expectancy of
55 to 65 years would probably benefit by expenditure on
one or two of the less expensive antibiotics. However,
the economic validity of using vaccines in such countries for the control of single diseases throughout the
entire population can be questioned and should be left
for the future. In summary, although most disease
control efforts for African countries are drawn from
the right hand side of Table 2, funding efforts would
more optimally be drawn primarily from the left half of
Table 2. It is also of importance to note that improvements in agriculture, listed in the left half of
Table 2, have a broad impact on all disease categories
whereas the purchase of vaccines, listed in the right
half of Table 2, has a limited impact that is disease-
specific and thus more costly.
     For the least developed African countries, im-
provements in agriculture and nutrition appear to be of
most importance. During the 18th century, as we have
seen, nutritional improvements appear to have had the
greatest impact on development. Unfortunately, detailed knowledge about these improvements is lacking. In
addition, we have only the sketchiest understanding of
other aspects of health development occurring during
this time period. In order to provide effective
systems for improving health in the least developed
African countries, further study into the details of
the early social development of the western world will
be required. For the time being, it appears that
improvements in local agricultural methods are the most
costeffective, appropriate, and developmentally functional health directed methodologies for the poorest
African countries.
     In the 18th century the role of hygiene in preven-
tion of infectious disease was not only unknown but
would have been unacceptable if introduced. Historically, societies at early levels of development
retained explanations for illness based in religious

contexts. To suggest to an individual whose thinking
was within such a framework that "illness" (not our
meaning of health) could be altered by doing something
different within his environment would have been equivalent to suggesting that his religious beliefs were
wrong. In order for behavioral changes to occur in
present-day African countries, changes must first be
preceded by alterations in the religious and social
custom framework of these countries or these changes
must take place within the context of these frameworks.
"Reason" as based on modern western paradigms is outside the framework of the average person of many
African countries: that is, logic and reason in the
western sense have no meaning or are controversial to
the rural African. In order for behavioral changes to
occur, such changes must be motivated not by western
scientific developments but by the beliefs of that
society. Although the most important advances in
health have come from influencing the behavior of
people, it is here that our capability is meager indeed. Changes in beliefs initiated by missionary work
may provide for major steps in development through
changes in underlying beliefs that are not conducive to
development.
    Introduction of health improvements in the areas
of hygiene and disease control also requires non-
behavioral inputs. While there is a great need to
provide clean water, soap, sewage disposal, and well-
ventilated housing, there is also a need for an industrial framework to support such disease control
efforts. The most common mistake made in developing
aid programs to supply needs is in the level of
technology supplied. For example, the rural African
farmer does not need a tractor but does need a plow and
an animal harness supplied by his nation's industry.
Appropriate or intermediate forms of technology and the
industrial framework to support them should be developed along the lines of the development that occurred in
North America and Europe during the 19th century (e.g.,
blacksmith, cabinetmaker, etc.).
    The historical development of the west provides
other insights into present health aid efforts in
Africa. During historical periods prior to 1800, the
average person's concept of "health" only went as far
as the absence of illness. When this average individual looked for help for a typical illness he was sent
to a "healer". Although such "healers" objectively
often provide only solace and perhaps relief from pain,
this was not the perception of the health seeker. Outside of each individual illness, "health" as it is
presently conceived in the developed west was neither
sought nor understood. This limited concept of health
and limited curative capability of "healers" is also

characteristic of present-day African countries. With
this in mind, the question could be raised whether it
is presently appropriate, developmentally functional,
or cost-effective to provide the "healers" of today's
poorest African countries with antibiotics and other
modes of modern medicine. Did not western healers of
the 18th century, as do the traditional healers of
today's African countries, have the most cost-effective
measures of healing (i.e., psychological support) for
health problems that had no solution then and have no
economic solution now?

The success of development work being carried out
within an appropriate historical framework could be
measured now as it was then: in terms of population
expansion. However, such a measure would not be appropriate for use in today's LDCs. Although current
population growth in LDCs is significant, there is a
difference between this expansion and that which occurred historically. Today's growth has largely been
induced by external aid focused on the mortality of
infectious diseases. Historically, population growth
was secondary to internal, self-induced improvements in
food supply and nutrition and in industry and production. The conflict between effective health care
efforts and the contribution of these efforts to
population growth has always presented a dilemma for
which there are no easy answers. For every forceful
argument for supporting modern health care programs, it
is also clear that such programs would add to the rate
of population growth by reducing mortality. Unless
declines in overall mortality and the associated
population expansion are closely linked to internal
improvements, a population's health and well-being
cannot be measured by a populations's growth rate.
Although it may not be morally acceptable to the
leaders of present-day LDCs or to the governing bodies
of aid agencies to allow population control by permit-
ting continued high disease mortality, it is illogical
to permit continued health expenditures with coincident
population expansion and associated increased demands
for health services without the coincident national
development to support them. Such orientations lead to
further underdevelopment and to continued suffering of
an even larger population. It is clear that such
methods lead to an overall decrease in health and an
increase in suffering. Such consequences far outweigh
the benefits of the transient improvements in disease
mortality that come with modern curative and preventive
medical care.

The real difference between modern day health
related development efforts and those that stem from
historically sound social frameworks can be seen in the
degree of economic stability found in present-day LDCs.

Those LDCs that are economically stable have developed
sufficiently to provide for their expanded populations;
those LDCs that are economically unstable have received
inappropriately directed development aid. The tremendous burdens of debt and economic instability found
among many LDCs today testify to inappropriate directions of development aid efforts.

We acknowledge the potential unpopularity of our
approach.   It is difficult for developed and less
developed nations alike to resist the lure of seemingly
easy solutions to chronic health problems. As western
civilizations evolved from approximately 1500 to the
present, there were no easy solutions, no advanced
cultures to provide answers and know-how. Mankind
learned "the hard way," so to speak. It is our belief
that while aid can speed up the development process, it
cannot succeed by passing over stages of development
and the inherent growth in cultural understanding
accompanying these stages. The earlier, more basic
impovements in nutrition, and later in hygiene, must
precede modern curative and preventive care both to lay
the foundation for and to enhance the effectiveness of
these latter approaches. Of course, these arguments
lose some of their force in nations with virtually
unlimited funds, such as the African oil countries.
But it is still true, even in these nations, that
agricultural and diet improvements will lead to more
significant and lasting developmental changes (for less
money) than will early introduction of antibiotics and
other curative care alone.

For any given amount of development aid expenditure there are a multitude of possible inputs. During
the time that developed countries have been rendering
international aid (approximately the last thirty
years), a greater understanding of the problems and
approaches to development has been acquired. Although
the goal of improving the average citizen's health has
been sought, the fact that this goal lies within the
context of overall social development has, we believe,
not been understood clearly. The historical context of
social development provides a simple model within which
appropriately aimed developmental inputs can be clearly
identified. Those inputs that are not well outlined
historically need to be studied in depth. Such study
is the job of the historical anthropologist. Anthropologists must seek suitable methods of putting both
food into the stomachs and new ideas into the thinking
of the average villager of today's African countries.
If this job is not done, the worldwide degradation of
mankind will continue to worsen. The goal of such
methods is soundly based development.

REFERENCES CITED

Baker, P. (ed.), Human Population Problems in the
    Bioshpere. Paris: UNESCO, 1977.
Basch, P. F., International Health. New York: Oxford
    University Press, 1978.
Brown, K. H., and W. C. MacLean, Nutritional management
    of acute diarrhea: an appraisal of the alterna-
    tives. Pediatrics, Vol. 73, No. 2, 1984.
Bryant, J. H., Health and the Developing World.
    Ithaca, New York: Cornell University Press, 1969.
Bulla, A., and K. L. Hitze, Acute respiratory infec-
    tions: a review. Bulletin of the World Health
    Organization, Vol. 56, No. 3, 1978.
Centers for Disease Control, Annual summary, reported
    morbidity and mortality in the United States.
    Morbidity Mortality Weekly Report, Vol. 29, No.
    54, 1981.
Cohen, I. B., Florence Nightingale. Scientific
    American, Vol. 250, No. 6, 1984.
De Buse, P. J., M. G. Lewis and J. W. Mugerwa,
    Pulmonary complications of measles in Uganda.
    Journal of Tropical Pediatrics, Vol. 16, 1970.
Denny, Floyd: Personal communication with Dr. Floyd
    Denny at the University of North Carolina, Chapel
    Hill.
Dyson, T., Levels, trends, differentials and causes of
    child mortality - a survey. World Health Status
    Report, Vol. 30, 1977.
Global Strategy for Health for All by the Year 2000.
    Geneva: World Health Organization, 1981.
Hall, C. B., and R. G. Douglass, Modes of transmission
    of respiratory syncytial virus. Journal of
    Pediatrics, Vol. 99, 1981.
Hall, C. B., J. M. Geiman, R. G. Douglass, Jr., and M.
    P. Mergher, Control of nosocomial respiratory
    syncytial viral infections. Pediatrics, Vol. 62,
    1978.
Health Hazards of the Human Environment. Geneva:
    World Health Organization, 1972.
Health United States and Prevention Profile.
    Washington, D.C.: United States Department of
    Health and Human Services, 1981.
Hobson, W. (ed.), The Theory and Practice of Public
    Health. New York: Oxford University Press, 1979.
Jelliffe, D. B., Infant Nutrition in the Subtropics and
    Tropics. Geneva: World Health Organization (2nd
    Ed.), 1968.
Kahn, H., and A. J. Weiner, The Year 2000. London:
    The MacMillan Company, 1967.
King, M. (ed.), Medical Care in Developing Countries.
    Nairobi: Oxford University Press, 1966.

McKeown, T., The Role of Medicine. Princeton:
    Princeton University Press, 1979.
Morley, D., Pediatric Priorites in the Developing
    World. London: Butterworth and Company, Ltd.,
    1973.
O'Donovan, C., and K. N. Barma, Measles pneumonia.
    American Journal of Tropical Medicine Hygiene,
    Vol. 22, No. 1, 1973
Pierce, N. F., and N. Hirschhorn, Oral fluid - a simple
    weapon against dehydration in diarrhea: how it
    works and how to use it. WHO Chronical, Vol. 31,
    1977.
Preston, S. H., Mortality Patterns in National
    Populations: with a Special Reference to Recorded
    Causes of Death. New York: Academic Press, 1976.
Schumacher, E. F., Small is Beautiful. New York:
    Harper and Rowe, 1973.
Scrimshaw, N. S., C. E. Taylor, and J. E. Gordon,
    Interactions of Nutrition and Infection. Geneva:
    World Health Organization, 1968
Sobeslovsky, O., S.R.K. Sibikori, P.S.E.G. Harland, V.
    Skertic, A. Foyinka and A. D. Soneji, The viral
    etiology of acute respiratory infections in
    children in Uganda. Bulletin of the World Health
    Organization, Vol. 55, No. 5, 1977.
Teadem, R., E. Burn, S. Cairncross, et al., Water,
    Health and Development. London: Tri-Med Books,
    1978.
Wagner, E. G., and T. N. Lanoix, Excreta Disposal for
    Rural Areas and Small Communities. Geneva:
    World Health Organization, 1958.
Wagner, E. G., and T. N. Lanoix, Water Supply for Rural
    Areas amd Small Communities. Geneva: World Health
    Organization, 1969.
Walsh, J. A., and K. S. Warren, Selective primary
    health care: an interim strategy for disease
    control in developing countries. New England
    Journal of Medicine, Vol. 301, No. 18, 1979.
Weinstein, L., Failure of chemotherapy to prevent the
    bacterial complications of measles. New England
    Journal of Medicine, Vol. 253, 1955.
Wittmann, W., and J. D. L. Hanson, Gastroenteritis and
    malnutrition. South African Medical Journal, Vol.
    39, 1965.
World Health Statistics - Annual. Geneva: World Health
    Organization, 1983.

LIST OF CONTRIBUTORS

ISMAIL H. ABDALLA is Assistant Professor of History at the College of William and Mary. He received his Ph.D. from the University of Wisconsin, where he wrote a dissertation on "Islamic Medicine and Its Influence of Hausa Practitioners in Northern Nigeria." His publications include "The Medicine of the Prophet Muhammad" (1983), "Medicine in 19th Century Arabic Literature in Northern Nigeria" (1979), and "The Choice of Khashim El-Girba" (1972). He is currently writing a book about Islamic medicine in sub-Saharan Africa.

ANN BECK is a professor emeritus of the University of Hartford's Department of History. She received her Ph.D in history at the University of Illinois in 1948. Among her publications are *A History of the British Medical Administration of East Africa, 1900-1950* (Harvard University Press, 1970); *Medicine and Society in Tanganyika, 1870-1930* (The American Philosophical Society, 1977); and *Medicine, Tradition and Development in Kenya and Tanzania, 1920-1970* (Crossroads Press, 1979). She has also published a number of articles on the social and economic impact of medicine and public health in eastern Africa and Zimbabwe. Professor Beck is presently working on a study of health, tradition, and society in eastern Africa and Tanzania, an assessment of the last twenty years.

LOUIS BRENNER is Honorary Lecturer at the School of Oriental and African Studies, University of London, and Research Associate at the African Studies Center, Boston University. His previous publications include *The Shehus of Kukawa: A History of the al-Kanemi Dynasty of Bornu* (Oxford: Clarendon Press, 1973) and *West African Sufi: The Religious Heritage and Spiritual Search of Cerno Bokar Saalif Taal* (London: C. Hurst & Co., Berkeley: University of California Press, 1984).

BRIAN M. DU TOIT is a Professor of Anthropology and a member of the African Studies faculty at the University of Florida. He received his Ph.D from University of Oregon. Among his numerous publications are *Cannabis in Africa: An Ethnography of Cannabis Use and Cannabis Users* (A.A. Blakema, 1980), *Ethnicity in Modern Africa* (editor; Westview Press, 1978), "The Anthropologist in South Africa" (1981), and "Religion, Ritual and Healing Among Urban Black South Africans" (1980). He is currently engaged in research on female aging in southern Africa.

THABO T. FAKO is a lecturer in the Department of Sociology at the University of Botswana. In 1979-80, he was appointed Acting Dean of Students at the University College of Botswana, and in the same year was Chairman of the Botswana Society and a member of the Advisory Council to the Ministry of Health on Health Education/Nutrition. In 1981 he worked as Consultant Lecturer at the National Health Institute. His publications include: "Traditional Medicine and Organisational Issues in Botswana", *National Institute for Research in Development and African Studies* (July 1978); "Development in Sub-Sahara Africa and the Decline of Folk Knowledge in Agriculture", in Lawrence Busch (ed.) *Science and Agricultural Development* (Allenheld Osmun and Co. Publisher, 1981); and "Current Issues in the Conceptualization of the Origins of African Agriculture", *Pula! Journal of Southern African Studies* (May 1984).

NANCY ELIZABETH GALLAGHER holds a Bachelor of Science degree in Public Health Microbiology from the University of California, Berkeley, and a Ph.D in History from the University of California, Los Angeles. She is currently Associate Professor of Middle East and Medical History at the University of California, Santa Barbara and has written *Medicine and Power in Tunisia, 1780-1900* (Cambridge University Press, 1983).

JOHN M. JANZEN is a Professor of Anthropology at the University of Kansas, was born in 1937. He received his B.A. from Bethel College (Kansas), a Certificate of African Studies from the Sorbonne, University of Paris, and his M.A. and Ph.D from the University of Chicago. His major anthropoligical fieldwork has been conducted in 1964-66, 1969, 1974 and 1982 in the Kikongo speaking region of Western Zaire; he has also made fieldwork trips to Central and Southern Africa in 1982-83. His major publications are on African health, healing, religion and society, including *The Quest for Therapy in Lower Zaire*, which won the Wellcome Price and Medal in 1978 from the Royal Anthropological Institute, and *Lemba 1650-1930: A Drum of Affliction in Africa and the New World*. He has served as a member of the Joint Committee on African Studies of the American Council of Learned Societies and the Social Science Research Council, as committee chair for three years, and as a co-director of the research planning project "Medicine and Society in Africa."

ALICE C. REUMAN is a Research Associate with the Center for Governmental Responsibility, affiliated with the Holland Law Center at the University of Florida. Mrs. Reuman obtained a degree in Urban and Regional Planning from the University of Florida and a law degree from the University of Wisconsin. She worked for the National Bureau of Resources and Land Use Planning in Tanzania and in a legal role in South America.

PETER D. REUMAN is an Assistant Professor of Pediatric Infectious Disease and Immunology at the University of Florida College of Medicine. Dr. Reuman has a Masters degree in Public Health from Harvard and a M.D. from the University of Chicago. He worked in Asia as a science teacher, was awarded a tropical medicine fellowship from Louisiana State University for work in South America, and taught Public Health in Tanzania for two years.

ARLAN L. ROSENBLOOM is Professor of Pediatrics, Chief of the Division Pediatric Endocrinology and Director of the Diabetes Research, Education, and Treatment Center at the University of Florida, where he has been on the faculty of the College of Medicine since 1968. Before that he served as Epidemiologist-Advisor in the African Smallpox Eradication and Measles Control Program while serving in the US Public Health Service, based in Yaounde, Cameroon from 1966-1968. His interest in international health dates from his work as a medical officer in Cambodia and Malaysia from 1960-1962 with MEDICO. Dr. Rosenbloom presently serves as consultant epidemiologist to the Project for Strengthening Health Delivery Systems in Central and West Africa, an AID Program contracted through Boston University's Health Policy Institute.

LAMIN SANNEH holds a Ph.D from the University of London and is at present Assistant Professor at Harvard University. He has previously taught at Ibadan, Nigeria, at Fourah Bay College, Freetown, Sierra Leone, and at the Universities of Ghana, Legon, and Aberdeen, Scotland. He is the author of two recent books and over twenty articles in scholarly journals.

CAROLYN SARGENT is Assistant Professor of Anthropology at Southern Methodist University. She received her M.A. (Econ.) at the University of Manchester, England, and her Ph.D. from Michigan State. She is the author of *The Cultural Context of Therapeutic Choice: Obstetrical Care Decisions Among the Bariba of Benin.*

NATALIE S. SMALL, M.S., Ed.S. is a licensed Mental Health Counselor in the Department of Social Work Services at Shands Hospital of the University of Florida where she counsels pediatric families adjusting to life-threatening illness. Her interest in cost-effective methods of counseling have led to the development of multi-media helath education presentations, a study tour of health and family life in China, consulting in Nigeria and work as a doctoral student in counseling at the University of Florida.

PARKER A. SMALL, JR., M.D. is Professor of Immunology and Medical Microbiology and Professor of Pediatrics at the College of Medicine, University of Florida. His research efforts are currently divided between the development and testing of new methods of teaching immunology. He has published over 100 articles, most in the area of immunology. His Patient Oriented Problem-Solving (POPS) system of teaching immunology is in use at over half the U.S. medical schools. The University of Lagos College of Medicine brought the Smalls to Nigeria in 1982 to advise them on immunology education and research and cost-effective counseling methods. In 1983 Dr. Small returned to Lagos, Kenya, and Saudi Arabia. The Smalls have three children.

ANITA SPRING is Associate Professor of Anthropology and Associate Dean, College of Liberal Arts and Sciences, and is affiliated with the Center for African Studies at the University of Florida. She received her Ph.D. from Cornell University, her M.A. from San Francisco State University and her B.A. from University of California, Berkeley. She has done work on health care, religion, and gender roles in Zambia, and in agricultural development and farming systems in Malawi and Cameroon. She co-edited *Women in Ritual and Symbolic Roles* (Plenum Press, 1978, with J. Hoch-Smith), and has written articles on population, symbolic systems, refugees, and women in farming. Most recently she directed a USAID project on women in agricultural development Malawi.

ROBERT STOCK is a medical geographer employed as a Postdoctoral Fellow in the Department of Geography, Queen's University. He has studied at the University of Western Ontario (B.A.), Michigan State University (M.A.) and the University of Liverpool (Ph.D.). He has undertaken considerable research on health care systems in Nigeria and the health care behaviour of the Hausa of Nigeria.